1st INTERNATIONAL CONGRESS OF NEUROENDOCRINOLOGY

Program and Abstracts

Wednesday, Thursday, Friday
July 9–11, 1986

Hilton Hotel
San Francisco, California

OFFICERS–INTERNATIONAL NEUROENDOCRINE SOCIETY

President	S.M. McCann
Vice President	M. Jutisz
Vice President	J.B. Martin
Vice President	W.O. Wuttke
Secretary-Treasurer	F. Labrie
Council	R.A. Gorski
	H. Imura
	Y. Koch
	B.S. McEwen
	B. Meyerson
	M. Motta
	R.I. Weiner

CONGRESS ORGANIZERS

Chairman	Richard Weiner	
Local Organizing Committee	Howard Bern	Robert B. Jaffe
	Mary Dallman	David Ramsy
	William F. Ganong	Ian Reid
	Paul C. Goldsmith	Judith Turgeon
Scientific Committee	Ivan Assenmacher	Jacob Kraicer
	Carl Denef	Fernand Labrie
	Alfredo Donoso	Joseph Martin
	J.W. Funder	Marcella Motta
	Tomas Hökfelt	Miklos Palkovits
	Hiroo Imura	James Roberts
	Yitschak Koch	Umberto Scapagnini
	Claude Kordon	Michael Thorner

SUSTAINING ORGANIZATIONS

The International Neuroendocrine Society expresses its warm appreciation for the contribution in support of Symposia Speakers and travel grants for the Meeting from the following organizations:

MAJOR DONORS

FIDIA S.P.A.
SANDOZ LTD.

BENEFACTORS

AYERST LABORATORIES
GENENTECH INC.
ORTHO PHARMACEUTICAL CORPORATION
ROUSSEL UCLAF
SCHERING

GENERAL INFORMATION

REGISTRATION

Location—East Lounge, Hilton Hotel

Hours:

Tuesday, July 8	3 PM– 8 PM
Wednesday, July 9	8 AM– 5 PM
Thursday, July 10,	8 AM– 5 PM
Friday, July 11	8 AM–12 PM

FEES

Members	$175
Non-Members	$225
Graduate Students & Postdoctoral Fellows	$100

POSTERS

Posters will be left in place from 8:30 AM until 5:00 PM. Authors will man their posters between 10:30 and 12:30 PM and 3:30 and 5:00 PM.

RECEPTION

On Tuesday evening from 6:00–8:00 PM a reception will be held in the Hilton Hotel. This is your chance to become familiar with the wines of California.

Wednesday, July 9, 1986

Time

8:30–11:00 *Session 1*
Plenary Session
Continental Ballrooms 5-6
Welcome: Samuel McCann, *President*
Harris Lecture: Tomas Hökfelt
Plenary Lectures: Wylie Vale and J. Joosse

8:00–5:00 *Session 2*
Poster Session
Continental Parlors 7–9
(posters will be manned from 10:30–12:30 PM and 3:30–5:00 PM)
Abstract numbers 2–88

1:30–3:30 **Slide Presentations**

Session 3
Neuroendocrine Regulation of Prolactin
Continental Ballroom 5
Abstract numbers 89–96

Session 4
Neuropeptides
Continental Ballroom 6
Abstract numbers 97–104

Session 5
Development and Aging
Teakwood
Abstract numbers 105–112

Thursday, July 10, 1986

Time

8:30–10:30 **Symposia**

Session 6
Expression and Processing of Neuroendocrine Peptides
Continental Ballroom 4
J. Funder and J. Martial, *chairpersons*
Abstract numbers 113–116

Session 7
Neuroregulatory Role of Peptides
Continental Ballroom 5
C. Kordon and M. Motta, *chairpersons*
Abstract numbers 117–120

Session 8
Integrative Neuroendocrinology
Continental Parlors 1–3
B. Halasz and J. Kraicer, *chairpersons*
Abstract numbers 121–124

8:00–5:00 *Session 9*
Poster Session
Continental Parlors 6–9
(posters will be manned from 10:30–12:30 PM and 3:30–5:00 PM)
Abstract numbers 125–200

1:30–3:30 **Slide Presentations**

Session 10
Mechanism of Action of Neurohormones
Continental Ballroom 4
Abstract numbers 201–208

Session 11
Neuroendocrine Regulation of ACTH
Continental Ballroom 5
Abstract numbers 209–216

Session 12
Regulation of Hormone Rhythms
Continental Parlors 1–3
Abstract numbers 217–224

5:00–6:00 **Business Meeting**
Continental Parlors 1–3

8:00 **Banquet**
Continental Ballrooms 4–5

Friday, July 11, 1986

Time

8:30–10:30 **Symposia**

Session 13
Mediation of Neuroendocrine Peptide Action
Continental Ballroom 4
K. Catt and Y. Koch, *chairpersons*
Abstract numbers 225–228

Session 14
Clinical Neuroendocrinology
Continental Ballroom 5
J. Martin and M. Grumbach, *chairpersons*
Abstract numbers 229–232

Session 15
Aminergic Regulation of Neuroendocrine Function
Continental Parlors 1–3
C. Sawyer and U. Scapagnini, *chairpersons*
Abstract numbers 233–236

8:00–5:00 *Session 16*
Poster Session
Continental Parlors 6–9
(posters will be manned from 10:30–12:30 PM and 3:30–5:30 PM)
Abstract numbers 237–331

1:30–3:30 **Slide Presentations**

Session 17
Neuroendocrine Regulation of LH
Continental Ballroom 4
Abstract numbers 332–339

Session 18
Neuroendocrine Regulation of GH
Continental Ballroom 5
Abstract numbers 340–347

Session 19
Expression and Processing of Peptides and Comparative Neuroendocrinology
Continental Parlors 1–3
Abstract numbers 348–355

SCIENTIFIC PROGRAMS

Wednesday AM **Continental Ballrooms 5–6**
8:30–11:00

SESSION 1:
Welcome:
Samuel McCann, *President*

8:30–9:30 **Harris Lecture:**
CHEMICAL NEUROANATOMY OF THE HYPOTHALAMO-PITUITARY AXIS—FOCUS ON MULTIMESSENGER SYSTEMS
Tomas Hökfelt

9:30–10:15 **Plenary Lecture:**
HYPOTHALAMIC AND GONADAL HORMONES MODULATING FUNCTIONS AND PROLIFERATION OF ANTERIOR PITUITARY CELLS
Wylie Vale

10:15–11:00 **Plenary Lecture:**
FUNCTIONAL AND EVOLUTIONARY PERSPECTIVES OF GENE CODING AND PROCESSING OF PEPTIDE PRECURSORS
Joos Joosse

Wednesday AM/PM **Continental Parlors 7–9**

SESSION 2: Neuroendocrine Regulation of LH; Action of Hypothalamic Hormones; Neuroendocrine Regulation of TSH; Neuroendocrinology of the Posterior Pituitary

Poster Session — Posters manned from 10:30–12:30 PM and 3:30–5:00 PM

Neuroendocrine Regulation of LH

Position

1 **2.** ANATOMICAL MAPPING OF PERIKARYA CONTAINING GONADOTROPIN-RELEASING HORMONE mRNA IN THE BRAIN OF THE MALE MONKEY, *MACACA FASCICULARIS,* BY *IN SITU* HYBRIDIZATION
L.A. Adams, L. Vician, L.J. Standish, D.K. Clifton, R.A. Steiner
University of Washington, Seattle, WA 98195

2 **3.** ESTROGEN AFFECTS CHEMOSENSITIVITY OF PARAVENTRICULAR NEURONS IN SLICES OF THE FEMALE RAT HYPOTHALAMUS
T. Akaishi, Y. Sakuma
Department of Physiology II, Niigata University School of Medicine, Niigata 951, Japan

3 **4.** POST-NEONATAL TESTICULAR SECRETIONS "ORGANISE" AND "ACTIVATE" NEURAL CIRCUITS INVOLVED IN THE OPIATERGIC CONTROL OF LH RELEASE IN RATS
O.F.X. Almeida, K.E. Nikolarakis, A. Herz
Department of Neuropharmacology, Max-Planck-Institut für Psychiatrie, D-8033 Martinsried, West Germany

4 **5.** ARE GONADOTROPINS AND PROLACTIN PITUITARY AND PLASMATIC LEVELS CORRELATED AFTER CHRONIC LHRH ANALOG (BUSERELIN) TREATMENT?
C. Alvarez Sanz, C. Bravo, C. Fdez Galaz, A. Tejero, P. Rodriguez, M.D. Vaticón
Dept. Physiol. Fac. Med. Univ. Complut. Madrid 28040. SPAIN

5 **6.** A ROLE FOR ORNITHINE DECARBOXYLASE IN THE PRO-OESTROUS LH SURGE IN RATS?
M. Aslam, S.A. Nicholson, B.B. Oon,** B. Gillham,** M.T. Jones*
Divisions of Gynaecology and Biochemistry** (St. Thomas') and Physiology* (Guy's), United Medical & Dental Schools London SE1 (U.K.)

6 **6a.** IN VITRO STUDIES OF INFLUENCES ON GONADOTROPIN-RELEASING HORMONE SECRETION FROM THE ISOLATED PERIFUSED GUINEA PIG HYPOTHALAMUS
P.E. Belchetz, P.E. McKibbin, H. Ainsworth
Department of Medicine, University of Liverpool, P.O. Box 147, Liverpool L69 3BX, U.K.

7 **7.** PHYSIOLOGICAL ATTRIBUTES OF LUTEINIZING HORMONE PULSES ASSESSED BY MULTIPLE-POINT (CLUSTER) ANALYSIS: STUDIES IN WOMEN AND ANALYSIS OF MALE VERSUS FEMALE PATTERNS
E. Christiansen, W.S. Evans, R.J. Urban, F.E. Barr, A.D. Rogol, D.L. Kaiser, M.L. Johnson, J.D. Veldhuis
University of Virginia Medical School, Charlottesville, Virginia 22908

8 **8.** EFFECT OF NEURAL PATHWAY BLOCKERS ON LHRH RELEASE FROM RAT HYPOTHALAMI PERFUSED/PERIFUSED IN VITRO
T.T. Chuang, M.T. Jones
Department of Gynaecology, United Medical and Dental Schools (St. Thomas's Campus), London SE1 7EH

9 **9.** THE ROLE OF LH IN THE AUTOFEEDBACK INHIBITION OF LH AND FSH SECRETION IN RATS
Sonya Conway, Samuel M. McCann
Northern Illinois University, DeKalb, Illinois and Dept. of Physiology, University of Texas Health Science Center, Dallas, Texas 75235

10 **10.** PULSATILE FSH SECRETION IS INDEPENDENT OF LHRH.
M.D. Culler, A. Negro-Vilar
Reprod. Neuroendo. Sec., Lab. Reprod. Dev. Tox., NIEHS-NIH, Res. Tri. Pk., NC 27709

11 **11.** PRL, FSH, LH RESPONSES TO OPIATE ANTAGONIST (NALOXONE) IN PATIENTS WITH ANOREXIA NERVOSA AND ISOLATED GONADOTROPHIN DEFICIENCY. PRELIMINARY DATA
S. Devescovi, G. Andreani, M.G. Toni, M. Rolla
1st Medical Clinic, Nuclear Medicine Service, CNR Institute of Clinical Physiology, Pisa-Italy

12 **12.** INFLUENCE OF GONADAL STEROIDS ON HUMAN AND MONKEY CEREBROSPINAL FLUID HOMOVANILLIC ACID CONCENTRATIONS
T. Di Paolo,[1] F. Bédard,[2] P. Bédard[2]

[1]School of Pharmacy, Laval University, Québec G1K 7P4 and Department of Molecular Endocrinology, Laval University Hospital Center, Québec G1V 4G2; [2]Neurobiology Research Center, Hôpital de l'Enfant-Jésus, Québec G1J 1Z4, Canada

13 **13.** IN VIVO MEASUREMENT OF LHRH AND NEUROTRANSMITTERS FROM THE ANTERIOR PITUITARY GLAND OF CASTRATED RATS WITH PUSH-PULL CANNULAE (PPC)
D.E. Dluzen, V.D. Ramirez
University of Illinois, Urbana

14 **14.** ESTROGEN-INDUCED DESENSITIZATION TO THE NEGATIVE ESTROGEN FEEDBACK
F. Döcke, W. Rohde, P. Gerber, R. Chaoui, G. Dörner
Institute of Experimental Endocrinology, Humboldt University, Berlin, GDR

15 **15.** A NEW METHOD TO PERFUSE THE RAT TESTES IN VIVO
E.-M Düker, B. Wolff, W. Wuttke
Div. Clin. Exp. Endocr., Dept. ObGyn., Univ. Göttingen, FRG

16 **16.** ADRENERGIC RECEPTORS MEDIATING STIMULATION OF CYCLIC AMP ACCUMULATION BY NOREPINEPHRINE IN HYPOTHALAMIC AND PREOPTIC AREA SLICES FROM OVARIECTOMIZED AND OVARIECTOMIZED, ESTRADIOL-PRIMED RATS
A.M. Etgen
Albert Einstein College of Medicine, Bronx, NY 10461

17 **17.** ACUTE EFFECT OF Δ^9-TETRAHYDROCANNABINOL ON THE PULSATILE RHYTHM OF BLOOD LH IN OVARIECTOMIZED RATS
G.I. Fujimoto, D.I. Whitmoyer
Laboratory of Neuroendocrinology, Brain Research Institute and Dept. of Anatomy, UCLA School of Medicine, Los Angeles, CA 90024

18 **18.** PULSATILE LH SECRETION IN HYPOGONADAL WOMEN: EFFECT OF CHRONIC BROMOCRIPTINE ADMINISTRATION
M. Gambacciani, G.B. Melis, A. Cagnacci, P. Fioretti
Dept. of Obstet. Gynecol., University of Pisa, Italy

19 **19.** HYPOTHALAMIC AREAS CONTROLLING LH PULSES IN THE RAT
R.L. Goodman
Department of Physiology, West Virginia University, Morgantown, WV

20 **20.** A NEW MODEL FOR THE IMITATION OF PROESTRUS-LIKE LH-SURGES AND CATECHOLAMINE TURNOVER FLUCTUATIONS IN OVARIECTOMIZED RATS
C. Hiemke, J. Hinze, A. Schmid, R. Ghraf
Institut für Physiologische Chemie, Universität Essen, Essen, F.R.G.

21 **21.** NEUROCHEMICAL CHARACTERIZATION OF THE NORADRENERGIC NEUROTOXIN, 5-ADMP, IN THE RAT HYPOTHALAMUS
H.D. Jarry, K.J. Lookingland, K.E. Moore
Dept. of Pharmacology and Toxicology, Michigan State Univ., East Lansing, MI 48824

22 **22.** HORMONAL REGULATION OF THE GONADOTROPIN SUBUNIT SYNTHESIS
M. Jutisz, R. Counis, A. Starzec, M. Corbani
Polypeptide Hormone Laboratory, CNRS, 91190 Gif-sur-Yvette, France

23 **23.** PULSATILE RELEASE OF LHRH IN THE MAMILLARY REGION OF THE HYPOTHALAMUS IN INFANT PIGS
S. Kanematsu, T. Hirata
Dept. of Animal Husbandry, Fac. of Agriculture, Iwate University, Morioka, 020, Japan

24 **24.** ESTROGEN MODULATION OF THE α_1-ADRENERGIC EXCITATION OF HYPOTHALAMIC PARVOCELLULAR NEURONS
M.J. Kelly, T.P. Condon, O.K. Ronnekleiv
Dept. of Physiology, Oregon Health Sci. U., Portland, Oregon 97201

25 **25.** THE EFFECT OF SEROTONIN DEPLETERS ON PROSTAGLANDIN D_2-INDUCED LH INHIBITION IN CASTRATED MALE RATS
T. Koh, Y. Nakai, F. Kinoshita, S. Tsujii, H. Takahashi, T. Usui, H. Imura
Second Division, Department of Medicine, Kyoto University, Kyoto, 606, Japan

26 **25a.** DOSE-DEPENDENT SUPPRESSION BY LHRH OF THE POSITIVE EFFECT OF ESTRADIOL ON THE PITUITARY GLAND
T.R. Koiter, H. Moes, G.A. Schuiling
Dept. of Obstetrics & Gynecology, University of Groningen, The Netherlands

27 **26.** EFFECT OF TRADITIONAL HERBAL MEDICINE ON HYPOTHALAMIC-PITUITARY-OVARIAN FUNCTION IN WOMEN WITH OVARIAN INSUFFICIENCY
T. Koyama, M. Ichimura, M. Ohara, Y. Kido, M. Saito
Department of Obstetrics and Gynecology, Tokyo Medical and Dental University, Tokyo, 113, Japan

28 **27.** THE EFFECT OF BARBITURATES ON PITUITARY SENSITIVITY TO LHRH IN THE OVARIECTOMIZED RAT
C.B. Lambalk, J.A.M.J. van Dieten, J. de Koning, J. Schoemaker, G.P. van Rees*
Dept of Pharmacology of the University of Leiden, P.O. Box 9503, 2300 RA Leiden, The Netherlands and *Dept. of Obstet./Gynaecology, Academic Hospital of the Vrije Universiteit, P.O. Box 7095, 1007 MB Amsterdam, The Netherlands.

29 **28.** THE EFFECTS OF HIGHLY SPECIFIC OPIATE RECEPTOR AGONISTS ON LH AND PROLACTIN SECRETION IN RATS
C.A. Leadem, S. Johnson
Department of Anatomy, University of Arizona, Tucson, AZ

30 **29.** HYPOTHALAMIC FACTOR THAT INHIBITS LH SECRETION: RELATIONSHIP WITH GnRH (1–5)
J. Leal, M. De la Lastra
Laboratorio Endocrinología, Facultad Ciencias Biológicas Pontificia Universidad Católica de Chile. Casilla 114-D. Santiago, Chile

31 **30.** INHIBITION OF LH AND PRL BY Δ^9-TETRAHYDROCANNABINOL IN MEDIAL BASAL HYPOTHALAMIC DEAFFERENTED OVARIECTOMIZED RATS
L.L. Murphy, C.D. Thomas, L. Tyrey
Dept. of Obstetrics and Gynecology, Duke University, Durham, NC 27710

32 **31.** USE OF POTENT LHRH ANALOGS IN THE CONTROL OF FERTILITY AND TREATMENT OF ENDOMETRIOSIS
R.M.G. Nair, G.K. Nambiar, M.A. Barnes, R.S. Mathur, M.R. Neff, G. Holtz, R.E. McIntosh
VA Medical Center & Depts. of Medicine and Obstetrics and Gynecology, Charleston, SC, School of Sciences & Technology, Savannah, GA, Mount Sinai Medical Center, Milwaukee, WI, and The Fertility Clinic, Seattle, WA

33 **32.** OPIOID PEPTIDE INHIBITION OF THE HYPOTHALAMIC-PITUITARY AXIS IN THE RABBIT
K.M. Orstead and H.G. Spies
Oregon Primate Research Center, Beaverton, Oregon 97006

34 **33.** THE EFFECT OF Δ^9-TETRAHYDROCANNABINOL ON SOMATOSTATIN AND LH-RH RELEASE FROM RAT MEDIAN EMINENCE "IN VITRO"
V. Rettori, C. Aguila, S. Dalterio, S.M. McCann*
Dept. of Physiology, University of Texas Health Science Center at Dallas, Texas 75235 and *Dept. of Pharmacology UTHSC at San Antonio, Texas 78284

35 **34.** PROCESSING OF PREPRO-LUTEINIZING HORMONE-RELEASING HORMONE IN THE HYPOTHALAMUS
O.K. Ronnekleiv, J. Adelman, W.E. Ellinwood, M.J. Kelly
Dept. Physiology and IABR, Oregon Health Sciences, U. Portland, Oregon

36 **35.** GONADAL MODULATION OF NEUROPEPTIDE Y RELEASE FROM THE MEDIOBASAL HYPOTHALAMUS (MBH) *IN VITRO*
A. Sahu, W.R. Crowley, T.L. O'Donohue, P.S. Kalra, S.P. Kalra
Dept. OB-Gyn, Univ. Fla. Col. Med., Gainesville, FL 32610 and Dept. Pharmacol., Univ. Tenn., Memphis, TN

37 **36.** PULSATILE RELEASE OF HYPOTHALAMIC LHRH INTO PITUITARY PORTAL BLOOD OF OVARIECTOMIZED RATS: EVIDENCE FOR AN AUTOFEEDBACK MECHANISM
D.K. Sarkar
University of California, San Diego, La Jolla, CA 92093

38 **37.** PATHOLOGIC EFFECTS OF ESTRADIOL ON THE HYPOTHALAMIC ARCUATE NUCLEUS
H.M. Schipper, J.R. Brawer
McGill University, Montreal, Canada

39 **38.** CHOLECYSTOKININ AND REPRODUCTION: CASTRATION ALTERS CCK LEVELS WITHIN CELLS OF THREE SEXUALLY DIMORPHIC NUCLEI
R.B. Simerly and L.W. Swanson
Howard Hughes Medical Institute and The Salk Institute, La Jolla, California, USA

40 **40.** QUANTITY, IN SITU ACTIVITY, AND PHOSPHORYLATION OF TYROSINE HYDROXYLASE IN THE MEDIAN EMINENCE AS A FUNCTION OF ESTROGEN AND PROGESTERONE
P.S. Wang, J.C. Porter
University of Texas Health Science Center, Dallas, Texas 75235

41 **41.** INTRAVENTRICULAR INJECTION OF OVINE FSH SUPPRESSES LH AND TO A LESSER EXTENT FSH RELEASE IN OVARIECTOMIZED RATS
W.H. Yu, S.M. McCann
Dept. of Physiol., University of Texas Health Science Center, Dallas, Texas, 75235

42 **42.** EFFECTS OF HORMONAL TREATMENT ON HYPOTHALAMIC LHRH CONTENT
M. Zanisi, E. Messi, M. Motta
Department of Endocrinology, University of Milano, Italy

Action of Hypothalamic Hormones

43 **43.** THE POSSIBLE ROLE OF CALMODULIN IN THE RELEASE OF SRIF INDUCED BY GRF
M.C. Aguila, S.M. McCann
Department of Physiology, Univ. of Texas Health Science Center at Dallas, Texas 75235

44 **44.** ANGIOTENSIN II (A_{II}) ACTS ON ANTERIOR PITUITARY (AP) CELLS TO INCREASE INTRACELLULAR FREE CALCIUM [Ca++]i AND STIMULATE PROLACTIN RELEASE
J.M. Anderson, M.J. Cronin
University of Virginia, Charlottesville, Virginia 22908

45 **45.** ACTH RELEASE IN RESPONSE TO CRF, FORSKOLIN, MAITOTOXIN, PHORBOL ESTER AND ATRIAL NATRIURETIC FACTOR (ANF)
A.J. Baertschi, T. Yasumoto, R. Pence, M.J. Cronin
University of Virginia, Charlottesville, VA 22908, Tohoku University, Sendai 980 Japan

46 **46.** INTERACTIONS BETWEEN STIMULATORY AND INHIBITORY NEUROHORMONES ON RAT ANTERIOR PITUITARY ADENYLATE CYCLASE ACTIVITY
P. Bertrand, J. Epelbaum, C. Kordon, A. Enjalbert
U. 159 INSERM, U. de Neuroendocrinologie, 2ter rue d'Alésia, 75014 Paris, France

47 **47.** SECRETION OF GROWTH HORMONE BY 5,6-EPOXY-EICOSATRIENOIC ACID IN NORMAL RAT PITUITARY CELLS
J.R. Cashman, D. Grandsaert, R.I. Weiner
University of California San Francisco, San Francisco, California

48 **48.** INOSITOL PHOSPHATES, DIACYLGLYCEROL, AND ARACHIDONIC ACID IN GnRH ACTION
J.P. Chang, R.O. Morgan, K.J. Catt
Endo. & Reprod. Res. Branch, NICHD, Bethesda, Maryland

49 **49.** LEUKOTRIENES C4 AND D4 ARE POTENT STIMULATORS OF LHRH RELEASE IN VITRO
K. Gerozissis, C. Rougeot, F. Dray
INSERM U. 207—Institut Pasteur, URIA, 75015 Paris

50 **50.** PITUITARY CYCLIC AMP RESPONSE TO CRF ADMINISTRATION IN VIVO
G.J. Kant, M.A. Oleshansky, D.D. Walczak, E.H. Mougey,

J.L. Meyerhoff
Dept. Medical Neurosciences, Walter Reed Army Institute of Research, Washington, DC 20307

51 **51.** SOMATOSTATIN RECEPTORS ON GH, TSH AND PRL CELLS: PHARMACOLOGICAL CHARACTERIZATION OF 125I NTyr SRIF BINDING SITES AND COUPLING TO ADENYLATE CYCLASE
S. Krantic, P. Bertrand, C. Shu, A. Enjalbert, C. Kordon, J. Epelbaum
U. 159 INSERM, 2 ter rue d'Alésia, 75014 Paris, France

52 **52.** ROLE OF Na^{+} AND Ca^{2+} IN DOPAMINE INHIBITION OF STIMULATED PROLACTIN RELEASE BY 7315a AND MtTW15 RAT PITUITARY TUMORS
J. Lafond, C. Bouvier, R. Collu
Research Unit on Reproductive and Developmental Biology, Pediatric Research Center, Hôpital Ste-Justine and University of Montreal, Montreal, Canada, H3T 1C5

53 **53.** SUPPRESSION OF TRH-INDUCED $^{45}Ca^{2+}$ FLUX IN 7315a TUMOR CELLS
I.S. Login, A.M. Judd, W.D. Jarvis, R.M. MacLeod
University of Virginia School of Medicine, Charlottesville, Virginia 22908

54 **54.** THYROLIBERIN (TRH) RELEASE IS DEPENDENT ON EXTRACELLULAR Ca^{+} AND PARTIALLY MEDIATED BY AN ACTIVATION OF PROTEIN KINASE C IN HYPOTHALAMIC CELLS GROWN IN SFM
C. Loudes, A. Faivre-Bauman, A. Barret, A. Tixier-Vidal
UA_CNRS 1115, Collège de France, Paris (FRANCE)

55 **55.** THE DESENSITIZATION PHASE OF GnRH STIMULATED LH RELEASE FROM SHEEP PITUITARY CELLS IN PERIFUSION
*R.P. McIntosh, J.E.A. McIntosh, L. Starling, W.R. Smith**
Wellington Clinical School of Medicine, University of Otago at Wellington, New Zealand and *University of Guelph, Ontario, Canada

56 **56.** SOMATOSTATINERGIC INHIBITION OF HYPOTHALAMIC AND ANTERIOR PITUITARY ADENYLATE CYCLASE ACTIVITY
G. Schettini, T. Florio, O. Meucci, E. Landolfi, M. Grimaldi, G. Magri
Dept. Pharmacol, II Medical School, 80131 Naples, ITALY

57 **57.** ADENOSINE MODULATION OF ANTERIOR PITUITARY ADENYLATE CYCLASE ACTIVITY
G. Schettini, E. Landolfi, O. Meucci, T. Florio
Dept. Pharmacol, II Medical School, 80131 Naples, ITALY

58 **58.** GROWTH INHIBITION OF PITUITARY TUMOR CELLS BY GM_1, PHORBOL ESTER, FORSKOLIN, AND BUTYRATE
M.A. Sortino, S.T. Summers, R. Steward, A. Fedson, M.J. Cronin
University of Virginia, Charlottesville, Virginia 22908

59 **59.** PROTEIN KINASE C ENHANCES GROWTH HORMONE RELEASING FACTOR (GRF) AND CORTICOTROPIN RELEASING FACTOR (CRF) STIMULATED CYCLIC AMP (cAMP) PRODUCTION IN ANTERIOR PITUITARY (AP) CELLS
S.T. Summers, A.J. Baertschi, J.R. Zysk, M.J. Cronin
University of Virginia, Charlottesville, Virginia 22908

60 **60.** CHARACTERIZATION OF PGE2 RECEPTORS IN PORCINE AND MURINE ANTERIOR PITUITARIES
C. Tiberghien, V. Fafeur, A. Wisner-Provost, M.C. Bommelaer, F. Haour, F. Dray
INSERM U. 207—Institut Pasteur, URIA, 75015 Paris

61 **61.** CHEMICAL CROSSLINKING OF A GROWTH HORMONE RELEASING FACTOR BINDING SITE IN ANTERIOR PITUITARY CELLS
J.R. Zysk, M.O. Thorner, J.M. Anderson, M.J. Cronin
University of Virginia, Charlottesville, Virginia 22908

Neuroendocrine Regulation of TSH

62 **62.** DUAL EFFECT OF GABA ON TRH-INDUCED TSH RELEASE FROM PERIFUSED RAT PITUITARIES
H. Astier, J.P. Roussel, L. Tapia-Arancibia
Lab. Neuroendocrinology, University of Montpellier II, 34060 Montpellier, France

63 **63.** OPIATE-THYROID HORMONE INTERACTIONS IN THE REGULATION OF TSH SECRETION IN THE RAT
L.A. Berglund, W.J. Millard, S.M. Gabriel, J.W. Simpkins
Department of Pharmacodynamics, College of Pharmacy, University of Florida, Gainesville, FL 32610

64 **63a.** THE SECRETION OF TSH IN ACROMEGALY MEASURED BY A SENSITIVE TSH ASSAY
P.C. Eskildsen, A. Kruse, C.B. Kirkegaard
Medical Dept. C, Neurosurg. Dept. H, Glostrup Hospital and Medical Dept. E, Frederiksberg Hospital, Copenhagen, Denmark

65 **64.** CHOLINERGIC SUPPRESSION OF TSH SECRETION: THERAPEUTIC APPLICATIONS
H.G. Fein, A.J. Ahmann, J.E. Hennessey, N.E. Butkus, D.M. Kornhauser, B.G. Petty, R.C. Smallridge
Depts. of Medicine, Walter Reed Army Institute of Research, Washington, D.C. 20307 and Johns Hopkins Medical Institutions, Baltimore, MD 21205

66 **65.** SERUM TSH REDUCTION IN RESPONSE TO hpGRF ADMINISTRATION IN PATIENTS WITH PITUITARY DWARFISM
T. Hashimoto, T. Sato, K. Kawai, N. Ohba, F. Matsubara
Central Clinical Laboratory and Department of Pediatrics, Kanazawa University Hospital, Ishikawa, 920, Japan

67 **66.** NEURO-HORMONAL REGULATION OF HUMAN TSH-SECRETING ADENOMA IN CELL CULTURE
P. Jaquet, G. Gunz, I. Pellegrini, J. Hassoun
INSERM U 297, UER de Médecine Nord 13326 Marseille Cedex 15 FRANCE

68 **67.** THYROID-HYPOPHYSO-HYPOTHALAMIC AXIS OF THE GENETICALLY HYPOPROLACTINEMIC RATS (IPL NUDE RATS)
D. Jordan (1), I. Sabbagh (2), P. Guillaumot (3), M. Veisseire (1), J. Bertrand (3), H. Cohen (3)
(1) INSERM U 197, Faculté de Médecine Alexis-Carrel, 69372 Lyon; (2) Institut Pasteur, Lyon; (3) INSERM U 34, Hôpital Debrousse, 69322 Lyon, France

69 **68** ANTERIOR PITUITARY HORMONE RESPONSES DURING EUGLYCEMIC INSULIN CLAMP
T. Hashimoto, I. Miyamoto, Y. Noto, F. Matsubara
Central Clinical Laboratory and the 1st Department of Internal

Medicine, Kanazawa University Hospital, Ishikawa, 920, Japan

70 **69.** HYPOTHALAMIC CONTROL OF 5'-DEIODINASE ACTIVITY IN RAT ANTERIOR PITUITARY
M. Murakami, K. Tanaka, M.A. Greer
Section of Endocrinology, Oregon Health Sciences University, Portland, Oregon 97201

71 **70.** DOPAMINE SYNTHESIS IN THE HYPOTHALAMUS AS WELL AS DOPAMINE AND PROLACTIN CONCENTRATIONS IN THE ADENOHYPOPHYSIS ARE INFLUENCED BY THYROID STATUS IN THE RAT
M.J. Reymond, Th. Lemarchand-Béraud
Division of Endocrinology, Department Internal Medicine, CHUV, 1011 Lausanne, Switzerland

Neuroendocrinology of the Posterior Pituitary

72 **71.** ARGININE-VASOPRESSIN MODULATES β-ENDORPHIN RELEASE FROM RAT BRAIN STRUCTURES
I. Barna, V.M. Wiegant, H.D. Veldhuis, D. De Wied
Rudolf Magnus Institute for Pharmacology, University of Utrecht, Utrecht, The Netherlands

73 **72.** OXYTOCIN RESPONSES TO STRESS IN LACTATING AND HYPERPROLACTINAEMIC RATS
D.A. Carter, S.L. Lightman
Medical Unit, Charing Cross & Westminster Medical School, Page St., London, SW1P 2AP

74 **73.** A CORRELATIVE NEUROPHYSIN IMMUNOHISTOCHEMICAL AND FINE STRUCTURAL STUDY OF NEUROSECRETORY AXON REGENERATION INTO INTRAHYPOTHALAMIC, NEURAL LOBE ALLOGRAFTS
H.-D. Dellmann, L.-F Lue, S.I. Bellin
Department of Veterinary Anatomy, Iowa State University, Ames, Iowa, 50011.

75 **74.** ARGININE VASOPRESSIN (AVP) AND CORTICOTROPIN RELEASING FACTOR (CRF) IN THE ANTERIOR PITUITARY: NO CORRELATION WITH PRESUMED SECRETION RATE
J. Dohanics,[1] E.A. Linton,[2] T. Janaky,[3] F.A. Laszlo,[3] G.B. Makara[1]
[1]Institute of Experimental Medicine, Hungarian Academy

76 **75.** CALCIUM IONS AND OXYTOCIN-INDUCED CONTRACTIONS OF THE MALE MOUSE ANOCOCCYGEUS
A. Gibson, M. Ginsburg
Dept. of Pharmacology, Kings College London, Chelsea Campus, London SW3 6LX, UK

77 **76.** CONVERGING EXCITATORY INPUTS TO PARVOCELLULAR PARAVENTRICULAR NEUROSECRETORY CELLS AFTER NOXIOUS AND HYPOVOLEMIC STIMULI
M. Hamamura, T. Onaka, K. Yagi
Dept. of Physiol., Jichi Med. Sch., Tochigi, Japan

78 **77.** VASOPRESSIN-STIMULATED TURNOVER OF PHOSPHATIDYLINOSITOL IN SENSORY GANGLIA OF THE RAT
A.M. Horn, S.L. Lightman
Medical Unit, Charing Cross & Westminster Medical School, Westminster Hospital, 17 Page Street, London, SW1P 2AP, UK.

79 **78.** HYPOTHALAMIC SARCOIDOSIS WITH PARTIAL HYPOPITUITARISM: A study of 3 cases
M. Kamelman Levitin, I. Molocznik, H.A. Ruggiero, J.E. Argonz, E. Caputti, A. Sanchez, R. Driollet Laspiur, R. Artese
Costa Buero Institute, Department of Neuroendocrinology, Medical School, U.B.A., Buenos Aires, Argentina

80 **79.** INHIBITORY INFLUENCE OF EXOGENOUS OXYTOCIN (OT) ON CORTISOL AND ACTH IN MAN: EVIDENCE FOR REBOUND EFFECT AND REPRODUCIBILITY
J.J. Legros, P. Chiodera, V. Geenen
Psychoneuroendocrine Unit, University of Liege, Sart Tilman, B23, B-4000 Liège, Belgium

81 **80.** THE ANTIBODY RAISED AGAINST NEUROPEPTIDE: IS IT A NEW MEAN TO ACT *IN VIVO* ON PEPTIDERGIC NEURONS?
A. Burlet, B. Leon-Henri, A. Arahmani, F. Robert, C. Burlet.
Laboratoire de Biologie cellulaire, Faculté de Médecine, BP 184-F-54505-Vandoeuvre-les-Nancy

82 **81.** VASOPRESSIN AND OXYTOCIN INCREASE ACTH BUT REDUCE PROLACTIN SECRETION. STUDY OF THE RECEPTOR(S) INVOLVED
P. Mormède,[1] J.D. Vincent,[2] B. Kerdelhue,[3] R. Dantzer,[1] M. Le Moal[1]
[1]INSERM-INRA U-259, [2]INSERM U-176, Domaine de Carreire rue Camille Saint-Saëns, 33077 Bordeaux, [3]CNRS Laboratoire des Hormones Polypeptides, 91190 Gif-sur-Yvette, France

83 **82.** OPOSITE EFFECTS OF ARGININE VASOTOCIN AND LYSINE VASOPRESSIN INJECTED INTO THE CEREBRAL VENTRICULES ON VISUAL EVOKED POTENITALS IN CAT
V. Neştianu, M[x)] Coculescu, M. Iancău, St. Mihăilescu
Dept. of Physiology, Craiova University School of Medicine and Dept.[x)] of Endocrinology, Bucharest Faculty of Medicine, Romania

84 **83.** HISTAMINE AS A NEUROMODULATOR OF THE VASOPRESSINERGIC SYSTEM
H. Niigawa, R. Cacabelos, A. Yamatodani, H. Wada*, K. Tada, S. Hariguchi, T. Nishimura*
Departments of Neuropsychiatry and Pharmacology II*, Osaka University Medical School, Osaka 553, Japan

85 **84.** EFFECTS OF LEU-ENKEPHALIN AND MET-ENKEPHALIN ON VASOPRESSIN RELEASE FROM PERIFUSED RAT HYPOTHALAMO-NEUROHYPOPHYSEAL COMPLEX
Y. Oki, I. Tanaka, S. Ohgo, Y. Ikeda, M. Sakamoto, M. Nanno, T. Yoshimi
Hamamatsu University School of Medicine, Hamamatsu, Japan

86 **85.** VASOPRESSIN RESPONSES TO CORTICOTROPIN-RELEASING FACTOR IN CONSCIOUS DOGS: GLUCOCORTICOID SUPPRESSION
H. Raff, D. Merrill, M. Skelton, A.W. Cowley, Jr.

Medical College of Wisconsin, Milwaukee, WI 53226 and St. Luke's Hospital, Milwaukee, Wi 53215

87 **86.** NEURAL GRAFTING IN THE THIRD CEREBRAL VENTRICULAR LUMEN OF THE BRATTLEBORO RAT WITH CHRONIC AUTOSOMOL DIABETES INSIPIDUS (DI)
D.E. Scott, R. Wolkowitz
Eastern Virginia Medical School, Norfolk, Virginia and University of Missouri-Columbia School of Medicine, Columbia, Missouri

88 **87.** VASOPRESSIN ACTIVATION OF PHOSPHATIDYLINOSITOL METABOLISM IN RAT ANTERIOR PITUITARY IS MODIFIED BY CHANGES IN THE HYPOTHALAMO-PITUITARY ADRENAL AXIS
K. Todd, S.L. Lightman
Medical Unit, Charing Cross & Westminster Medical School, Westminster Hospital, 17 Page Street, London, SW1P 2AP, UK

89 **88.** β-ENDORPHIN AND DYNORPHIN SUPPRESS VASOPRESSIN RELEASE IN RATS UNDER VARIOUS CONDITIONS
Tj.B. Van Wimersma Greidanus, J.A. Ten Haaf
Rudolf Magnus Institute for Pharmacology, University of Utrecht, Vondellaan 6, 3521 GD Utrecht, The Netherlands

Wednesday PM **Continental Ballroom 5**

SESSION 3: Neuroendocrine Regulation of Prolactin
Chairpersons: **R. MacLeod**
A. Enjalbert

1:30 **89.** MODULATION OF HORMONE SECRETION BY FOLLICULO-STELLATE CELLS IN RAT ANTERIOR PITUITARY CELL AGGREGATES
W. Allaerts, C. Denef
Laboratory of Cell Pharmacology, School of Medicine, University of Leuven, Belgium

1:45 **90** ARTERIES ARE PRESENT IN HUMAN PROLACTINOMAS
J.E. Schechter, R.I. Weiner
University of Southern California, School of Medicine, Los Angeles, California and University of California San Francisco, School of Medicine, San Francisco, California

2:00 **91.** DOPAMINE (DA) D_2 RECEPTORS IN DA-RESISTANT PROLACTIN-SECRETING RAT PITUITARY TUMORS 7315a AND MtTW15: STRUCTURAL STUDIES
C. Bouvier, J. Lafond, G. Beauregard, M. Potier, R. Collu
Research Unit on Reproductive and Developmental Biology, and Section of Medical Genetics, Hôpital Sainte-Justine and University of Montreal, Montreal, Canada, H3T 1C5

2:15 **92.** THE PROLACTIN RELEASING ACTION OF TRH BUT NOT VIP IS POTENTIATED FOLLOWING THE BRIEF INTERRUPTION OF DA INHIBITION
G. Martinez-Escalera, J. Guthrie, R. Weiner
Reprod. Endo. Center, UCSF, San Francisco, CA 94143

2:30 **93.** LIVER FACTOR(S) STIMULATES CASEIN RELEASE *IN VITRO* IN THE ABSENCE OF ADDED PROLACTIN
J.P. Hoeffler, L.S. Frawley
Zoology Dept. Iowa State University, Ames, IA 50011

2:45 **94.** SIMULTANEOUS BILATERAL COLLECTION OF BLOOD FROM INFERIOR PETROSAL SINUSES OF PATIENTS WITH PROLACTIN-SECRETING ADENOMAS
L. Annunziato, B. Merola, P. Miletto, A.M. Colao, M. Taglialatela, C. Nappi, G. De Chiara, G. Lombardi
Institute of Endocrinology, Pharmacology and Gynecology, 2nd School of Medicine, University of Naples, Via S. Pansini 5, 80131 Naples, Italy

3:00 **95.** CONCORDANCE BETWEEN LH AND PRL PULSES IN OVARIECTOMIZED RATS IN THE PRESENCE AND ABSENCE OF DOPAMINE INHIBITION
C.R. Pohl, R.I. Weiner, M.S. Smith
University of Pittsburgh, Pittsburgh, PA 15261 and University of California at San Francisco, San Francisco, CA 94143

3:15 **96.** EFFECT OF PLACENTAL LACTOGEN ON CIRCULATING PROLACTIN AND HYPOPHYSIAL STALK PLASMA DOPAMINE LEVELS
J.L. Voogt, W.J. deGreef, J.T.M. Vreeburg
Univ. of Kansas Med. Ctr., Kansas City, KS 66103 and Erasmus Univ., Rotterdam, Netherlands

Wednesday PM **Continental Ballroom 6**

SESSION 4: Neuropeptides
Chairpersons: **P. Goldsmith**
D. Pfaff

1:30 **97.** CENTRAL NERVOUS SYSTEM SITES OF ACTION OF ATRIAL NATRIURETIC FACTOR
W.K. Samson, J. Antunes-Rodrigues, C.A. Dudley and R.L. Moss
Southwestern Medical School, Dallas, Texas 75235

1:45 **99.** PRESENCE OF AN ENKEPHALIN-CONVERTING ENZYME (ENDO-OLIGOPEPTIDASE A) IN ENDOCRINE TISSUES
E.B. Oliveira, M.S. Medeiros,* A.C.M. Camargo,* K.M. Metters[+], J. Rossier[+]*
*Instituto Ciências Biomédicas-USP, São Paulo, Brasil
[+]Laboratorie de Physiologie Nerveuse, C.N.R.S. 91190 Gif-sur-Yvette, France

2:00 **100.** EVIDENCE FOR PROGNRH IN RAT PERIPHERAL TISSUES: IMMUNOSTAINING WITH ANTIBODIES AGAINST GNRH AND THE GNRH-ASSOCIATED PEPTIDE
C.A. Padula, K. Nikolics, P.H. Seeburg, P.C. Goldsmith
Reproductive Endocrinology Center, Dept. of Ob/Gyn and Repro. Sci., University of Calif., San Francisco, CA 94143

2:15 **101.** IMMUNOHISTOLOGICAL STUDIES ON NEUROPEPTIDES IN THE RAT OVARY
T.J. Gorcs,[1] A. Arimura,[1] D.H. Coy[2]
U.S.-Japan Biomedical Research Laboratories, LMNED,

Tulane University Hebert Center, Belle Chasse, LA 70037[1] and Department of Medicine, Tulane University School of Medicine, New Orleans, LA 70112[1,2]

2:30 **102.** HYPOTHALAMIC CYCLIC AMP AND cGMP RESPONSE TO INTRAVENTRICULAR SUBSTANCE P AND/OR NEUROTENSIN IN THE RAT
E. Vijayan, Anahita Mistry
School of Life Sciences, University of Hyderabad, Hyderabad 500134, India

2:45 **103.** HYPOTHALAMO-HYPOPHYSIAL SYSTEM: HIDDEN MICROVASCULAR BLOOD FLOW PATTERNS REVEALED *IN VIVO* BY FLUORESCENT MICROSPHERES
A.J. Baertschi
University of Virginia, Charlottesville, VA 22908

3:00 **104.** SELECTED NEUROPEPTIDES IN AMYOTROPHIC LATERAL SCLEROSIS PATIENTS
J. Szulc-Kuberska, H. Stepien, A. Klimek, D. Cieslak
Dept. Neurology and Inst. Endocrinology, Medical Academy in Lodz, Poland

Wednesday PM **Teakwood**

SESSION 5: DEVELOPMENT AND AGING
Chairpersons: **W. Lichtensteiger**
C. Finch

1:30 **105.** SIMULTANEOUS DISTRIBUTION OF OVARIAN LHRH AND β-ADRENERGIC RECEPTORS DURING SEXUAL MATURATION IN THE RAT: ROLE OF OVARIAN INNERVATION
*B. Marchetti, M. Cioni, U. Scapagnini, *G. Pelletier*
Dept. Pharmacology, Catania University, 95125 Italy and *Molecular Endocrinol. Laval University, Quebec, Canada

1:45 **106.** ANGIOTENSIN II: A GROWTH HORMONE RELEASING FACTOR IN THE DEVELOPING RAT?
Wim Robberecht, Carl Denef
Laboratory of Cell Pharmacology, School of Medicine, University of Leuven, Belgium

2:00 **107.** DEVELOPMENTAL CHANGE IN THE SENSITIVITY TO SOMATOSTATIN IN THE OVINE FETUS AND LAMB
J. Daaboul, F. de Zegher, S.L. Kaplan, M.M. Grumbach
Dept. of Pediatrics, University of California San Francisco, San Francisco, CA 94143

2:15 **108.** DIFFERENTIAL EFFECTS OF THE PERINATAL STEROID ENVIRONMENT ON SEXUALLY DIMORPHIC PARAMETERS IN THE RAT BRAIN
A. Siddiqui, D.P. Gilmore, J.S. Clark
Institute of Physiology, University of Glasgow, Glasgow, G12 8QQ

2:30 **109.** AROMATASE ACTIVITY IN BRAIN REGIONS OF STANLEY-GUMBRECK PSEUDOHERMAPHRODITE MALE RATS AND NORMAL LITTERMATES
C.E. Roselli, R.L. Salisbury, J.A. Resko
Oregon Health Sci. Unv., Portland, Oregon and the Univ. of Akron, Akron, OH

2:45 **110.** APPRAISING THE INSTANTANEOUS SECRETORY RATES OF LUTEINIZING HORMONE AND TESTOSTERONE IN RESPONSE TO SELECTIVE MU OPIATE RECEPTOR IN LATE PUBERTAL BOYS
N. Mauras, A.D. Rogol, J.D. Veldhuis
The University of Virginia Medical Center, Charlottesville, Virginia 22908

3:00 **111.** REMOVAL OF A CENTRAL INHIBITORY COMPONENT AND HYPOTHALAMIC MATURATION AT THE ONSET OF PUBERTY
N.J. Schultz, E. Terasawa
Wis. Reg. Primate Res. Ctr., Univ. WI, Madison, WI 53715

3:15 **112.** β-ENDORPHIN AND DYNORPHIN-17 LEVELS IN RAT PITUITARY AND HYPOTHALAMUS: AGE STUDIES
Elizabeth M. Dax, Coral Reichman, Meryl Fullerton, John W. Funder*
National Institutes of Aging, Francis Scott Key Medical Center, Baltimore 21224, and Medical Research Centre, Prince Henry's Hospital, Melbourne 3004, Australia

Thursday AM **Continental Ballroom 4**

SESSION 6: Symposium on Expression and Processing of Neuroendocrine Peptides
Chairpersons: **J. Funder**
J. Martial

8:30 **113.** Peter Seeburg (USA)—Structure and Activity of the GnRH Precursor

9:00 **114.** James Roberts (USA)—Transcriptional Regulation of Proopiomelanocortin Gene Expression in Neuroendocrine Cells

9:30 **115.** Shigetada Nakanishi (Japan)—Structure and Regulation of the Preprotachykinin Gene

10:00 **116.** Edward Herbert (USA)—How Gene Transfer Methods Help Us to Understand Regulation of Expression of Opioid Peptides

Thursday AM **Continental Ballroom 5**

SESSION 7: Symposium on Neuroregulatory Role of Peptides
Chairpersons: **C. Kordon**
M. Motta

8:30 **117.** Michel Ferin (USA)—Endogenous Opiates and Gonadotropin Secretion in the Non-Human Primate

9:00 **118.** Sami Said (USA)—Peptides Common to the Brain, Gastrointestinal Tract and Other Organs

9:30 **119.** Miklos Palkovits (Hungary)—Neuropeptides in the Median Eminence

10:00 **120.** Leo Renaud (Canada)—Intrinsic and Synaptic Regulation of Vasopressinergic Neurons

Thursday AM **Continental Ballrooms 1–3**

SESSION 8: Symposium on Integrative Neuroendocrinology

Chairpersons: **B. Halasz**
J. Kraicer

8:30 **121.** Detlev Ganten (Germany)—The Renin Angiotensin System (RAS) in the Brain

9:00 **122.** Carl Denef (Belgium)—Modulation of Pituitary Hormone Secretion by Intercellular Communication

9:30 **123.** Bruce McEwen (USA)—Stress, Adrenal Steroids and the Hippocampus

10:00 **124.** George Hedge (USA)—Functional Significance of Peptidergic Thyroid Nerves

Thursday AM/PM **Continental Parlors 6–9**

SESSION 9: Neuroendocrine Regulation of Prolactin; Comparative Neuroendocrinology; Neuroendocrine Regulation of GH; Expression and Processing of Neuroendocrine Peptides

Poster Session **Posters manned from 10:30–12:00PM and 3:30–5:00PM**

Neuroendocrine Regulation of PRL

Position

1 **125.** EFFECTS OF GONADAL STEROIDS AND BROMOCRYPTINE ON LACTATION AND SUCKLING-INDUCED PROLACTIN SECRETION
S. El Arab, M.I. El-Ghamry, B. Abou Hozaifa, J.W. Simpkins
Department of Pharmacodynamics, College of Pharmacy, Univ. of Florida, Gainesville, FL 32610

2 **126.** FEMALE PROLACTINOMAS: A STUDY OF 77 CASES
J.E. Argonz, R. Artese, I. Molocznik, H. Benencia, E. Raida, R. Driollet Laspiur
Costa Buero Institute, Department of Neuroendocrinology, Medical School, U.B.A., Buenos Aires, Argentina (1121)

3 **127.** GALACTORRHEA AS ONLY SYMPTOM OF HYPOTHALAMIC-CHIASMATICAL GLIOMA
J.E. Argonz, A. Martino, I. Molocznik, S. Damilano, A. Mosto

4 **128.** MALE INVASIVE PROLACTINOMAS: A STUDY OF 15 CASES
J.E. Argonz, I. Molocznik, R. Artese, J. Razumny, S. Damilano, M. Kamelman Levitin, J. Oviedo
Costa Buero Institute, Department of Neuroendocrinology, Medical School, U.B.A., Buenos Aires, Argentina

5 **129.** P-TYRAMINE INHIBITS PROLACTIN SECRETION "IN VITRO"
D. Becu-Villalobos, M.I. Vacas, C. Libertun
IBYME and CEFAPRIN; Obligado 2490, (1428) Buenos Aires, Argentina

6 **130.** PITUITARY REGIONS DIFFER IN THE PROPORTIONS OF CELLS THAT RELEASE PROLACTIN (PRL) ALONE OR BOTH GROWTH HORMONE (GH) AND PRL
F.R. Boockfor, L. Stephen Frawley
Zoology Dept., ISU, Ames, IA 50011

7 **131.** DOPAMINERGIC CONTROL OF PRL SECRETION IN THE RAT VARIES DURING THE ESTROUS CYCLE IN RELATION TO ESTRADIOL AND PROGESTERONE LEVELS
A.M. Brandi, D. Bression, M. Michard, M. Le Dafniet, F. Peillon
INSERM U. 223, Faculté de Médecine Pitié-Salpétrière, 105 Boulevard de l'Hôpital, 75013 Paris, France

8 **132.** EVIDENCE THAT OPIATE STIMULATION OF PROLACTIN SECRETION INVOLVES VASOACTIVE INTESTINAL POLYPEPTIDE (VIP)
G. Burns, B.L. Brown, P.R.M. Dobson
Department of Human Metabolism & Clinical Biochemistry, University of Sheffield Medical School, Beech Hill Road, Sheffield S10 2RX, UK

9 **133.** EVIDENCE FOR AN INTRINSIC CHOLINERGIC SYSTEM IN THE ANTERIOR PITUITARY
Peter Carmeliet, Carl Denef
School of Medicine, University of Leuven, Belgium

10 **134.** MONOCLONAL ANTIBODY RECOGNIZING BOTH MAMMOTROPHS AND SOMATOTROPHS OF THE RAT
H.T. Chen, C.S. Pittman
Univ. of Alabama at Birmingham, Birmingham, AL 35294

11 **134a.** CEREBROSPINAL FLUID PROLACTIME AND GONADOTROPINS IN HUMAN FOETUSES
M. Coculescu,[1] C. Poiană,[1] D. Alessandrescu[2]
[1]Dept. Endocrinology and [2]Dept. Obstetrics-Ginecology, Faculty of Medicine, Bucharest, Romania.

12 **135.** EVIDENCE FOR A DIRECT ACTION OF CORTICO-LIBERIN ON PROLACTIN RELEASE
A. Enjalbert, L. Proulx, G. Pelletier,* P.M. Dubois,** G. Morel***
INSERM U. 159, 2ter rue d'Alésia, 75014 PARIS, France; *MRC Endocrinology Moléculaire, CHUL, Québec, Canada; **CNRS UA 559, Fac. Méd., 69600 Oullins, France

13 **136.** PROLACTIN IN THE CNS OF HYPOPHYSECTOMIZED RATS: COMPARISON WITH PITUITARY PROLACTIN
N.V. Emanuele, L. Metcalfe, L. Wallock, J. Tentler, T.C. Hagen, C. Beer, D. Martinson, P. Gout, L. Kirsteins, A.M. Lawrence
Hines Veterans Administration Hospital, Hines, Illinois 60141, Loyola University of Chicago Stritch School of Medicine, Maywood, Illinois 60152, Zablocki Veterans Administration and Medical Center, Milwaukee, Wisconsin 53202, and Cancer Control Agency of British Columbia, Vancouver, B.C.

14 **137.** FOLLICULAR CELLS OF THE BOVINE ANTERIOR PITUITARY HAVE BETA ADRENOCEPTORS THAT STIMULATE ADENYLATE CYCLASE
P.R. Findell, M. Jacobs, R.I. Weiner

15 **138.** Specific Effect of CV 205-502, a Potent Dopamine Agonist, on Prolactin Secretion Combined Pituitary Function Test With TRH, CRH, GRH and LHRH
R.C. Gaillard,[1] J. Brownell,[2] K. Abeywickrama[2]
University Hospital Medical Clinic, Geneva[1] and Clinical Research Department[2], SANDOZ LTD., Basle, Switzerland

16 **139.** INTERACTION OF CHLORDIAZEPOXIDE WITH TRH BINDING AND BIOLOGICAL EFFECTS IN GH3/B6 RAT PITUITARY CELL STRAIN
D. Gourdji, J.M. Sequier, N. Buisson, A. Tixier-Vidal
Groupe de Neuroendocrinologie Cellulaire et Moléculaire UA CNRS 1115, Collège de France, PARIS, France

17 **140.** NEUROCHEMICAL AND ENDOCRINE INDICES OF TUBEROINFUNDIBULAR DOPAMINERGIC NEURONAL ACTIVITY FOLLOWING STIMULATION OF THE ARCUATE NUCLEUS
J.W. Gunnet, K.J. Lookingland, K.E. Moore
Dept. Pharmacology/Toxicology, Michigan State Univ., East Lansing, MI 48824

18 **141.** CYTOSKELETAL ORGANIZATION IN LACTOTROPHS
J. Guthrie, G. Martinez-Escalera, R. Weiner
Reprod. Endo. Center, UCSF, San Francisco, CA 94143

19 **142.** EFFECTS OF DEXAMETHASONE AND MORPHINE ON PLASMA PROLACTIN LEVELS: A RAT MODEL FOR ENDOCRINE TESTS IN DEPRESSION RESEARCH
J.L. Haracz, E.G. Zimmermann
Brain Research Institute, UCLA, Los Angeles, CA 90024

20 **142a.** AN INCREASE IN THE RATIO OF SEROTONINERGIC TO DOPAMINERGIC ACTIVITY IN THE MEDIAN EMINENCE PRECEDES PREOVULATORY PROLACTIN AND LUTEINIZING HORMONE SURGES IN CYCLING FEMALE RATS
B. Kerdelhué,[a] Ph. Lesieur,[b] A. El Abed,[a,c] F. Bojda,[a] C. Pasqualini[a], V. Lenoir,[a] P. Douillet,[b] C.C. Chiueh,[b] M. Palkovits[b,d]
[a]Unité Neurobiol. Reprod., INRA-CNRS, 78350 Jouy-en-Josas; [b]Lab. Clin. Sci. and Cell Biol., Natl, Inst. Mental Health, Bethesda, Md. 20014, USA; [c]Ecole Ntle d'Ingénieurs, 3038 Sfax, Tunisie; [d]First Dpt. Anatomy, Semelweiss Univ., Medical School, H-1450 Budapest, Hungary.

21 **143.** HISTAMINERGIC MEDIATION OF THE STRESS-INDUCED RELEASE OF PROLACTIN
Ulrich Knigge, Steen Matzen, Jørgen Warberg
Inst. of Medical Physiology C, The Panum Inst., University of Copenhagen, Copenhagen, Denmark

22 **143a.** MECHANISMS INVOLVED IN THE REGULATION OF PROLACTIN GENE TRANSCRIPTION BY THYROLIBERIN
Laverrière JN, Tixier-Vidal A. Buisson N, Gourdji D.
UA CNRS 1115, College De France, Paris, France.

23 **144.** EFFECTS OF PROLACTIN AND STRESS ON DOPAC CONCENTRATIONS IN THE MEDIAN EMINENCE: EVIDENCE THAT DOPAMINE METABOLISM REFLECTS THE ACTIVITY OF TUBEROINFUNDIBULAR NEURONS
K.J. Lookingland, H.D. Jarry, K.E. Moore
Dept. of Pharmacology and Toxicology, Michigan State Univ., East Lansing, MI 48824

24 **145.** NEUROENDOCRINE EFFECTS OF DIHYDROERGOKRYPTINE (DEKP) AND DIHYDROERGOCRISTINE (DECS): EVIDENCE FOR A DOPAMINOMIMETIC ACTION
F. Mailland, L. Fiore, M. Poli,** U. Scapagnini, P.L. Canonico*
Inst. Pharmacology, University of Catania; *Poli Research Center, Milan; **2nd Dept. Internal Medicine, S. Paolo Hospital, Milan, Italy

25 **146.** EGF RECEPTORS PRESENT IN NORMAL RAT AND HUMAN PITUITARIES ARE ABSENT IN HUMAN PRL-, GH- AND NON-SECRETING PITUITARY ADENOMAS
M. Michard, P. Birman, F. Peillon, D. Bression
INSERM U. 223, Faculté de Médecine Pitié-Salpétrière, 105 Boulevard de l'Hôpital, 75013 Paris, France

26 **147.** PITUITARY ADNEOMAS: IN VIVO STUDY WITH POSITRON EMISSION TOMOGRAPHY (PET) OF DOPAMINE RECEPTORS AND METABOLISM
C. Muhr, M. Bergström, P.O. Lundberg, K. Bergström, H. Lundqvist, B. Langstöm
Department of Neurology, Uppsala University, Akademiska sjukhuset, Uppsala, Sweden

27 **148.** MULTIPLE METASTATIC PROLACTINOMA: IN VIVO STUDIES WITH POSITRON EMISSION TOMOGRAPHY (PET) DEMONSTRATING DOPAMINE RECEPTORS AND EFFECT OF BROMOCRIPTINE TREATMENT
C. Muhr, M. Bergström, P.O. Lundberg, M. Hartman, K. Bergström, B. Langström, L. Pellettieri
Department of Neurology, Uppsala University, Akademiska sjukhuset, Uppsala, Sweden

28 **149.** EVIDENCES FOR AND AGAINST THE EXISTENCE OF A HYPOTHALAMIC PRL-INHIBITING PEPTIDE
R.M.G. Nair, M.A. Barnes, M. Somasundaran, P. Subramaniam, J. Sagel, P. Pritchard
VA Medical Center and Depts. of Medicine and Neurology, Medical University of South Carolina, Charleston, SC

29 **150.** SYNERGISTIC POTENTIATION OF NOXIOUS STIMULI-INDUCED PROLACTIN SECRETION BY HYPOVOLEMIA
T. Onaka, M. Hamamura, K. Yagi
Dept.of Physiol. Jichi Med. Sch. Tochigi, Japan

30 **151.** CHANGES IN TUBEROINFUNDIBULAR DOPAMINERGIC NEURONS ACTIVITY DURING THE RAT ESTROUS CYCLE. CORRELATION WITH THE PRL SURGE AND ALTERATION BY A MAMMARY CARCINOGEN
C. Pasqualini, F. Bojda,* E. Teissier,° B. Guibert,· V. Leviel,· R. Rips,° B. Kerdelhué**
*U. Neurobiol. Reprod. INRA-CNRS, 78350 Jouy-en-Josas; °INSERM, U. 98 Pharmacol. Chim., 17 rue Fer à Moulin, 75005 Paris; •Lab. Physiol. Nerv., CNRS, 91190 Gif-sur-Yvette, France

31 **152.** NATURE OF PATHOLOGICAL AND PHARMACOLOGICAL HYPERPROLACTINEMIA INFLUENCES OPIOID CONTROL OF LH SECRETION IN WOMEN
F. Petraglia, V. DeLeo, C. Nappi,** F. Facchinetti, A. Volpe, A.R. Genazzani*
Depts. Obstetrics and Gynecology, Univ. of Modena, *Siena and **Naples, Schools of Medicine, Italy

32 **153.** PROLACTIN LOWERING EFFECT OF CQP201-403; A NEW DOPAMINE AGONIST
R. Rolland, P.F.M. van der Heijden, J. Brownell, J. van Gennep***
Dept. of Obstetrics and Gynecology, St. Radboud Hospital, Nijmegen, The Netherlands and *Clinical Research Dept. Sandoz, Basle, Switzerland, and **the Netherlands.

33 **154.** THE BENZODIAZEPINE RECEPTOR LIGANDS REGULATE THE CELL PROLIFERATION OF THE RAT ANTERIOR PITUITARY GLAND IN ADRENALECTOMIZED RATS
H. Stepień, J. Kunert-Radek, M. Pawlikowski
Institute of Endocrinology Medical Academy of Lódź, 91-425 Lódź

34 **155.** A NEW DOPAMINE AGONIST IN THE TREATMENT OF HYPERPROLACTINAEMIA
K.T. Stokke, L.E. Hanssen, S. Reinli, S. Stray-Pederson, J. Halse, J. Jervell*
Rikshopitalet, N-0027 Oslo 1, Norway and Ulleval Hospital,* N-0407 Oslo 4, Norway

35 **156.** THE ESTRADIOL-INDUCED INCREASE IN ANTERIOR PITUITARY DOPAMINE IS NOT MEDIATED BY PROLACTIN
N. Telford, Y.N. Sinha
Univ. of So. Calif., Los Angeles, CA 90089-0191

36 **157.** INVESTIGATION OF THE ROLE OF DOPAMINE AS THE PROLACTIN INHIBITING FACTOR IN SHEEP
G.B. Thomas, J.T. Cummins, G.A. Smythe,+ R. Gleeson and I.J. Clark
Medical Research Centre, Prince Henry's Hospital, Melbourne and +Garvan Institute of Medical Research, St. Vincent's Hospital, Sydney, Australia

37 **158.** PHARMACOLOGICAL ASPECTS OF TERGURIDE AND ITS CLINICAL ROLE IN PRL SECRETION
P.L. Venturini, V. Fasce, F. Gorlero, M. Valenzano, S. Constantini, R. Horowski, E. Rainer, L. De Cecco
Clinica Ostetrica e Ginecologica, University of Genoa, V. le Benedetto XV, 16132, Genova, ITALY

38 **159.** BROMOCRIPTINE AS PRIMARY TREATMENT FOR PROLACTIN SECRETING MACROADENOMAS: A RADIOLOGICAL, OPHTHALMOLOGICAL AND ENDOCRINOLOGICAL STUDY
J.W van't Verlaat, R.J.M. Croughs, M.J. Hendriks, N.J. Bosma, J.W.R. Nortier, J.H.H. Thijssen
Departments of Neurosurgery, Endocrinology and Radiology, University Hospital Utrecht, Utrecht, The Netherlands

39 **160.** CRITERIA TO PREDICT THE OUTCOME OF DRUG THERAPY IN PATIENTS WITH PROLACTINOMA
W. Winkelmann, B. Allolio, U. DeuB, D. Heesen
Dept. Internal Med. II, Univ. of Köln, FRG

Comparative Neuroendocrinology

40 **161.** ASSESSMENT OF THE REPRODUCTIVE AND ANTLER PERFORMANCE OF THE MALE WHITE-TAILED DEER BY GN-RH STIMULATION TEST.
G.A. Bubenik, D. Schams, A.J. Sempere*
Dept. of Zoology, Univ. of Guelph, Guelph, Ontario, Canada, NIG 2W1 and Dept. of Physiology, TU-Univ. Munchen-Weihenstephan, D-805 Freising, FRG.*

41 **162.** NPY AND GABA ACT AS α-MSH-RELEASE INHIBITING FACTORS ON FROG MELANOTROPHS
J.M. Danger, M. Lamacz, M.C. Tonon, E. Leneveu, S. Adjeroud, M. Tappaz, M.E. Stoeckel,** G. Pelletier,*** and H. Vaudry*
UA CNRS 650, Unité Alliée INSERM, Univ. Rouen, 76130 Mt-St-Aignan, France; *INSERM U171, Hôp. Ste Eugenie, 69001 Lyon, France; **UA CNRS 309, Univ. L. Pasteur, 67084 Strasbourg, France; ***Grp. MRC, CHU Laval Québec, Canada

42 **163.** HYPOTHALAMIC AND EXTRAHYPOTHALAMIC MESOTOCIN-LIKE IMMUNOREACTIVITY IN THE BULLFROG (*RANA CATESBEIANA*)
G.C. Gonzalez, K. Lederis
University of Calgary, Calgary, Alberta, Canada, T2N 4N1

43 **163a.** GABAERGIC INNERVATION OF THE MEDIANEMINENCE PITUITARY COMPLEX: A COMPARATIVE IMMUNOCYTOCHEMICAL STUDY IN MAMMALS AND FISH
O. Kah, C. Decavel, M. Rabhi, M.G. Martinoli, P. Dubourg, B. Onteniente, M. Geffard, A. Calas*
Lab. Physiologie des Interactions Cellulaires, UA 339 CNRS and *Lab. Neuroimmunologie, Bordeaux, France

44 **163b.** EFFECTS OF INSULIN-LIKE GROWTH FACTOR I (IGF-I) ON GROWTH HORMONE-RELEASING FACTOR (GRF) AND THYROTROPIN-RELEASING HORMONE (TRH) STIMULATION OF GH SECRETION IN THE DOMESTIC FOWL
F.C. Buonomo, T.J. Lauterio, C.A. Baile, W.H. Daughaday**
Monsanto Co., Anim. Sci. Div. and *Washington University School of Medicine, St. Louis, MO, USA

45 **164.** CHARACTERIZATION OF UROTENSIN I AND CRF-LIKE PEPTIDES IN *CATOSTOMUS* BRAIN AND PITUITARY BY HPLC AND RADIOIMMUNOASSAY
D. McMaster, K. Lederis
University of Calgary, Calgary, Alberta, Canada T2N 4N1

46 **165.** PINEAL, RETINAL AND SERUM MELATONIN AND N-ACETYL-SEROTONIN (NAS) RHYTHMS ON LIGHT PHASE SHIFTING AND BLINDING
*I. Nir, *S.F. Pang, *A.E. Allen*
Hebrew University-Hadassah Medical School, Jerusalem, *Hong Kong University Faculty of Medicine, Hong Kong

47 **166.** ALTERNATIVES TO DOPAMINE: WHAT CONTROLS PROLACTIN SECRETION IN SOME FISHES?
R.S. Nishioka, H.A. Bern, K. Kelley, E.G. Grau, R. Rivas, G. Young*
University of California, Berkeley, CA 94720 and *University of Hawaii, Honolulu, HI 96744

48 **167.** THE EFFECT OF HYDROCORTISONE, VASOPRESSIN (AVP) AND CRF ADMINISTRATION ON ACTH, αMSH AND AVP PULSATILE SECRETION IN THE PITUITARY VENOUS EFFLUENT OF THE HORSE
*C. Redekopp, *C.H.G. Irvine, R.A. Donald, J.H. Livesey, *S.L. Alexander*
Dept. of Endocrinology, The Princess Margaret Hospital,

*Dept. of Veterinary Science, Lincoln College, Christchurch, New Zealand

49 **168.** COMPARATIVE ASPECTS OF HYPOTHALAMIC α-MSH-LIKE IMMUNOREACTIVE SYSTEMS
M. Vallarino
Istituto Anatomia Comparata, Università di Genova, Genova, Italy

50 **169.** EFFECTS OF [D-ALA^{6}, PRO^{9}-NEt]-LHRH AND CATECHOLAMINERGIC DRUGS ON GONADOTROPIN SECRETION AND OVULATION IN THE CHINESE LOACH
G. Van Der Kraak,[1] H.R. Lin,[2] C. Peng,[2] R.E. Peter[1]
[1]Department of Zoology, University of Alberta, Edmonton, Alberta, Canada; and [2]Department of Biology, Zhongshan University, Guangzhou, China

51 **170.** COMPARISON OF *IN VITRO* EFFECTS OF DIFFERENT SPECIES SPECIFIC GnRH AND THEIR ANALOGUES IN A DISPERSED CELL SUPERFUSION SYSTEM
S. Vigh, A. Horváth, C. Kéri, T. Gulyás, V. Csernus,* K. Nikolics, I. Teplán, B. Flerkó**
1st Institute of Biochemistry, Semmelweis University Medical School, 1444 Budapest, Hungary; and *Department of Anatomy, University Medical School of Pécs, 7643 Pécs, Hungary

Neuroendocrine Regulation of GH

52 **171.** THE EFFECTS OF TESTOSTERONE ON METABOLIC CLEARANCE RATE OF GH IN FEMALE RATS
T.M. Badger, D. O'Sullivan, J. LaRovere, W.J. Millard, J.B. Martin
Massachusetts General Hospital, Boston, MA 02114

53 **172.** GROWTH HORMONE SECRETION IN ACROMEGALY: EFFECTS OF SOMATOSTATIN ANALOGUE SMS 201-995 (SANDOZ)
A. Barkan, R. Lloyd, W. Chandler, R. Kelch, I. Beitins, N. Hopwood
Departments of Medicine, Pathology, Neurosurgery and Pediatrics, University of Michigan, Ann Arbor, MI 48109, U.S.A.

54 **173.** THE PRESENCE OF NEURAL PATHWAYS INHIBITING THE EXCITEMENT OF HYPOTHALAMIC GH-RH-NEURONS IN THE RATS
K. Chihara, Y. Okimura, T. Kita, Y. Kashio, M. Sato, T. Fujita
Kobe University School of Medicine, Kobe, Japan

55 **174.** ARCUATE hGHRF MAINLY OCCURS IN AN EXTRA-INFUNDIBULARLY PROJECTING MULTIPEPTIDERGIC NEURONAL SYSTEM
Ph. Ciofi, G. Tramu
INSERM U156, place de Verdun, 59045 LILLE Cedex, France

56 **175.** FEEDBACK: EFFECT OF GROWTH HORMONE ON HYPOTHALAMIC OPIOID AND GHRH PRODUCING NEURONS
D. Cocchi, I. Ganzetti, F. Petraglia, E.E. Müller
Department of Pharmacology, School of Medicine, University of Milan and Department of Obstetrics and Gynecology, University of Modena, ITALY

57 **176.** ETHANOL AND GROWTH HORMONE SECRETION IN THE FEMALE RAT
W.L. Dees, V. Rettori, S. Kentroti
Department of Physiology, Univ. of Texas Health Science Center, Dallas, Texas 75235

58 **177.** HUMAN FETAL CORTICAL NEURONES IN CULTURE: A MODEL FOR THE STUDY OF THE NEUROSECRETORY ACTIVITY OF THE HUMAN BRAIN
R. Elli, V. Silani, A. Pizzuti, G. Toffano, G. Scarlato, G. Faglia
Departments of Endocrinology and Neurology, School of Medicine, University of Milan, Italy

59 **178.** AUTOINHIBITION OF HYPOTHALAMIC SOMATOSTATIN RELEASE: LOCALIZATION BY IN VITRO RELEASE EXPERIMENTS AND ULTRASTRUCTURAL EVIDENCE
J. Epelbaum, L. Tapia-Arancibia, G. Alonso,* H. Astier,* C. Kordon*
U 159 INSERM, 2ter rue d'Alésia, 75014 Paris and *ERA 85 CNRS, Montpellier, France

60 **179.** IMPACT OF INTENSIVE VENOUS SAMPLING ON DETECTION OF GROWTH HORMONES PULSES IN NORMAL MEN
W.S. Evans, A.C.S. Faria, E. Christiansen, K.Y. Ho, J. Weiss, A.D. Rogol, M.L. Johnson, R.M. Blizzard, J.D. Veldhuis, M.O. Thorner
University of Virginia Medical Center, Charlottesville, Virginia 22908

61 **180.** THE GHRH-INDUCED GH RELEASE IS MODULATED BY THE CHOLINERGIC SYSTEM
E. Ghigo, E. Mazza, V. Locatelli, E.E. Müller,* F. Camanni, F. Massara*
Department of Biomedicine, University of Turin and Department of Pharmacology, University of Milan,* Italy.

62 **180a.** RAPID PROGRESSION OF A GROWTH HORMONE PRODUCING TUMOR DURING BROMOCRIPTINE TREATMENT
A-L Hulting, K. Heidvall, B. Isberg, L. Fredstorp, S. Werner
Dept. of Endocrinology, Karolinska Hospital, Stockholm

63 **181.** OPIOID AND ADRENERGIC RECEPTORS INVOLVING IN THE NEURAL REGULATION OF GROWTH HORMONE SECRETION ARE CHANGED BY GLUCOCORTICOIDS
B. Kanyicska, B. Kacsoh, M.I.K. Fekete, E. Stark*
Inst. Exptl. Med., Hung. Acad. Sci., Semmelweis Univ., Med. School, 2nd Dept. Anatomy, Budapest, Hungary

64 **182.** DISTRIBUTION OF GASTRIN-RELEASING PEPTIDE (GRP) IN THE RAT BRAIN CONCURS WITH ITS PROPOSED MECHANISM OF ACTION ON GH RELEASE
S. Kentroti, L. Dees
Department of Physiology, Univ. of Texas Health Science Center, Dallas, TX 75235

65 **183.** GROWTH HORMONE RELEASE INDUCED BY ELECTRICAL STIMULATION OF THE BASOLATERAL AMYGDALA, OBSERVED IN PENTOBARBITAL AN-

ESTHETIZED RATS
N. Koibuchi, M. Kato, T. Kakegawa, M. Suzuki
Department of Physiology, Institute of Endocrinology, Gunma University, Maebashi, Japan

66 **184.** LONG-LASTING DOPAMINERGIC STIMULATION OF PITUITARY SECRETION
Ioana Lancranjan, L. Portmann, C. Felley, J.P. Felber
Department of Endocrinology, University Hospital, Lausanne, Switzerland

67 **185.** INFLUENCE OF THEOPHYLLINE ADMINISTRATION ON BASAL AND GHRH STIMULATED GH SECRETION IN ACROMEGALY
M. Losa, J. Schopohl, J. Alba-Lopez, S. Sobieszczyk, Y. Spiess, O.A. Müller, K. von Werder
Med. Klin. Innenstadt, University of Munich, FRG

68 **186.** THE MANNER OF GHRH INVOLVEMENT IN GH STIMULATION TESTS IN MAN
A. Masuda, T. Shibasaki, T. Imaki, H. Demura, K. Shizume
Dept. of Medicine, Tokyo Women's Medical College, Tokyo 162, Japan

69 **187.** THE HYPOTHALAMO-INFUNDIBULAR GROWTH HORMONE RELEASING FACTOR (GRF) SYSTEM OF THE RAT
I. Merchenthaler, A. Arimura, P. Petrusz
University Medical School, Pécs, Hungary; Tulane University, New Orleans,Louisiana, U.S.A.; University of North Carolina, Chapel Hill, North Carolina, U.S.A.

70 **188.** GROWTH HORMONE (GH) SECRETION DURING A CONTINUOUS 6-HOUR INFUSION OF GH-RELEASING FACTOR (GRF) IN MONOSODIUM GLUTAMATE (MSG) TREATED RATS
*S. Minami, I. Wakabayashi, H. Sugihara, S. Akira, F. Takahashi, A. Motoyama, N. Ling**
Nippon Medical School, Tokyo, Japan and *The Salk Institute, San Diego, California, U.S.A.

71 **189.** CHOLINERGIC MUSCARINIC RECEPTOR BLOCKADE WITH PIRENZEPINE ABOLISHES SLOW WAVE SLEEP-RELATED GH RELEASE IN NORMAL AND INSULIN DEPENDENT DIABETIC SUBJECTS
M.D. Page, H.P.F. Koppeschaar, C. Dieguez, J.R. Peters, M.F. Scanlon
Neuroendocrine Unit, University of Wales College of Medicine, Cardiff

72 **190.** IN VITRO SIMULTANEOUS RELEASE OF ENDOGENOUS SOMATOSTATIN AND GROWTH HORMONE FROM HUMAN ADENOMATOUS PITUITARY CELLS
F. Peillon, C. Liapi,** P. Garnier,*** A.M. Brandi,* D. Evain-Brion,*, D. Bression,* H. Scheerer,**** M. Donnadieu***
*INSERM U. 223, **INSERM U. 188, ***Fondation de Recherches en Hormonologie, ****Service d'Endocrinologie la Pitié, Paris, France

73 **191.** PREVENTION BY SOMATOSTATIN OF THE DESENSITIZATION OF hpGRF-INDUCED GH RELEASE FROM RAT ANTERIOR PITUITARY *IN VITRO*
H. Soya, M. Suzuki
Department of Physiology, Institute of Endocrinology, Gunma University, Maebashi 371, Japan

74 **192.** INTERACTION OF GROWTH HORMONE (GH) RELEASING FACTOR (GRF) AND SOMATOSTATIN (SS) TO ESTABLISH PULSATILE GH RELEASE *IN VITRO*
J. Weiss, M.O. Thorner, M.J. Cronin
University of Virginia, Charlottesville, Virginia 22908

75 **193.** SECRETION OF GHRH IN PATIENTS WITH HYPERSOMATOTROPISM
R. Yamasaki, S. Saito, H. Saito, K. Kameyama, S. Mitsuhashi, E. Hosoi, T. Sano
School of Medicine, The University of Tokushima, Tokushima, Japan

Expression and Processing of Neuroendocrine Peptides

76 **194.** MOLECULAR CHARACTERIZATION OF A NEUROPHYSIN-COPEPTIN PRECURSOR FROM GUINEA PIG NEURO-INTERMEDIATE PITUITARY
R. Acher, J. Chauvet, M.T. Chauvet, D. Sunde,[+] A.N. Thorn[+]
Lab. of Biol. Chemistry, Univ. of Paris VI (France) and Inst. Med. Physiol., Univ. of Copenhagen (Denmark)

77 **195.** CONCOMITANT DOPAMINERGIC AND GLUCOCORTICOID CONTROL OF ANTERIOR AND INTERMEDIATE LOBE β-ENDORPHIN
D.J. Autelitano, I. Nikolaidis, J.A. Clements, J.W. Funder
Medical Research Centre, Prince Henry's Hospital, Melbourne, Australia 3004

78 **196.** GLUCOCORTICOID REGULATION OF PRO-OPIOMELANOCORTIN (POMC) mRNA CONTENT OF RAT HYPOTHALAMUS AND AMYGDALA
S. Beaulieu, B. Gagné, N. Barden
MRC Group in Molecular Endocrinology, CHUL, Laval University, Quebec, Canada, G1V 4G2

79 **197.** HORMONAL REGULATION OF POMC GENE TRANSCRIPTION IN INDIVIDUAL CELL NUCLEI OF THE RAT PITUITARY
R.T. Fremeau, Jr., J. Lundblad, D. Pritchett, J. Wilcox, J.L. Roberts
Columbia Univ. College of Physicians & Surgeons, New York, NY

80 **198.** THE PROHORMONE FOR UROTENSIN II FROM THE CAUDAL NEUROSECRETORY COMPLEX OF THE GOBY
D. Pearson, Y. Cheers, D. Atmani, J.E. Shively, D. Hawk, I. Ishida, T. Deguchi, R.S. Nishioka, H.A. Bern

81 **198a.** OXYTOCIN AND UROKINASE SPECIFIC mRNA IN GRANULOSA CELLS
K.H. Scheit, R. Einspanier
Max-Planck-Institut für Biophysikalische Chemie, 3400 Göttingen, W. Germany

82 **199.** β-ENDORPHIN PROCESSING: DIFFERENCES BETWEEN SLAUGHTERHOUSE AND UNSTRESSED SHEEP
A.I. Smith, C.A. Wallace, I.J. Clarke, J.W. Funder
Medical Research Centre, Prince Henry's Hospital, Melbourne, Australia 3004

83 **200.** CIRCULATION OF NEURALLY DERIVED CALCITONIN GENE-RELATED PEPTIDE
M. Zaidi, P.J.R. Bevis, J. Diez Guerra, C. Lynch, S.J. Wimalawansa, P.C. Emson, I. MacIntyre
Endocrine Unit, Department of Chemical Pathology, Royal Postgraduate Medical School, London W12 and MRC Neurochemical Pharmacology Unit, Babraham, Cambridge (UK).

Thursday PM **Continental Ballroom 4**

SESSION 10: Mechanism of Action of Neurohormones

Chairpersons: **P. Conn**
M. Chretien

1:30 **201.** GnRH ACTIVATES A RAPID CA^{2+}-INDEPENDENT PHOSPHODIESTER HYDROLYSIS OF POLYPHOSPHOINOSITIDES IN PITUITARY GONADOTROPHS
Zvi Naor
Department of Hormone Research, The Weizmann Institute of Science, Rehovot 76100, Israel

1:45 **202.** PROTEIN KINASE C ACTIVATION ATTENUATES SECRETAGOGUE-INDUCED INOSITOL PHOSPHATE GENERATION IN NORMAL PITUITARY AND 7315a TUMOR CELLS
A.M. Judd, W.D. Jarvis, R.M. MacLeod
Dept. of Internal Medicine, University of Virginia School of Medicine, Charlottesville, Virginia 22908

2:00 **203.** EFFECTS OF ESTRADIOL ON RECEPTORS COUPLED TO ADENYLATE CYCLASE AND ON PHOSPHOLIPID METHYLATION OF ANTERIOR PITUITARY CELLS
A. Enjalbert, S.V. Drouva, P. Bertrand, S. Krantic, J. Epelbaum, E. Laplante, E. Rerat, C. Kordon
INSERM U. 159, 2ter rue d'Alésia, 75014 PARIS, France

2:15 **204.** A NOVEL SERINE PROTEASE FROM HUMAN AND PORCINE PITUITARY CLEAVING AT PAIRS OF BASIC RESIDUES IN PRO-OPIOMELANOCORTIN AND PRO-ATRIAL NATRIURETIC FACTOR RELATED PEPTIDES: A CANDIDATE PROCESSING ENZYME?
N.G. Seidah, J.A. Cromlish, G. Thibault, M. Chrétien
Clinical Research Institute of Montreal, Montreal, Quebec, Canada

2:30 **205.** MECHANISM OF ACTION OF GROWTH HORMONE-RELEASING FACTOR (GHRF): ROLE OF CYCLIC AMP AND CALCIUM ION
J. Kraicer, B. Lussier, M.S. Sheppard, B. Moor, N. Narayanan
Department of Physiology, University of Western Ontario, London, Ontario

2:45 **206.** COPPER-AMPLIFIED PGE_2, STIMULATION OF LHRH RELEASE FROM MEDIAN EMINENCE (ME) EXPLANTS: A POST-RECEPTOR EVENT AT THE LEVEL OF THE ADENYLATE CYCLASE SYSTEM
Ayalla Barnea, Gloria Cho
Debts. Ob-Gyn. & Physiol., Green Ctr. Reprod. Biol., University of Texas Health Science Center, Dallas, TX 75235

3:00 **207.** CYCLIC AMP AND PROSTAGLANDIN F2α STIMULATE GnRH SECRETION BY HUMAN PLACENTAL CELL CULTURES
F. Petraglia, A.T.W. Lim, W. Vale
The Clayton Foundation Laboratories for Peptide Biology, The Salk Institute, La Jolla, CA

3:15 **208.** ARACHIDONATE EPOXIDES ARE POTENT STIMULATORS OF PROLACTIN SECRETION IN NORMAL RAT PITUITARY CELLS
D. Grandsaert, J.R. Cashman, R.I. Weiner
University of California San Francisco, San Francisco, California

Thursday PM **Continental Ballroom 5**

SESSION 11: Neuroendocrine Regulation of ACTH

Chairpersons: **I. Assenmacher**
H. Imura

1:30 **209.** IDENTIFICATION AND SORTING OF ANTERIOR PITUITARY CELLS THAT BIND CORTICOTROPIN-RELEASING FACTOR: ABSENCE OF ADRENOCORTICOTROPIN RESPONSE TO VASOPRESSIN IN SORTED CELLS
J. Schwartz, J. Trotter, J. Rivier, W. Vale
The Clayton Foundation Laboratories for Peptide Biology and Flow Cytometry Laboratory, The Salk Institute, La Jolla, CA 93037

1:45 **210.** ULTRASTRUCTURAL ANALYSIS OF THE CATECHOLAMINERGIC INNERVATION OF THE HYPOTHALAMIC PARAVENTRICULAR NUCLEUS WITH SPECIAL REFERENCE TO CORTICOTROPIN RELEASING FACTOR SYNTHESIZING NEURONS
Zs. Liposits, C. Phelix, W.K. Paull
Department of Anatomy, University of Missouri-Columbia, Columbia, Mo.

2:00 **211.** CHARACTERIZATION OF HUMAN PLACENTAL CORTICOTROPIN RELEASING HORMONE
G.K. Stalla, H. Bost, T. Kaliebe, M. Huber, J. Stalla, K. von Werder, O.A. Müller
Med. Klinik Innenstadt, Univ. of Munich, FRG

2:15 **212.** INHIBITION OF CRF RELEASE IN HYPOPHYSIAL PORTAL BLOOD AFTER 6-OHDA-LESION OF THE VENTRAL NORADRENERGIC BUNDLE
V. Guillaume, B. Conte-Devolx, A. Szafarczyk, N. Pares-Herbute, M. Grino, I. Assenmacher, C. Oliver
Lab. Neuroendoc. INSERM U 297 Fac. Med. Nord F. 13326 Marseilles and CNRS UA 639 Univ. Montpellier F. 34060, Montpellier, France.

2:30 **213.** HISTAMINERGIC MODULATION OF THE NEUROENDOCRINE SYSTEM
R. Cacabelos, H. Niigawa, A. Miyake, S. Hariguchi, T. Nishimura*
Departments of Neuropsychiatry and Gynecology,* Osaka University Medical School, Osaka 553, Japan

2:45 **214.** REEVALUATION OF THE ROLE OF DIRECT beta-ADRENERGIC STIMULATION OF ACTH RELEASE FROM THE ANTERIOR PITUITARY
G.B. Makara,[1] K. Kovács,[1] I. Kakucska,[1] D. Ježova,[2] R. Kvetnansky[2]

[1]Institute of Experimental Medicine, Hung. Acad. Sci., Budapest, Hungary, [2]Institute of Experimental Endocrinology, Slovak Acad. Sci., Bratislava, Czechoslovakia

3:00 **215.** EVIDENCE THAT CHRONIC PREDNISOLONE TREATMENT INHIBITS PITUITARY RESPONSIVENESS BY A DUAL MECHANISM
S.A. Nicholson
Division of Physiology, United Medical and Dental Schools (Guy's) London, SE1 9RT, U.K.

3:15 **216.** DIFFERENCES IN RNA ABUNDANCE IN RAT HIPPOCAMPUS IN RESPONSE TO ENDOGENOUS AND HIGH DOSE ADMINISTERED CORTICOSTERONE
N.R. Nichols, J.N. Masters, P.C. May, S.L. Millar, C.E. Finch
University of Southern California, Los Angeles, California

Thursday PM **Continental Parlors 1–3**

SESSION 12: Regulation of Hormone Rhythms
Chairpersons: **R. Reiter**
T. Hiroshige

1:30 **217.** LIGHT AND MOTOR ACTIVITY IN THE FERRET
B.T. Donovan
Department of Physiology, Institute of Psychiatry, De Crespigny Park, London SE5 8AF, England

1:45 **218.** EFFECT OF LOCAL PHARMACOLOGICAL DESTRUCTION OF THE SEROTONINERGIC INNERVATION OF THE HYPOTHALAMIC SUPRACHIASMATIC REGION OF YOUNG RATS ON CIRCADIAN HORMONE RHYTHMS
B. Halász, Zs. Bánky
2nd Department of Anatomy, Semmelweis Medical University, Budapest, Hungary

2:00 **219.** NYCTOHEMERAL INCREASE IN THE SENSITIVITY OF THE PINEAL GLAND OF THE SYRIAN HAMSTER TO NOREPINEPHRINE
R.J. Reiter, G.M. Vaughn, S. Oaknin, M.E. Troiani
Department of Cellular and Structural Biology, University of Texas Health Science Center, San Antonio, Texas 78284

2:15 **220.** HYPOTHALAMIC SITE OF ACTION OF MELATONIN IN RATS
F. Gibbs, J. Corcoran, L. Petterborg, K. Rudeen
Dept. of Anatomy, Univ. of Missouri, Columbia, MO 65212

2:30 **221.** THYROXINE ACTIVATION AND ITS CIRCADIAN RHYTHMICITY IN RAT PINEAL GLAND
K. Tanaka, M. Murakami, M.A. Greer
Section of Endocrinology, Oregon Health Sciences University, Portland, Oregon 97201

2:45 **222.** THE PRESENCE OF BIOLOGICALLY ACTIVE DOPAMINE RECEPTORS IN THE PITUITARIES OF LONG AND SHORT PHOTOPERIOD-EXPOSED MALE HAMSTERS
D.M. Burns, C.A. Leadem, B. Benson
Department of Anatomy, University of Arizona, Tucson, AZ

3:00 **223.** THE EFFECT OF PINEALECTOMY AND LIGHT CYCLE ON SPONTANEOUS AND PROSTAGLANDIN E_2-INDUCED RELEASE OF LH IN PROESTROUS RATS
J. Warberg, L.D. Wogensen, M. Møller
Departments of Medical Physiology C and Medical Anatomy B, University of Copenhagen, Copenhagen, Denmark

3:15 **224.** PINEALECTOMY-INDUCED NUMERICAL INCREASE IN MITOCHONDRIA AND EXOCYTOSIS IN PERIVASCULAR COMPARTMENTS IN ADRENOMEDULLARY ADRENALINE CELLS
T. Kachi, T.K. Banerji, W.B. Quay
Asahikawa Medical College, Asahikawa 078, Japan, Univ. of Texas Medical Branch, Galveston, Texas, Univ. of California, Berkeley, California

Friday AM **Continental Ballroom 4**

SESSION 13: Symposium on Mediation of Neuroendocrine Peptide Action
Chairpersons: **K. Catt**
Y. Koch

8:30 **225.** Andrée Tixier-Vidal (France)—Pathways Involved in the Stimulation by Thyroliberin of Prolactin Release and of Prolactin Gene Transcription in GH_3 Cells

9:00 **226.** Thomas Martin (USA)—Regulated Phospholipid Hydrolysis as a Transduction Mechanism for Neuropeptides and Peptide Hormones

9:30 **227.** Karl Bauer (Germany)—Enzymatic Degradation and Biological Inactivation of Neuropeptides

10:00 **228.** Pierlugi Canonico (Italy)—Hormone-Receptor Coupling Mechanism in the Anterior Pituitary: Modulation by Protein Kinase C Activators and Cyclic AMP (cAMP)

Friday AM **Continental Ballroom 5**

SESSION 14: Symposium on Clinical Neuroendocrinology
Chairpersons: **J. Martin**
M. Grumbach

8:30 **229.** Michael Thorner (USA)—Growth Hormone Releasing Hormone (GHRH)

9:00 **230.** Kalman Kovacs—Pathology of Pituitary Adenomas

9:30 **231.** William F. Crowley (USA)—GnRH Pulses

10:00 **232.** Fernand Labrie (Canada)—Combination Therapy with Flutamide and an LHRH Agonist in Advanced Prostate Cancer

Friday AM **Continental Parlors 1–3**

SESSION 15: Symposium on Aminergic Regulation Neuroendocrine Action
Chairpersons: **C. Sawyer**
U. Scapagnini

8:30 **233.** Eva Mezey (Hungary)—Catecholamines and ACTH Release

9:00 **234.** Wolfgang Wuttke (Germany)—Involvement of GABA in the Neuroendocrinology of Reproduction

9:30 **235.** Phyllis Wise (USA)—Changing Hypothalamic Function and its Role in Aging of the Female Reproductive System

10:00 **236.** William R. Crowley (USA)—Control of Luteinizing Hormone Secretion by Ovarian Hormone-Monoamine-Neuropeptide Interactions

Friday AM/PM **Continental Parlors 6–9**

SESSION 16: Neuropeptides; Neuroendocrine Regulation of ACTH; Development and Aging; Regulation of Hormone Rhythms; Immunology; Behavior

Poster Session **Posters manned from 10:30–12:00 PM and 3:30–5:00 PM**

Neuropeptides

Position

1 **237.** LOCALIZATION OF β-ENDORPHIN (β-END), METENKEPHALIN (MET-ENK) AND NEUROTENSIN (NT) IN THE RAT HYPOTHALAMUS: AN IMMUNOHISTOCHEMICAL STUDY
K. Ajika, K. Arai, S. Okinaga
Teikyo University School of Medicine, Tokyo, Japan

2 **238.** SUBSTANCE P- BUT NOT CHOLECYSTOKININ-IMMUNOREACTIVE HYPOTHALAMIC CELLS CONCENTRATE ESTROGEN
T.R. Akesson, A. Coquelin, P.E. Micevych
Dept. of Anatomy, CHS-UCLA, Los Angeles, CA 90024

3 **239.** ADENOSINE 3',5'-CYCLIC MONOPHOSPHATE STIMULATES DOPAMINE SYNTHESIS IN THE MEDIAN EMINENCE OF RAT HYPOTHALAMIC SLICES
J. Arita, F. Kimura
Yokohama City University School of Medicine, Yokohama

4 **240.** REGIONALIZATION OF THE DIRECT ARTERIAL BLOOD SUPPLY AND PRL CONTENT OF THE ANTERIOR PITUITARY OF RABBITS
M. Bamat, G. Martinez-Escalera, R. Weiner
Reprod. Endo. Center, UCSF, San Francisco, CA 94143

5 **240a.** PITUITARY-ADRENAL AXIS RESPONSE TO NALOXONE IN NORMALS AND IN PATIENTS WITH DEXAMETHASONE SUPPRESSIBLE HYPERALDOSTERONISM
M. Boscaro, F. Fallo, N. Sonino, A. Rampazzo, F. Mantero
Institute of Semeiotica Medica, University of Padua, Italy

6 **241.** EFFECTS OF CYSTEAMINE ON THE *IN VIVO* INCORPORATION OF [^{35}S]-CYSTEINE INTO SOMATOSTATIN-14, SOMATOSTATIN-28, ARGININE VASOPRESSIN, AND OXYTOCIN IN RAT HYPOTHALAMUS
J.L. Cameron, J.D. Fernstrom
Department of Psychiatry and Center for Neuroscience, University of Pittsburg, Pittsburg, PA 15213

7 **241a.** POSSIBLE PHYSIOLOGICAL SIGNIFICANCE OF GLUCOCORTICOID INDUCED CHANGES OF OPIATE SENSITIVITY
M.I.K. Fekete, Do Tanh Kiem, B. Kanyicska, E. Stark
Inst. Exptl. Med., Hung. Acad. Sci., Budapest, Hungary

8 **242.** ANGIOTENSIN II SPECIFIC BINDING IN THE SUBCOMMISSURAL ORGAN OF NEWBORN MALE RATS
P. Ghiani, B. Uva
Istituto di Anatomia Comparata, Università di Genova, 16126 GENOVA, ITALY

9 **243.** UROTENSIN II IS VASODEPRESSOR IN RATS
A. Gibson, M. Ginsburg, H.A. Bern
Kings College, University of London, UK and University of California, Berkeley, USA

10 **244.** HYPOTHALAMIC REGULATION OF PLASMA RENIN ACTIVITY: EFFERENT PATHWAYS
E. Gotoh, K. Murakami, R. Golin, W.F. Ganong
Department of Physiology, University of California, San Francisco, California 94143, U.S.A

11 **245.** CENTRAL EFFECTS OF CORTICOTROPIN-RELEASING FACTOR (CRF) ON PENTOBARBITAL-INDUCED ANESTHESIA AND HYPOTHERMIA IN RAT
T. Imaki, T. Shibasaki, A. Masuda, H. Demura, K. Shizume
Institute of Clinical Endocrinology, Tokyo Women's Medical College, Tokyo 162, Japan

12 **246.** POSSIBLE ROLE OF LEUMORPHIN, AN OPIOID PEPTIDE, IN CENTRAL REGULATION OF FLUID BALANCE IN RATS
H. Imura, N. Nakao, T. Yamada, H. Itoh, S. Shiono, M. Sakamoto, N. Morii, A. Sugawara, Y. Saito
Kyoto University Faculty of Medicine, Kyoto, Japan

13 **247.** LINKAGE OF ADRENAL MEDULLARY OPIOID RECEPTORS TO GTP-BINDING PROTEINS, PERTUSSIS TOXIN SUBSTRATES
K. Kamikubo, H. Murase, M. Niwa, K. Miura, M. Nozaki,* K. Tsurumi**
Departments of Internal Medicine (III) and *Pharmacology Gifu University School of Medicine, Gifu 500, Japan

14 **248.** EFFECT OF CENTRAL LHRH MANIPULATION ON THE SKIN TEMPERATURE RESPONSE IN AN ANIMAL MODEL FOR THE HOT FLUSH
Michael J. Katovich, J.W. Simpkins, J. O'Meara
Department of Pharmacodynamics, University of Florida, Gainesville, FL 32610

15 **249.** HYPOTHALAMIC MU OPIOID RECEPTORS DURING PREGNANCY AND AFTER PARTURITION
P. Limonta, D. Dondi, R. Maggi, M. Motta, F. Piva
Department of Endocrinology, University of Milano, Italy

16 **250.** *IN VIVO* ACTH TREATMENT ALTERS *IN VITRO* RESPONSE TO TESTICULAR INTERSTITIAL CELLS TO HCG
D.R. Mann, M.M. Smith, C. Nelson, C.L. Free
Morehouse School of Medicine, Atlanta, GA 30310

17 **251.** EFFECTS OF CHOLECYSTOKININ ON RENAL FUNCTION IN SHEEP
J.G. McDougall, A.R. Coker, J.P. Coghlan, D.A. Denton, B.A. Scoggins
Howard Florey Institute of Experimental Physiology & Medicine, Parkville, Vic. 3052 Australia

18 **251a.** POSSIBLE ROLE OF DYNORPHIN IN THE PATHOPHYSIOLOGY OF TRAUMATIC BRAIN INJURY
T.K. McIntosh, A.I. Faden
University of California, San Francisco

19 **252.** EXISTENCE OF PEPTIDERGIC NERVES AND MORPHOLOGICAL CHANGES OF THE SMOOTH MUSCLES IN THE CONGENITAL AGANGLIONIC INTESTINE OF RATS
M. Oki, T. Domoto, T. Gonda, K. Inoue, S. Note
Shimane Medical University, Shimane, Japan

20 **253.** HETEROGENEITY OF OXYTOCIN RECEPTORS ON RAT AND SHEEP MYOMETRIAL CELLS
V. Pliška, J. Heiniger, H. Albertin-Kohlhauf
Institute of Animal Science, Swiss Federal Institute of Technology, ETH Zentrum, CH-8092 Zürich, Switzerland

21 **254.** THE ACTION OF THE LATERAL HYPOTHALAMIC AREA ON NEURONS IN THE REGION OF THE SUBFORNICAL ORGAN WITH EFFERENT PROJECTIONS TO THE HYPOTHALAMIC PARAVENTRICULAR NUCLEUS IN THE RAT
H. Saito, J. Tanaka, H. Kaba, K. Seto
Kochi Medical School, Nankoku, Kochi, Japan

22 **254a.** EFFECTS OF LONG-ACTING SOMATOSTATIN ANALOGUE IN A CASE OF MULTIPLE ENDOCRINE NEOPLASIA WITH αSUBUNIT-SECRETING PITUITARY ADENOMA, ZOLLINGER-ELLISON AND HYPERPARATHYROIDISM
G. Sassolas, J.C. Souquet, J.A. Chayvialle, C. Partensky, B. Loras
Centre Médecine Nucléaire, Hop Cardiologique, Lyon, France

23 **255.** NUTRITIONAL MODULATION OF THE EXERCISE-INDUCED INCREASE OF HYPOTHALAMIC NOREPINEPHRINE TURNOVER
U. Schweiger, J. Leifeld, M. Seidl, K.M. Pirke
Max-Planck-Institut für Psychiatrie. D-8000 München 40, F.R.G.

24 **256.** GNRH PROHORMONE IMMUNOREACTIVITY IN THE PRIMATE FOREBRAIN AND HYPOTHALAMUS
T. Song, K. Nikolics, P.H. Seeburg, P.C. Goldsmith
Reproductive Endocrinology Center, Dept. of Ob/Gyn and Repro. Sci., Univ. of Calif., San Francisco, CA 94143

25 **257.** MORPHOMETRIC AND TOPOGRAPHICAL ORGANIZATION OF CAPILLARIES WITHIN THE RAT SUBFORNICAL ORGAN
N.M. Sposito, P.M. Gross, J.D. Fenstermacher
Dept. Neurol. Surg., SUNY Stony Brook, NY 11794

26 **258.** PHENCYCLIDINE AND OPIATE BINDING SITES IN HYPOTHALAMUS AND PITUITARY CELLS
S.S. Stojilkovic, M.L. Dufau, K.J. Catt
Endo. & Reprod. Res. Branch, NICHD, Bethesda, Maryland

27 **259.** THE EFFECT OF HIGH POTASSIUM ON ATRIAL NATRIURETIC FACTOR RELEASE FROM RERIFUSED RAT HYPOTHALAMUS
I. Tanaka, Y. Oki, M. Sakamoto, T. Inagami, H. Imura,** K. Nakao,** T. Yoshimi*
Hamamatsu University School of Medicine, Hamamatsu, Kyoto University School of Medicine,** Kyoto, Japan, Vanderbilt University School of Medicine,* Nashville, Tennessee

28 **260.** SUBFORNICAL ORGAN AND HYPOTHALAMIC PARAVENTRICULAR NUCLEUS CONNECTIONS WITH MEDIAN PREOPTIC NUCLEUS NEURONS IN RATS
J. Tanaka, H. Kaba, H. Saito, K. Seto
Kochi Medical School, Nankoku, Kochi, Japan

29 **261.** ACCUMULATION OF SEROTONIN AND COEXISTENCE WITH TYROSINE HYDROXYLASE IN HYPOTHALAMIC NEURONS OF ACUTELY STALK-SECTIONED BABOONS
K.K. Thind, J.E. Boggan, T. Song, P.C. Goldsmith
Reproductive Endocrinology Center, Dept. of Ob/Gyn and Repro. Sci., University of Calif., San Francisco, CA 94143

30 **262.** INFLUENCE OF PROSTAGLANDINS ON PITUITARY PORTAL BLOOD FLOW (PPBF)
W.Z. Traczyk, U. Szkudlarek
Department of Physiology, School of Medicine, Lodz, Poland

31 **263.** RENIN-RELEASING FACTOR IN RAT AND BOVINE HYPOTHALAMUS
L.D. Van de Kar, J.H. Urban
Loyola Univ. of Chicago, Sch. Med. Dept. Pharmacol., Maywood, IL 60153

32 **264.** IN VIVO RELEASE RATES OF ADRENAL NEUROPEPTIDES IN THE RAT MEASURED BY A NOVEL DIALYSIS METHOD
R. Vaupel, H. Jarry, E.-M. Düker, W. Wuttke
Div. Clin. Exp. Endocr., Dept. ObGyn., Univ. Göttingen, FRG

33 **265.** USE OF EVOKED POTENTIALS (EEG) FOR EVALUATION OF NEUROPEPTIDE FUNCTIONS IN MAN
K. Voigt, U. Bickel, J. Born, H.L. Fehm
Institute of Clinical Pharmacology, Free University of Berlin, Hindenburgdamm 30, 1000 Berlin 45

34 **266.** METABOLISM OF DEHYDROEPIANDROSTERONE BY DISCRETE BRAIN REGIONS AND HYPOPHYSIS OF THE RAT
J. Weidenfeld, H. Schiller, I. Chowers
Laboratory of Experimental Endocrinology, Dept. of Neurology, Hadassah University Hospital and Dept. of Internal Medicine, Bikur Cholim Hospital-Hebrew University Medical School, Jerusalem, Israel

Neuroendocrine Regulation of ACTH

35 **267.** COMPARISON OF IMMEDIATE AND DELAYED REPLACEMENT OF CORTICOSTERONE AFTER ADRENALECTOMY ON ACTH
S.F. Akana, C.S. Cascio, L. Jacobson, N. Levin, J. Shinsako, M.F. Dallman
UCSF, San Francisco, CA 94143, USA

36 **268.** ACETYLCHOLINE AND SEROTONIN REGULATION OF HYPOTHALAMIC CRH RELEASE *IN VITRO*
A.E. Calogero, R. Bernardini, L. Tamarkin, T. Tomai, A. Luger, P.W. Gold, D.L. Loriaux, G.P. Chrousos
DEB, NICHD, NIH and CPB and BPB, NIMH, Bethesda, MD

37 **270.** THE ROLE OF GABA IN THE HYPOTHALAMO-PITUITARY ADRENAL (HPA) AXIS IN THE RAT
*E.A. Campbell, *P.R. Scraggs, *A.R.H. Altaher, B. Gillham, *M.T. Jones*
Departments of Biochemistry and *Gynaecology, United Medical and Dental Schools (St. Thomas's Campus), London

38 **271.** THE EFFECTS OF DEXAMETHASONE ON CENTRAL AND PERIPHERAL ACTH SYSTEMS IN RATS
M. Carnes, C.M. Barksdale, N.H. Kalin, M.S. Brownfield, S.J. Lent
Wm. S. Middleton Veterans Hospital and University of Wisconsin, Madison, Wisconsin

39 **272.** SEROTONIN-OPIOID INTERACTIONS ARE NOT MEDIATED THROUGH $5HT_2$ RECEPTOR SUBTYPE
F. Facchinetti, °E. Martignoni, °°S. Marini, A.R. Genazzani
Dept. of Obstetrics and Ginecology, University of Modena, °Dept. of Neurology, University of Pavia, °°Janssen Italia, Roma-Italy

40 **273.** EFFECT OF CHRONIC HYPERPROLACTINEMIA ON CATECHOLAMINE CONTENT AND RELEASE FROM ADRENAL TISSUE
J.J. Fernández Ruiz, M. Cebeira, C. Agrasal, J.A.F. Tresguerres, J.A. Ramos, A.I. Esquifino*
Department of Biochemistry and Human Physiology.* F. Medicine. U. Complutensis. Madrid. Spain.

41 **274.** EFFECT OF PASSIVE IMMUNIZATION AGAINST CORTICOTROPIN RELEASING-FACTOR (CRF) ON THE POST-ADRENALECTOMY CHANGES IN CRF BINDING SITES IN THE RAT ANTERIOR PITUITARY GLAND
M. Grino, V. Guillaume, E. Castanas, B. Conte-Devolx, C. Oliver
Laboratoire de Neuroendocrinologie Expérimentale, INSERM U 297, Faculté de Médecine Nord, Bd P. Dramard, 13326 Marseille Cédex 15, FRANCE

42 **275.** EFFECTS OF OVINE CRF, VASOPRESSIN AND METYRAPONE UPON PLASMA LEVELS OF ACTH AND CORTISOL IN STRESS-SENSITIVE AND STRESS-RESISTANT PIGS
J. Hari, V. Pliška
Institute of Animal Science, Swiss Federal Institute of Technology, ETH Zentrum, 8092 Zürich, Switzerland

43 **276.** EFFECT OF SYNTHETIC ATRIAL NATRIURETIC PEPTIDE ON ACTH AND CORTICOSTERONE SECRETION IN RATS
K. Hashimoto, S. Suemaru, T. Hattori, M. Sugawara, H. Inoue, T. Takao, J. Kageyama, Z. Ota
Third Department of Internal Medicine, Okayama University Medical School, Okayama 700, Japan

44 **277.** EFFECTS OF BACLOFEN ON HYPOTHALAMO-PITUITARY-ADRENOCORTICAL (HPA) FUNCTION IN RATS
A. Häusler
Res. Dept., Pharm. Div., CIBA-GEIGY Ltd., 4002 Basel, SWITZERLAND

45 **278.** THE EFFECT OF CORTISOL ON MEMBRANE POTENTIAL OF THE HIPPOCAMPUS CELLS IN VITRO
S.Y. Hua, Y.Z. Chen
Second Military Medical College, Shanghai, China

46 **279.** A NOCTURNAL RISE IN CORTICOSTERONE MAY BE REQUIRED FOR NORMAL ACTH RESPONSES TO STRESS IN RATS
L. Jacobson, S.F. Akana, M.F. Dallman
Department of Physiology, UC San Francisco, CA 94143

47 **280.** COORDINATE ENDOCRINE ROLES FOR ADRENAL MEDULLA AND CORTEX IN STRESS
D. Jefferys, J.W. Funder
Medical Research Centre, Prince Henry's Hospital, Melbourne, Australia 3004

48 **281.** THE ROLE OF THE ADRENAL MEDULLA IN MODULATING THE STRESS-INDUCED RELEASE OF PITUITARY HORMONES
O. Khorram, S.M. McCann
Department of Physiology, Univ. of Texas Health Science Center, Dallas, Texas 75235

49 **282.** STRESS-INDUCED RELEASE OF β-ENDORPHIN, ACTH AND CATECHOLAMINES: MEDIATION VIA THE HISTAMINERGIC SYSTEM
U. Knigge, S. Matzen, F.W. Bach, P. Bang, J. Warberg
Inst. of Medical Physiology C, University of Copenhagen, and Dept. of Clinical Chemistry, Gentofte Hospital, Denmark

50 **283.** DEXAMETHASONE FEEDBACK TO CRF AND AVP AT THE PARAVENTRICULAR NUCLEUS
K. Kovács, J.Z. Kiss, G.B. Makara
Institute of Experimental Medicine, Hungarian Academy of Sciences, Budapest, Hungary

51 **284.** ENDORPHIN MODULATION OF THERMAL ADAPTATION TO EMOTIONAL STRESS
K. Kubo, S. Tsuzuki, T. Sasaki
Dept. Bioregulation, Inst. Med. Gen., Kumamoto Univ. Med. Sch., Kumamoto 862, Japan

52 **285.** CORTICOTROPES ARE INSENSITIVE TO STEROID FEEDBACK SIGNAL *IN VIVO*
N. Levin, M. Blum, C. Cascio,* J.L. Roberts, M.F. Dallman.**
*UC San Francisco, CA 94143 USA and Columbia Univ. College of Phys. & Surg., New York, NY 10032 USA

53 **286.** EFFECTS OF ETHANOL ON NALTREXONE INDUCED STIMULATION OF ANTERIOR PITUITARY, ADRENAL AND GONADAL HORMONES IN WOMEN
J.H. Mendelson, N.K. Mello
Harvard Medical School-McLean Hospital, Belmont, MA

54 **287.** PVN LESIONS COMPLETELY ABOLISH STRESS-INDUCED INCREASES IN PITUITARY CYCLIC AMP IN VIVO
J.L. Meyerhoff, G.J. Kant, E.H. Mougey
Neuroendo. Branch, Dept. Medical Neurosciences, Walter Reed Army Institute of Research, Washington, D.C. 20307-5100

55 **288.** INFLUENCE OF RESTRAINT STRESS ON THE NOCTURNAL PROLACTIN SURGE OF PSEUDO-PREGNANT ANIMALS
M. Morehead, R.R. Gala
Dept.of Physiology, Wayne State Univ., Detroit, MI 48201

56 **289.** POMC-DERIVED HORMONE RESPONSES TO MAXIMAL TREADMILL EXERCISE

M. Oleshansky, J. Zoltick, R. Herman, E. Mougey, J. Meyerhoff
Dept. Medical Neurosciences, Walter Reed Army Institute of Research, Washington, D.C. 20307-5100

57 **290.** CHOLINERGIC AND SEROTONERGIC STIMULATION OF HYPOTHALAMIC CRF RELEASE IN VITRO
M.J. Owens, M.A. Smith, C.B. Nemeroff
Departments of Pharmacology and Psychiatry, Duke University Medical Center, Durham, N.C., USA

58 **291.** DOPAMINERGIC MODULATION OF THE SEPTO-HIPPOCAMPAL CHOLINERGIC SYSTEM UNDER STRESS
J.M. Rabey, V.H. Gilad, G.M. Gilad
The Center for Neurosciences and Behavioral Research, The Weizmann Institute of Science, Rehovot, Israel

59 **292.** PLASMA CORTISOL AND BETA ENDORPHIN AFTER DEXAMETHASONE IN PARKINSON DISEASE
J.M. Rabey, M. Zohar, Z. Oberman, E. Graff
Department of Neurology, and Department of Chemical Pathology, Tel Aviv Medical Center, Sackler School of Medicine, Tel Aviv University, Israel

60 **293.** EFFECT OF ETHANOL ON CRF RELEASE *IN VITRO*
E. Redei, B. Branch, A.N. Taylor
Dept. of Anatomy, UCLA and West LA/Brentwood VA, Los Angeles, CA 90024

61 **294.** ALDOSTERONE SELECTIVITY OF TYPE I CORTICOID RECEPTORS IN RAT ANTERIOR PITUITARY
K. Sheppard, J.W. Funder
Medical Research Centre, Prince Henry's Hospital, Melbourne, Australia 3004

62 **295.** STRESS-INDUCED ALTERATIONS IN NEUROTENSIN-LIKE IMMUNOREACTIVITY (NTLI) IN RAT BRAIN AND ADRENALS
M.A. Smith, A.Y. Deutch, P.B. Chappell, G. Bissette, L. O'Connor, R.H. Roth, C.B. Nemeroff
Dept. of Psychiatry, Duke Univ. Med. Ctr., Durham, N.C. and Yale Univ., New Haven, CT

63 **296.** BRAIN CORTICOTROPIN-RELEASING FACTOR (CRF) AND PITUITARY-ADRENAL RESPONSIVENESS IN CHRONICALLY STRESSED RATS
S. Suemaru, K. Hashimoto, T. Takao, T. Hattori, M. Sugawara, H. Inoue, J. Kageyama, Z. Ota
Third Department of Internal Medicine, Okayama University Medical School, Okayama, Japan

64 **297.** DIFFERENCES IN (3H) CORTICOSTERONE AND (3H) DEXAMETHASONE BINDING CHARACTERISTICS TO HYPOTHALAMUS, HIPPOCAMPUS AND ANTERIOR PITUITARY GLAND
W. Sutanto, B.D. Allen
Human Physiology, Royal Holloway and Bedford New College, Egham Hill, Egham, Surrey TW20 OEX, ENGLAND

65 **298.** CENTRAL ADRENERGIC AND NORADRENERGIC STIMULATORY CONTROL OF THE CRH-ACTH AXIS IN THE RAT
A. Szafarczyk, G. Alonso, F. Malaval, R. Gibaud, I. Assenmacher
Neuroendocrinology Lab., UA 1197 CNRS, Dept. of Physiology, Univ. Montpellier II, F 34060, Montpellier, France

66 **299.** RELEASE OF CORTICOTROPIN-RELEASING FACTOR FROM RAT HYPOTHALAMUS IN VITRO
T. Takao, K. Hashimoto, S. Suemaru, T. Hattori, J. Kageyama, Z. Ota
Third Department of Internal Medicine, Okayama University Medical School, Okayama 700, Japan

67 **300.** EFFECT OF STRESS ON NEUROPEPTIDES AND THEIR RECEPTORS OF RAT CNS
H. Takayama, H. Kuroda, N. Ogawa, Z. Ota
Third Department of Internal Medicine and Institute for Neurobiology, Okayama University Medical School, Okayama, Japan

68 **301.** ACTH RESPONSE TO CHRONIC INTRAVENTRICULAR ADMINISTRATION OF ANTI-CORTICOSTERONE IN THE RAT
J.E. Van Zuylen, A.N. Taylor, S. Gholami, E. Redei
Dept. of Anatomy, UCLA, Los Angeles, CA 90024

69 **302.** QUANTITATIVE ANALYSIS OF ADRENOCORTICAL SECRETION IN RESPONSE TO ACTIVATION OF PERIPHERAL NERVE FIBER GROUPS OF DIFFERENT DIAMETERS
Z.Z. Wang, Y.Z. Chen
Second Military Medical College, Shanghai, China

70 **303.** PLASMA CORTICOTROPIN-RELEASING FACTOR, CORTISOL, AND CORTISOL-BINDING GLOBULIN DURING THIRD TRIMESTER PREGNANCY
C.D.A. Wolfe, E.A. Linton,[2] P.R. Scraggs, E.A. Campbell,[1] M.T. Jones
Department of Gynaecology and [1]Biochemistry, St. Thomas's Hospital Medical School and [2]Protein Hormone Unit, St. Bartholomew's Centre for Clinical Research, London

71 **304.** INHIBITION OF PLASMA RENIN ACTIVITY BY CORTISOL
C.E. Wood, J. Silbiger
Department of Physiology, University of Florida College of Medicine, Gainesville, FL 32610

Development and Aging

72 **305.** HYPOTHALAMIC LHRH CONTENT IN NEONATALLY ESTROGENIZED-STERILE FEMALE RATS IS HIGHER THAN THAT IN INTACT CYCLING RATS
M. Aihara (1), S. Hayashi(2), K. Wakabayashi(3), H. Kobayashi(1)
(1)Dept. Biol., Toho Univ., Funabashi, Chiba 274, (2)Dept. Anat./Embryol., Tokyo Metropol. Inst. Neurosci., Fuchu, Tokyo 183, (3) Inst. Endocr., Gunma Univ., Maebashi, Gunma 371, Japan

73 **306.** IS THERE A DEFECTIVE CENTRAL COORDINATION OF OVARIAN ACTIVITY IN AGING RATS?
M. Cioni, L. Greco, H. Zachi Pour, U. Scapagnini, B. Marchetti
Dept. of Pharmacology, Catania University, 95125 Italy

74 **307.** DELAYED SEXUAL MATURATION DURING PREPUBERTAL CHRONIC CANNABINOID TREATMENT: ASSOCIATED REDUCTION IN SERUM PROLACTIN

E. Field, L. Tyrey
Duke University, Durham, N.C. 27710

75 **308.** DECREASED IMMUNOREACTIVE GNRH AND PROGNRH HYPOTHALAMIC NEURONS IN JUVENILE PRIMATES
P.C. Goldsmith, K.K. Thind, T. Song, S.E. Monroe
Reproductive Endocrinology Center, Dept. of Ob/Gyn and Repro. Sci., Univ. of Calif., San Francisco, CA 94143

76 **309.** DIFFERENTIAL EFFECTS OF NEONATAL AND ADULT ANDROGEN EXPOSURE ON THE GROWTH HORMONE (GH) SECRETORY PATTERN IN THE MALE RAT
J-O Jansson, L.A. Frohman
Div. of Endocrinology and Metabolism, University of Cincinnati College of Medicine, Cincinnati, OH 45267

77 **310.** DEVELOPING NEUROENDOCRINE SYSTEMS AS TARGETS FOR DRUGS AND PEPTIDE HORMONES
W. Lichtensteiger, M. Schlumpf, U. Ribary
Inst. of Pharmacology, University of Zürich, Zürich, Switzerland

78 **311.** ELECTRICAL STIMULATION OF THE HYPOTHALAMUS INDUCES DIFFERENTIAL LH RELEASE AT TWO DEVELOPMENTAL STAGES IN IMMATURE FEMALE GUINEA PIGS
M.D. Loose, E. Terasawa
Wis. Regional Primate Research Ctr., Univ. of Wisconsin, Madison, WI 53715-1299

79 **312.** AGING AND BRAIN K OPIOID RECEPTORS
R. Maggi, D. Dondi, F. Piva
Department of Endocrinology, University of Milano, Italy.

80 **313.** SELECTIVE INCREASE OF TYPE I CORTICOSTEROID RECEPTORS IN HIPPOCAMPUS OF SENESCENT RATS AFTER CHRONIC TREATMENT WITH A BEHAVIORALLY POTENT $ACTH_{4-9}$ ANALOG
J.M.H.M. Reul, J.A.D.M. Tonnaer, E.R. de Kloet
Rudolf Magnus Institute for Pharmacology, Utrecht, and Organon Scientific Development Group, Oss, The Netherlands

81 **314.** AGE-RELATED CHANGES IN MOLECULAR FORMS OF POMC-DERIVED PEPTIDES IN THE BRAIN OF RATS
C.W. Wilkinson, D.M. Dorsa
Geriatric Research, Education and Clinical Center, American Lake and Seattle VA Medical Centers, and University of Washington, Seattle, Washington

82 **315.** AGE- AND STRAIN-RELATED DIFFERENCES IN VASOPRESSIN AND OXYTOCIN RELEASE
V. Zbuzek, A.R. Fuchs,+ V.K. Zbuzek,* W. Wu**
*UMDNJ, New Jersey Medical School, Newark, New Jersey 07103 and +Cornell University Medical Center, New York, New York 10021

Regulation of Hormone Rhythms

83 **316.** MODULATION OF CIRCADIAN AND PULSATILE THYROTROPIN-RELEASE BY THYROID HORMONES, GLUCOCORTICOIDS AND SOMATOSTATIN
G. Brabant, A. Esslinger, R.D. Hesch, A. von zur Mühlen
Dept. Clin. Endocrinol, Med. Hochschule D-3 Hannover F.R.G.

84 **317.** POSSIBLE PROLACTIN MEDIATED EFFECT OF MELATONIN ON REPRODUCTIVE AXIS IN FEMALE RATS
A.I. Esquifino, M.A. Villanúa, J.A.F. Tresguerres*
Depts. of Biochem. and Physiol. Faculty of Medicine. Complutense University. 28040 Madrid. SPAIN

85 **318.** CHRONIC ADMINISTRATION OF METHAMPHETAMINE DISORGANIZES THE CIRCADIAN LOCOMOTOR RHYTHM IN THE RAT
T. Hiroshige, K. Honma, S. Honma, Y. Katsuno, T. Nagasaka, Y. Noe
Hokkaido University School of Medicine, Department of Physiology, Sapporo, 060 Japan

86 **318a.** RELATIONSHIP BETWEEN SLEEP, MELATONIN AND GROWTH HORMONE IN NORMAL YOUNG MEN
B. Roussel, P. Garry, B. Claustrat, R. Cohen, R. Amalberti, G. Sassolas
Centre Médecine Nucléaire, Hop. Cardiologique, Lyon, France

87 **319.** DAILY PATTERN OF SOMATOSTATIN CONCENTRATION IN HUMAN CEREBROSPINAL FLUID: CONNECTION WITH DISEASE ACTIVITY IN MULTIPLE SCLEROSIS
K.V. Sørensen,[1] T. Alslev,[1] S.E. Christensen,[2] N.B. Jensen,[1] H. Ørskov[3]
Departments of Neurology, Aarhus, Odense, Viborg.[1]- Second Clinic of Internal Medicine, Aarhus[2]- Institute of Exp. Clinical Research, University of Aarhus, Denmark

88 **320.** INFLUENCE OF MELATONIN ON THE TESTICULAR REGRESSION INDUCED BY TESTOSTERONE PELLETS IN MALE RATS KEPT IN LONG OR SHORT PHOTOPERIOD
M.K. Vaughan, S. Oaknin, B. Cozzi, K. Li, R.J. Reiter
Cellular & Structural Biology, Univ. Texas Health Science Center, San Antonio, Texas

89 **321.** ESTRADIOL REGULATES MELATONIN ACTIVITY IN THE FEMALE RAT BRAIN
N. Zisapel, M. Laudon
Dept. of Biochemistry, Tel-Aviv University, Tel-Aviv 69978, Israel.

Immunology

90 **322.** INTERLEUKIN-1 MODULATES SECRETION BY RAT PITUITARY CELLS IN MONOLAYER CULTURE
J.E. Beach, E.W. Bernton, J.W. Holaday, R.C. Smallridge, H.G. Fein
Divs. of Medicine and Neuropsychiatry, Walter Reed Army Institute of Research, Washington, D.C. 20307-5100

91 **323.** NEUROENDOCRINE REGULATION OF RAT SPLEEN LYMPHOCYTES
R. Bernardini, G. Paciotti, R. Skwerer, L. Tamarkin
CPB/NIMH, Bethesda, MD 20892

92 **324.** THYMOSIN REGULATES HORMONE SECRETION OF MOUSE CORTICOTROPHIC TUMOR CELLS
J.M. Farah, N.R. Hall, A.L. Goldstein, J.F. Bishop, T.L O'Donohue

Experimental Therapeutics, N.I.N.C.D.S. N.I.H., Bethesda, MD 20892 & Department of Biochemistry, The George Washington University, Washington, DC 20037

93 **325.** NEURO-ENDOCRINE AND IMMUNOLOGICAL EFFECTS OF PHOSPHATIDYLSERINE
E. Galbiati, G. Calderini, E. Boarato, L. Mietto, A. Bruni
Fidia Neurobiological Research Laboratories, 35031 Abano Terme, Italy

94 **326.** THE THYMUS AS A NEUROENDOCRINE ORGAN
V. Geenen, J.J. Legros, M.P. Defresne, J. Boniver
University of Sart Tilman, B-23, B-4000 Liège, Belgium

95 **327** HUMAN INTERLEUKIN 1 β.STIMULATES ACTH RELEASE FROM RAT ANTERIOR PITUITARY CELLS IN A CAMP AND PROSTAGLANDIN E_2 INDEPENDANT-MANNER
Ph. Kehrer,[1] R.C. Gaillard,[1] J-M. Dayer,[2] A.F. Muller[1]
Clinique Médicale[1] et Division d'Immunologie[2] et d'Allergie. Dept. of Medecine, University Hospital CH-1211 Geneva 4/Switzerland.

Behavior

96 **328.** NEUROPEPTIDE Y (NPY)-INDUCED SUPPRESSION OF MALE SEXUAL BEHAVIOR: NEURAL LOCI
J.T. Clark, S.P. Kalra, P.S. Kalra
Dept. OB-Gyn. Univ. Fla. Col. Med., Gainesville, FL 32610

97 **329.** DIET-INDUCED THERMOGENESIS (DIT) IN DEPRESSION: EFFECT OF IMIPRAMINE TREATMENT
M.H. Fernstrom, M. Massoudi, D.J. Kupfer
Department of Psychiatry and Center for Neuroscience, University of Pittsburgh School of Medicine, Pittsburg, PA USA

98 **330.** ROLL OF SEPTUM AND PREOPTIC AREA IN MASCULINE AND FEMININE SEXUAL BEHAVIORS IN MALE RATS
*Y. Kondo, A. Shinoda, *K. Yamanouchi, *Y. Arai*
Department of Psychology, Faculty of Letters, Gakushuin University, Tokyo, and *Department of Anatomy, Juntendo University School of Medicine, Tokyo, Japan

99 **331.** VASOACTIVE INTESTINAL POLYPEPTIDE (VIP) IN HUMAN CEREBROSPINAL FLUID OF DEMENTIA WITH CEREBRAL ATROPHY IN JAPAN
K. Nakamura, H. Kaneko, M. Hayashi, T. Shimizu, T. Ihara, S. Kanto, M. Kusakabe, J. Itoh, C. Yanaihara,[1] N. Yanaihara,[1] M. Irie
Toho University School of Medicine, Tokyo 143, [1]Shizuoka College of Pharmacy, Shizuoka 422, Japan

Friday PM **Continental Ballroom 4**

SESSION 17: Neuroendocrine Regulation of LH
Chairpersons: **S. Kalra**
M. Ginsberg

1:30 **332.** NOREPINEPHRINE STIMULATES AND DOPAMINE INHIBITS PULSATILE LHRH RELEASE *IN VIVO* IN OVARIECTOMIZED RHESUS MONKEYS
E. Terasawa, C. Krook, G.A. Davis, G. Watanabe
Wis. Reg. Primate Research Ctr., Univ. of Wisconsisn, Madison, WI 53715-1299

1:45 **333.** EPINEPHRINE & ESTRADIOL PRETREATMENT ENHANCE NOREPINEPHRINE-MEDIATED SECRETION OF GnRH BY RAT HYPOTHALAMIC CELL CULTURES.
A.T.W. Lim, F. Petraglia, W. Vale
The Clayton Foundation Laboratories for Peptide Biology, The Salk Institute, La Jolla, CA

2:00 **334.** CRF INHIBITION OF LH IS MEDIATED BY OPIOIDS: ROLE OF TESTOSTERONE
K.E. Nikolarakis, O.F.X. Almeida, A. Herz
Department of Neuropharmacology, Max-Planck-Institut für Psychiatrie, D-8033 Martinsried, West Germany

2:15 **335.** ESTROGEN-DEPENDENT EFFECTS OF NOREPINEPHRINE ON HYPOTHALAMIC GnRH RELEASE IN THE RABBIT
K.-Y.F. Pau, H.G. Spies
Oregon Regional Primate Research Center, Beaverton, Oregon 97006

2:30 **336.** CENTRAL EFFECTS OF LHRH ANALOGS INDICATE AN INHIBITORY ROLE OF LHRH TO MODULATE ITS OWN SECRETION
M. Valenca, M. Ching, A. Negro-Vilar
Reprod. Neuroendo. Sec., Lab. Reprod. Dev. Tox., NIEHS-NIH, Res. Tri. Pk., NC 27709

2:45 **337.** PREOVULATORY LH SURGE IN THE RAT: PULSE ANALYSIS AND ADVANCEMENT BY OPIOID RECEPTOR BLOCKADE
L.G. Allen, D. Caton, S.P. Kalra
Depts. of OB-Gyn and Anesthesiology, Univ. of Fla. Col. of Med., Gainesville, FL 32610

3:00 **338.** EVIDENCE AGAINST A COMMON RELEASE SIGNAL FOR PROLACTIN AND LH IN WOMEN
L.A. Marshall, M.C. Martin, R.B. Jaffe
U of Calif., San Francisco, San Francisco, CA

3:15 **339.** OVARIAN FACTORS ANTAGONIZE THE SELF PRIMING ACTION OF LUTEINIZING HORMONE RELEASING HORMONE (LH-RH)
J. de Koning, A.M.I. Tijssen, G.W. Hilberath, H. Kamsteeg, G.P. van Rees
Dept. of Pharmacology, Univ. of Leiden, The Netherlands

Friday PM **Continental Parlor 5**

SESSION 18: Neuroendocrine Regulation of GH
Chairpersons: **D. Cocchi**
J. Apelbaum

1:30 **340.** MODULATION OF β-ADRENERGIC STIMULATION OF GROWTH HORMONE RELEASE BY STIMULATORY AND INHIBITORY INTERCELLULAR COMMUNICATIONS
M. Baes, C. Denef
Laboratory of Cell Pharmacology, School of Medicine, University of Leuven, Belgium

1:45 **341.** EVIDENCE THAT GH DEPLETION AND N_s UNCOUPLING BOTH CONTRIBUTE TO THE DESENSITISATION OF GH RESPONSES TO GRF
C. Dieguez, C.A.E. Edwards, J.R. Peters, R. Hall, M.F. Scanlon

Neuroendocrine Unit, University of Wales College of Medicine, Cardiff

2:00 **342.** RELEASE OF IMMUNOREACTIVE GROWTH HORMONE-RELEASING FACTOR (GRF) AND SOMATOSTATIN FROM INCUBATED HYPOTHALAMUS IN YOUNG AND OLD MALE RATS
M. Ono, N. Miki, K. Shizume
Department of Medicine, Institute of Clinical Endocrinology, Tokyo Women's Medical College, Shinjuku-ku, Tokyo 162, Japan

2:15 **343.** MECHANISMS UNDERLYING THE EFFECTS ON GROWTH HORMONE SECRETION OF PHARMACOLOGIC MANIPULATION OF α-ADRENOCEPTOR OR CHOLINERGIC RECEPTOR AGONISTS AND ANTAGONISTS IN THE NEONATAL RAT
V. Locatelli, S.G. Cella, V. De Gennaro, W. Wehrenberg, E.E. Müller
Department of Pharmacology, University of Milan, Italy, and Department of Health Sciences, University of Wisconsin, Milwaukee U.S.A.

2:30 **344.** EXOGENOUS GROWTH HORMONE (GH) INHIBITS BOVINE BUT NOT MURINE PITUITARY GH SECRETION
S.M. Rosenthal, B.L. Silverman, W.B. Wehrenberg, S.L. Kaplan, M.M. Grumbach*
Dept. of Pediatrics, Univ. of California—San Francisco, San Francisco, CA; *Dept. of Health Sciences, University of Wisconsin—Milwaukee, Milwaukee, WI

2:45 **345.** ARE HYPOTHALAMIC GRF AND SRIF INVOLVED IN HYPOTHYROIDISM-INDUCED GROWTH FAILURE?
N. Miki, M. Ono, T. Tsushima, K. Shizume
Dept. of Medicine, Tokyo Women's Medical College, Tokyo 162, Japan

3:00 **346.** COMPARISON OF THE EFFECTS OF ACUTE GROWTH HORMONE (GH) AND CLONIDINE (CLON) ADMINISTRATION ON THE GH RHYTHM
M. Zorza, L.C. Terry
Univ. of Mich. and VA Medical Centers, Ann Arbor, MI

3:15 **347.** EFFECT OF TESTOSTERONE ON GROWTH HORMONE (GH) SECRETION IN FEMALE RATS DURING A CONTINUOUS INFUSION OF GH-RELEASING FACTOR (GRF)
*H. Sugihara, I. Wakabayashi, S. Akira, S. Minami, F. Takahashi, A. Motoyama, N. Ling**
Nippon Medical School, Tokyo, Japan and *The Salk Institute, San Diego, U.S.A.

Friday PM **Continental Parlors 1–3**

SESSION 19: Expression and Processing of Peptides and Comparative Neuroendocrinology

Chairpersons: **K. Lederis**
H. Kobayashi

1:30 **348.** REGULATION OF TH GENE TRANSCRIPTION IN THE FEMALE RAT HYPOTHALAMUS
M. Blum[+°], B.S. McEwen,[°] J.L. Roberts[+]
[+]Columbia University, College of Physicians & Surgeons, and [°]Rockefeller University, New York, NY

1:45 **349.** POST-TRANSLATIONAL PROCESS OF CRF IN THE OVINE MEDIAN EMINENCE
J.W. Funder, A.I. Smith, F.J. Morgan, M. Fullerton, I.J. Clarke, D. Engler
Medical Research Centre, Prince Henry's Hospital and St. Vincent's Institute of Medical Research, Melbourne, Australia 3004

2:00 **350.** CHARACTERISATION OF CALCITONIN GENE-RELATED PEPTIDE RECEPTORS IN RAT NERVOUS SYSTEM
S.J. Wimalawansa, H.R. Morris, I. MacIntyre*
Royal Postgraduate Medical School, London; *Imperial College, London

2:15 **351.** PROOPIOMELANOCORTIN (POMC) GENE EXPRESSION AND PEPTIDE PROCESSING DURING EARLY STAGES OF RAT PITUITARY DEVELOPMENT
J.E. Pintar, A.S. Liotta, D.I. Lugo
Columbia P&S and Mt. Sinai Medical School, NYC, 10032

2:30 **352.** DOUBLE IMMUNOFLUORESCENCE REVEALS PARTIAL COLOCALIZATION OF UROTENSINS I AND II IN A TELEOST CAUDAL NEUROSECRETORY SYSTEM
B.A. Larson, H.A. Bern, R.J. Lin, R.S. Nishioka
Wichita State University, Wichita, KS 67208 and University of California, Berkeley, CA 94720

2:45 **353.** FURTHER EVIDENCE THAT SOMATOSTATIN-14 IS A GROWTH HORMONE RELEASE-INHIBITING FACTOR IN THE GOLDFISH
T.A. Marchant, J.G. Dulka, R. Fraser, R.E. Peter
Department of Zoology, University of Alberta, Edmonton, Alberta, Canada T6G 2E9

3:00 **354.** STEREOSPECIFICITY OF DOPAMINE INHIBITION OF GONADOTROPIC HORMONE GtH SECRETION IN GOLDFISH (*Carassius auratus*) *IN VIVO*
R.J. Omeljaniuk, S.H. Shih, R.E. Peter
Dept. Zoology, Univ. Alberta, Edmonton, Alberta, CANADA

3:15 **355.** PROLACTIN SECRETION IN RAINBOW TROUT: EFFECT OF OSMOTIC PRESSURE AND CHARACTERIZATION OF A HYPOTHALAMIC PRL RELEASING ACTIVITY
P. Prunet, F. Gonnet
INRA, Laboratoire de Physiologie des Poissons—Campus de Beaulieu 35042 RENNES FRANCE

Abstracts

FUNCTIONAL AND EVOLUTIONARY PERSPECTIVES OF GENE CODING AND PROCESSING OF PEPTIDE PRECURSORS 1

J. Joosse
Biological Laboratory, Vrije Universiteit, P.O.B. 7161, 1007 MC Amsterdam, The Netherlands

Peptides function as neuronal messengers in all animals, even in the most simply organised ones such as polyps. Some of these peptides have molecular structures and/or functions which are unique for specific groups (insects, molluscs), others have identical or nearly identical structures throughout the animal kingdom, including man. Examples of both categories will be presented.

Gene directed synthesis of polyprotein precursors and proteolytic processing of these precursors is probably basically uniform in vertebrates and invertebrates. Detailed knowledge is availabe from two species of invertebrates, the marine snail *Aplysia* and the freshwater snail *Lymnaea*. The precursors of their egg laying hormones each give rise to about 10 neuropeptides which act as neurotransmitter, neuromodulator and/or neurohormone. The multiple release of these peptides results in a coordinated program of covert and overt egg laying behaviours. Although these snails have a separate history for about 400 million years, the genes coding for these peptides show highly conserved regions, besides completely diverged regions.

Intragenic duplication, wellknown from pro-enkephalin and TRH genes of vertebrates, is also found in molluscs. The most extreme case is represented by the gene coding for the tetrapeptide FMRFamide, originally identified in a mollusc and now known to occur in all animal groups, including mammals. This gene contains about 20 times the code for this peptide. Intragenic duplication is suggested to serve not only amplification of product formation, but also evolutionary stability.

The persistent presence of (neuro)peptides in animals irrespective of the degree of development of their brains, raises the question of the specific roles of these messengers, in addition to those of the classical transmitters and steroids. This problem will be discussed.

ANATOMICAL MAPPING OF PERIKARYA CONTAINING GONADOTROPIN-RELEASING HORMONE mRNA IN THE BRAIN OF THE MALE MONKEY, MACACA FASCICULARIS, BY IN SITU HYBRIDIZATION 2

L.A. Adams, L. Vician, L.J. Standish, D.K. Clifton, R.A. Steiner
University of Washington, Seattle, WA 98195

Gonadotropin-releasing hormone (GnRH) plays a major role in the regulation of mammalian reproduction. The physiologic functions of GnRH are well characterized, but very little is known about the genetic elements which control its biosynthesis. Using the recently developed technique of in situ hybridization, we have localized cell bodies containing the messenger RNA (mRNA) coding for GnRH production in the basal forebrain and hypothalamus of the male monkey, Macaca fascicularis. An adult male monkey was anesthetized, then perfused with 4% paraformaldehyde. A block of tissue containing the hypothalamus and preoptic /septal area was frozen and 20 micra coronal sections cut from this block were mounted on slides. Sections were incubated overnight at 37 C with an 35-S-labeled synthetic oligonucleotide probe (DNA*) complementary to the proGnRH mRNA. After incubation, sections were washed, dipped in photographic emulsion, and exposed for 2 weeks. The slides were then developed, counterstained with cresyl violet, and read blindly by light and dark-field illumination. Cells containing GnRH mRNA/ DNA* hybrids were identified in the medial and triangular septal nucleus, the horizontal and vertical limbs of the diagonal band of Broca, medial preoptic area, lateral hypothalamus, infundibulum, and the infundibular lip.This study demonstrates the presence of GnRH mRNA in neuroanatomic regions previously shown to include perikarya containing immunoreactive GnRH and establishes the feasibility of using in situ hybridization as a quantitative tool to study the development and regulation of GnRH gene expression in the primate brain.

(Supported in part by NIH Grant HD 12625)

ESTROGEN AFFECTS CHEMOSENSITIVITY OF PARAVENTRICULAR NEURONS IN SLICES OF THE FEMALE RAT HYPOTHALAMUS 3

T. AKAISHI, Y. SAKUMA
Department of Physiology II, Niigata University School of Medicine, Niigata 951, Japan

In superfused slices of the hypothalamus (frontal section, 400-500 μm thick) taken from ovariectomized female rats, extracellular action potentials were recorded from 126 neurons in the magnocellular region of the paraventricular nucleus (PVN). Effects of 17β-estradiol (E_2)(10^{-8}M) were observed on their spontaneous as well as induced discharges, the latter followed infusion of either noradrenaline (NA), dopamine (DA) or acetylcholine. Biologicaly inactive 17α-E was used as control. Twenty-one among the recorded cells were antidromically identified from the PVN-neurohypophyseal tract. Estrogen altered spontaneous activity in 19 of 26 PVN neurons, including the 6 identified cells. Nineteen cells were consisted of those responded with excitation (n=7, latency 82.3±11.6 sec) and those with inhibition (n=12, latency 89.3±7.4 sec). None of 5 cells in this group responded to 17 -E . In other PVN neurons, perfusion with medium containing either α or β anomer of E_2 resulted in varying magnitudes of excitatory or inhibitory responses induced by NA (n=5) or DA (n=3). These data suggest that estrogen or its catechol derivatives exerts an immediate action on some groups of PVN neurons directly or by modifying their responsiveness to other chemicals.

POST-NEONATAL TESTICULAR SECRETIONS "ORGANISE" AND "ACTIVATE" NEURAL CIRCUITS INVOLVED IN THE OPIATERGIC CONTROL OF LH RELEASE IN RATS 4

O.F.X. Almeida, K.E. Nikolarakis & A. Herz,
Department of Neuropharmacology, Max-Planck-Institut für Psychiatrie, D-8033 Martinsried, West Germany.

Male rats were castrated either pre-pubertally (26d.o.) or post-pubertally (59d.o.), and their LH and PRL responses to morphine (5mg/kg; 30min.) were studied for up to 120 days post-castration. Rats castrated when 26d.o. showed a progressively decreasing susceptibility to the inhibitory effects of the opiate upon LH secretion for up to 28 days after gonadectomy, but thereafter morphine again caused an almost total inhibition of LH secretion; the minimum inhibition found at 28 days after castration (age 54 days) occurred at the time at which male rats normally reach puberty. A different pattern of response was observed in rats castrated when 59 days old. Morphine maximally suppressed serum LH levels 2 and 5 days after castration, but it did not significantly reduce LH levels in these animals when administrated beyond 28 days post-castration. In contrast to the different LH responses in rats castrated pre- and post-pubertally, morphine application consistently elevated serum PRL levels in gonadectomised rats of all ages, regardless of the time elapsed after gonadectomy.

These data indicate that there is a transient fall in the inhibitory opioidergic tone upon LH secretion as the normal age of puberty approaches and that the ability of opiates to alter LH secretion in adulthood may depend upon the presence of the gonads at the age of puberty. In addition, the results demonstrate that the LH responses do not reflect general changes in the neuroendocrine response to opiates following castration since the PRL response to morphine remained intact after both pre- and post-pubertal castration.

This work was supported by SFB 220 of the Deutsche Forschungsgemeinschaft, Bonn.

ARE GONADOTROPINS AND PROLACTIN PITUITARY AND PLASMATIC LEVELS CORRELATED AFTER CHRONIC LHRH ANALOG (BUSERELIN) TREATMENT? 5

C.Alvarez Sanz, C.Bravo, C.Fdez Galaz, A.Tejero, P.Rodriguez, M.D.Vaticón. Dept.Physiol. Fac.Med. Univ.Complut. Madrid 28040. SPAIN

The chronic administration of a potent agonist analog D-Ser-(TBU)^6-LHRH-EA^{10} (HOE766, buserelin) suppresses ovarian cyclicity. We studied the effect of buserelin chronic treatment on pituitary and plasmatic concentrations of gonadotropins and prolactin in adult female Wistar rats. Animals were divided into 4 groups. Beginning on estrous a daily s.c. injection of buserelin was administered at doses of 1 ug/day for 7 days, or 0.5 ug/day for 14 days. Control groups received saline on the same days. Trunk blood was collected by decapitation the day following treatment withdrawal.

Buserelin treated group showed constant vaginal diestrous and depressed pituitary levels of LH and Prolactin respect to the values obtained in saline group ($p < 0.01$ in both cases). No change in plasma LH and a slight rise in plasma Prolactin ($p < 0.05$) was found in these animals. No significant changes in pituitary FSH were found in buserelin 7 or 14-days treated rats in respect to saline animals. This effect is concomitant with a dramatic rise in plasma FSH after buserelin chronic treatment ($p < 0.001$).

These results suggest that a dissociated control of gonadotropin secretion is expressed after buserelin chronic stimulation. A paradoxical effect on synthesis and/or release of pituitary gonadotropins is revealed after treatment with this LHRH analog.

Funded by F.I.S.S. grant #85/889. Buserelin was kindly supplied by Hoechst Iberica S.A.

A ROLE FOR ORNITHINE DECARBOXYLASE IN THE PRO-OESTROUS LH SURGE IN RATS? 6

M. Aslam, S.A. Nicholson*, B.B. Oon**, B. Gillham** and M.T. Jones
Divisions of Gynaecology and Biochemistry**(St. Thomas') and Physiology* (Guy's), United Medical & Dental Schools London SE1 (U.K.)

Putrescine and the catalytic activity of the enzyme that forms it, ornithine decarboxylase (ODC), have been found to be massively increased in the anterior pituitary gland during pre-oestrus in rats (1). In the current study, pro-oestrous anterior pituitary fragments were perifused and exposed to hourly volleys of six, 1-min. pulses of LHRH (10^{-8} M). LH release showed a characteristic pattern of progressive (over 5h) sensitisation to the releasing hormone. The addition of 2mM difluoromethyl-ornithine (DFMO), a specific inhibitor of ODC, to the perifusion medium completely inhibited the response to all volleys of LHRH. The inability to respond to the peptide was reversed by the concurrent addition of 2mM putrescine to the medium. Whereas, putrescine had no significant enhancing effect on basal or LHRH-induced LH secretion from control tissue.

To measure the activity of ODC, tissues were loaded with 1-^{14}C-ornithine (25nCi/ml) and $^{14}CO_2$ in the perifusate was determined. Pulsatile LHRH stimulation caused a progressive increase in the amount of $^{14}CO_2$ coming from the tissues. In the absence of LHRH pulses or with such pulses in the presence of DFMO, no comparable increase in $^{14}CO_2$ output was noted. Pituitary glands taken from rats given DFMO(50 mg) at pro-oestrus, contained significantly less putrescine and LH than those from control animals and the surge of plasma LH was blunted by the drug.

These results suggest that putrescine may act as a 2nd or 3rd messenger to regulate the pro-oestrous LH surge.

1. Persson, L., Nilsson, M. and Rosengren E.:J.Endocr. 107, 83-87 (1985)

(DFMO was a gift from Merrell Dow Research Institute, Strasbourg)

IN VITRO STUDIES OF INFLUENCES ON GONADOTROPIN-RELEASING HORMONE SECRETION FROM THE ISOLATED PERIFUSED GUINEA PIG HYPOTHALAMUS 6a

P.E. Belchetz, P.E. McKibbin, H. Ainsworth
Department of Medicine, University of Liverpool, P.O. Box 147, Liverpool L69 3BX, U.K.

Studies in primate species indicate that sexually mature gonadal function depends on regular, pulsatile secretion of gonadotropin-releasing hormone (GnRH). This primes gonadotropin release and permits negative and positive feedback actions of estradiol at the pituitary level. The rhythm appears to originate in the medial basal hypothalamus (MBH). Deafferentation of the MBH interferes with neither pulsatile release of LH nor ovulation in primates or guinea pigs, in sharp contrast to the laboratory rat.

The isolated guinea pig MBH, rapidly removed after sacrifice, consisting of a block bounded by the posterior border of the optic chiasm, lateral hypothalamic sulci, mamillary bodies and 2mm depth of tissue cut parallel to the floor of the diencephalon, is capable of pulsatile secretion of GnRH, which may be augmented by 60mM KCl, for upto 72h when perifused with Krebs-Ringer solution, pH 7.4, gassed with 95% O_2 5% CO_2, at 37°C and containing bacitracin 20mM to inhibit hypothalamic peptidases. In keeping with the permissive role hypothesized for GnRH in primates and the guinea pig, there was no difference in mean levels or patterns of GnRH released from hypothalami removed from intact or longterm ovariectomized animals. Progesterone is suggested to have an action at the pituitary level which is supported by the immediate slowing of GnRH pulses when progesterone (50 and 10nM) was added to the perifusing medium. Opioid systems operate powerfully in vivo to inhibit pulsatile GnRH release in the guinea pig, this involvement is supported by the use of opiate agonists and antagonists including naloxone and the specific delta-receptor antagonist ICI 154,129.

These studies suggest that the isolated perifused guinea pig MBH is an appropriate model for studying directly influences on pulsatile secretion of GnRH, whereas in vivo methods may not distinguish reliably between hypothalamic and pituitary tiers of action.

This work was supported by the MRC and ICI.

PHYSIOLOGICAL ATTRIBUTES OF LUTEINIZING HORMONE PULSES ASSESSED BY MULTIPLE-POINT (CLUSTER) ANALYSIS: STUDIES IN WOMEN AND ANALYSIS OF MALE VERSUS FEMALE PATTERNS 7

E. Christiansen, W.S. Evans, R.J. Urban, F.E. Barr, A.D. Rogol, D.L. Kaiser, M.L. Johnson, and J.D. Veldhuis
University of Virginia Medical School, Charlottesville, Virginia 22908

Pulsatile LH release was characterized in the early follicular phase in normal women (n=8) using a comprehensive pulse detection algorithm (Cluster) in combination with intensive sampling (every 5 minutes for 24 hours) and the results compared to those obtained in an identical manner in normal men (n=8). Cluster analysis is unique in comparison to other pulse analysis algorithms in that it: (1) uses multiple-point criteria for pulse detection, (2) is not affected by non-uniform pulse amplitude or an unstable baseline, (3) measures error intrinsic to replicates within the experimental series, and (4) allows statistical definition of upstroke and downstroke bounds of an individual pulse. No differences between the sexes were found for several pulse properties (mean ± SEM; women vs men) including mean interpulse interval (58 ± 2.7 vs 61 ± 2.9 min), peak area (84 ± 12 vs 67 ± 7 mIU/ml x min), peak width (44 ± 1.9 vs 51 ± 2.6 min) or interpulse valley width (23 ± 1.3 vs 23 ± 1.4 min). However, mean LH pulse amplitude in women was greater compared to men as defined by both peak height (12 ± 0.8 vs 7.7 ± 1.1 mIU/ml; p = 0.006) or peak increment (4.4 ± 0.32 vs 2.7 ± 0.44 mIU/ml; p = 0.010). Interpulse valley means were also higher in women versus men (8.6 ± 0.80 vs 5.2 ± 0.072 mIU/ml; p = 0.012). Circulating levels of testosterone correlated negatively with pulse frequency in women (r = -0.833; p = 0.0061) but not in men. No other significant correlations between concentrations of testosterone or 17-beta-estradiol and any other pulse properties were documented in women or men. These data suggest that the GnRH pulse generator may be firing at similar rates in men and early follicular phase women, but that factors which relate to LH pulse amplitude and LH baseline concentrations differ between the sexes.

EFFECT OF NEURAL PATHWAY BLOCKERS ON LHRH RELEASE FROM RAT HYPOTHALAMI PERFUSED/PERIFUSED IN VITRO. 8

T. T. Chuang and M. T. Jones
Department of Gynaecology, United Medical and Dental Schools(St. Thomas's Campus), London SE1 7EH.

Atropine, hexamethonium, naloxone and picrotoxin have been used to investigate the possible presence of tonic neuronal inhibitory pathways involved in the control of LHRH release. Since these inhibitory pathways may be acting *via* axo-axonal, axosomatic or axodendritic sites, care was taken to include the main LHRH neuronal cell bodies i.e. the preoptic area, arcuate nucleus as well as the median eminence(ME) in the hypothalamic preparation used. By using the perfused/perifused hypothalamic preparation described previously(1), addition of the muscarinic blocker atropine (10^{-7}-10^{-5}M) or the nicotinic blocker hexamethonium (10^{-6},10^{-4}M) to the perfusion/perifusion medium were shown not to effect LHRH release. However the specific opiate receptor blocker, naloxone(10^{-5}-10^{-4}M), and/or the GABAergic blocker, picrotoxin(10^{-4}M) produced a pronounced increase in LHRH release.

These observations suggest the presence in this preparation of tonic opioidergic and GABAergic inhibition of the LHRH releasing activity. Such inhibitory tone may influence the secretory activity of LHRH neurone terminals in the ME, as was suggested by Negro-Vilar *et al*(2), and may also explain the differing results obtained when comparing medio-basal hypothalamus(MBH) and ME preparations. For example Negro-Vilar *et al*(2) found that while norepinephrine and dopamine had no effect on the incubated MBH they stimulated LHRH release from the isolated ME, which consists mainly of nerve terminals. Similar results have also been found for the release of somatostatin from the hypothalamus(3).

We therfore suggest that when investigating the hormonal releasing activity of putative secretagogues on *in vitro* hypothalamic preparations, the presence of intrinsic overriding excitatory or inhibitory tones may mask the effects of the secretagogues.

1. T.T.Chuang *et al*, J. Endoc.(Suppl) 108, Abs.132(1986)
2. A. Negro-Vilar *et al*, Endocrinol. 104, 1749 (1979)
3. L.C.Terry *et al*, Endocrinol. 107, 794 (1980)

THE ROLE OF LH IN THE AUTOFEEDBACK INHIBITION OF LH AND FSH SECRETION IN RATS. 9

Sonya Conway and Samuel M. McCann
Northern Illinois University, DeKalb, Illinois and Dept of Physiology, U of Texas Health Science Center, Dallas, Texas 75235.

The present study was initiated to examine the role of exogenous LH in the autofeedback regulation of LH and FSH release in the rat. In this study female rats were implanted with third ventricular cannulae three weeks after ovariectomy and fitted with silastic jugular cannulae one week later. Baseline hormone levels were established on the day of experimentation in conscious, unrestrained animals. Thereafter, experimental animals received intraventricularly (IVT) either a 9 µg or 20 µg dose of a purified preparation of human (h)LH (NIH) that did not crossreact in our rLH RIA. In response to 20 µg, but not 9 µg of LH plasma levels of both LH and FSH were significantly reduced during the following one hour period compared to values in controls receiving buffer IVT. On the other hand administration of oLH (6 µg, IVT), a preparation which crossreacts in our rLH RIA, significantly elevated plasma levels of detectable LH during the experimental period indicating that LH reached the blood stream from the third ventricle and, thus, may affect endogenous hormone release at either the pituitary or hypothalamic levels. However, in animals preinjected with 9 µg or 20 µg of hLH IVT one hour previously the surge of both LH and FSH in response to LHRH (25 ng iv) was not different from controls receiving LHRH alone. The results of this study indicate that the inhibitory short-loop feedback of LH on endogenous LH and FSH secretion in the rat occurs at the level of the hypothalamus.

Supported by NIH grant HD 07062.

PULSATILE FSH SECRETION IS INDEPENDENT OF LHRH. 10

M. D. Culler and A. Negro-Vilar.
Reprod. Neuroendo. Sec., Lab. Reprod. Dev. Tox., NIEHS-NIH, Res. Tri. Pk., NC 27709.

We recently reported (Endo. 118:609, 1986) that passive immunoneutralization of endogenous LHRH in castrate male rats completely abolishes pulsatile LH secretion and, within 1 hr, lowers mean plasma LH by 86%. While pulsatile FSH secretion is not affected, mean plasma FSH is gradually lowered, but only by 48.5% after 24 hr. In the present study, we have examined the effect of replacing LHRH activity on LH and FSH secretion in castrate male rats in which endogenous LHRH has been immunoneutralized by anti-LHRH serum #772 (A772). A772 is specific for the 3-10 amino acid sequence of LHRH including the amidated C-terminus. In order to circumvent the antiserum, we utilized the LHRH agonist, [Des-Gly^{10}]-LHRH ethyl amide (DG-LHRH) which crossreacts <0.01% with A772 compared with LHRH and which possesses 2.7 times the bioactivity of LHRH. Twenty-four hours after injecting 500µl A772 into cannulated, castrate male rats, sequential blood samples were taken every 10 min for 4 hrs. Bolus, 3 ng injections of DG-LHRH or saline were given i.v., either every 30 min during the 4 hr collection period or every 60 min for 10 hr prior to the initiation of and during the 4 hr collection period. Each DG-LHRH injection stimulated the release of a single pulse of LH (mean amplitute= 220.4 ± 11.8 ng/ml), while pulsatile FSH secretion was unaffected. No synchroneity was observed between the DG-LHRH stimulated LH pulses and the endogenous FSH pulses. Short-term DG-LHRH treatment partially restored, while the long-term DG-LHRH treatment completely restored mean plasma FSH to the level observed in non-antiserum treated, castrate rats. The mean plasma level of LH was entirely dependent on the frequency of the DG-LHRH injections. The results of the present study substantiate that pulsatile FSH secretion is independent of LHRH but demonstrate that LHRH is required to maintain elevated mean plasma FSH levels. Basal (trough) LH levels, however, are dependent on the frequency of LHRH induced pulsatile LH secretion.

PRL,FSH,LH RESPONSES TO OPIATE ANTAGONIST(NALOXONE)IN PATIENTS WITH ANOREXIA NERVOSA AND ISOLATED GONADOTROPHIN DEFICIENCY.PRELIMINARY DATA. 11

S.Devescovi,G.Andreani,M.G.Toni,M.Rolla.
1st Medical Clinic,Nuclear Medicine Service,CNR Institute of Clinical Physiology,Pisa-Italy.

It is known that opiate peptides are involved in the regulation of appetite and body weight as well as in the neuroendocrine controls of hormonal secretions.Particularly some authors have hypothesized that opiate system releases PRL through a dopamine system interaction.The aim of our study is to evaluate the effects of naloxone (an opiate antagonist) on the release of LH,FSH, PRL in patients(pts) with anorexia nervosa(AN) and with isolated gonadotrophin deficiency(IGD). We evaluate 5 pts with AN,5 pts with I.G.D. and 7 control subjects.The diagnosis of AN was estabilished according to the criteria of Feighner and Russell.AN and IGD pts were tested with GnRH test(25 mcg i.v.)to evaluate basal and stimulated gonadotrophin levels.FSH,LH and PRL values were estimated by RIA methods at 15',30',45',60' 90',120',150',180' minutes following naloxone administration(10 mg i.v.);the same procedure was carried out after the administration of placebo(0.9% saline).No effect of naloxone administration on FSHand LH levels was found in any group.In IGD pts and in controls we observed a decrease of PRL values as compared to the basal levels after naloxone administration.On the contrary we have a significant increase of PRL levels after naloxone in AN pts as compared to the levels after placebo(Δmax 10ng/ml vs 0 ng/ml $p<0.02$).This paradoxical PRL response in AN pts could be related to a modified opiate activity, at least in the more severe stages of the disease.

INFLUENCE OF GONADAL STEROIDS ON HUMAN AND MONKEY CEREBROSPINAL FLUID HOMO-VANILLIC ACID CONCENTRATIONS. 12

T. Di Paolo[1], F. Bédard[2] and P. Bédard[2]
[1]School of Pharmacy, Laval University, Québec G1K 7P4 and Department of Molecular Endocrinology, Laval University Hospital Center, Québec G1V 4G2; [2]Neurobiology Research Center, Hôpital de l'Enfant-Jésus, Québec G1J 1Z4, Canada.

The influence of gonadal steroids on central dopaminergic function was assessed by measuring concentrations of the dopamine metabolite homovanillic acid (HVA) in cerebrospinal fluid (CSF) in humans and monkeys. CSF HVA and 5-hydroxyindoleacetic acid (5-HIAA) concentrations were measured by HPLC with electrochemical detection. 13 maccaca facicularis intact adult female monkeys and 6 ovariectomized monkeys had a lumbar puncture to collect CSF. Ovariectomized monkeys had higher HVA concentrations in their CSF (intact = 55.63 ± 3.70 and ovariectomized = 81.79 ± 7.05 ng/ml, $p < 0.05$) while 5-HIAA levels remained unchanged (intact = 26.77 ± 3.37 and ovariectomized = 30.31 ± 3.02 ng/ml). In a second experiment, 40 persons were divided in six groups as follows: I- women with menses; II- menopaused or ovariectomized women taking estrogens; III- hysterectomized women; IV- menopaused or ovariectomized women; V- women taking drugs or showing signs of Parkinsonism; VI- men, and CSF collected by lumbar puncture. 5-HIAA levels (I = 47.6 ± 6.0; II = 44.0 ± 17.6; III = 43.0 ± 7.0; IV = 47.0 ± 4.9; V = 49.5 ± 8.9; VI = 41.0 ± 5.6 ng/ml) were constant. Hysterectomized (III) as well as menopaused or ovariectomized (IV) women had significantly ($p < 0.05$) higher CSF HVA concentrations compared to men (I = 30.4 ± 5.8; II = 28.1 ± 5.5; III = 50.7 ± 15.9; IV = 46.6 ± 4.7; V = 106.8 ± 33.6; VI = 20.7 ± 2.9 ng/ml) while women in group IV were older, those of group III were of the same age as men (I = 34.0 ± 2.3; II = 44.5 ± 0.5; III = 43.0 ± 1.4; IV = 57.0 ± 2.9; V = 60.0 ± 10.0; VI = 37.6 ± 3.6 years old). These results provide further evidence for the role of endogenous ovarian factors as modulators of central dopaminergic activity. Estimation of central dopaminergic activity, by measurement of HVA in CSF may be useful in improving therapeutic regimen for reducing neuroleptic-induced tardive dyskinesia.

IN VIVO MEASUREMENT OF LHRH AND NEUROTRANSMITTERS FROM THE ANTERIOR PITUITARY GLAND OF CASTRATED RATS WITH PUSH-PULL CANNULAE (PPC). 13

D. E. DLUZEN and V. D. RAMIREZ
University of Illinois, Urbana

The amplitude of in vivo LHRH output from castrated rats as estimated with PPC implanted in the medial hypothalamus was markedly diminished as compared to intacts (J. Endocr. 107: 331, 1985). To better characterize the in vivo release process of LHRH in castrated animals we have incorporated the following modifications in our push-pull procedure: 1) A reduction in the size of the PPC, 2) Implantation of cannulae aiming along the midline of the median eminence(ME) and anterior pituitary and 3) Addition of bacitracin to the medium. Perfusate samples were also analyzed with HPLC-EC to determine neurotransmitter output. In long term castrate rats (>1 yr) with PPC implanted in the midline of the anterior ME (3 females, 1 male), LHRH levels during a 4-5 h perfusion were very low (.397±.056 pg/10min) with only 25% of the samples detected in the RIA. Some neurotransmitter output was detected, including FPI,5HIAA,DA and DOPAC, however, no consistent pattern could be discerned. In 3 long term castrate males with PPC located either in the midline of the posterior ME (2) or in the anterior pole of the pituitary (1), LHRH output was much greater (.944±.105 pg/10min, amplitude = 1.2±.04 pg) with almost all samples detectable. There was a tendency for increased LHRH frequency from these animals, particularly in the rat with the PPC in the pituitary (33 min) compared to our previously reported LHRH frequency in intact males (77 min). There appeared to be higher and pulsatile release of DOPAC and NE in these animals, while 5HIAA remained fairly stable.

These results demonstrate that push-pull perfusion can be performed with cannulae located at the midline of the posterior ME or in the anterior pituitary and suggest that this latter location may be a better site for determination of neuropeptide and neurotransmitter release. Moreover, the results lend support to the idea that the frequency of LHRH release may be an important factor in determining LH output in castrated rats.

ESTROGEN-INDUCED DESENSITIZATION TO THE NEGATIVE ESTROGEN FEEDBACK 14

F. Döcke, W. Rohde, P. Gerber, R. Chaoui, G. Dörner
Institute of Experimental Endocrinology, Humboldt University, Berlin, GDR

In several female mammals a simultaneous rise of circulating estrogen and basal LH levels has been recorded both prepubertally and during the preovulatory phase of the ovarian cycle. To study the neurohormonal mechanism(s) underlying this phenomenon, experiments were performed in immature and adult female rats.
The following results were obtained:

(1) The sensitivity to the LH-inhibiting effect of estradiol benzoate (EB) decreased significantly in respectively immature and cyclic females during the last week before the onset of puberty and during the preovulatory phase. (2) Bilateral lesioning of the medial preoptic area (MPOA) reduced the gonadotropic response to estrogen in ovariectomized prepubertal and adult rats. (3) A similar effect was recorded after the implantation of very small quantities of EB into the MPOA, but not into the hypothalamic ventromedial-arcuate region. (4) Findings obtained after the implantation of dopamine agonists and antagonists suggest that lowering of the medial preoptic dopaminergic activity is involved in the desensitizing effect of estrogen. (5) Spontaneous desensitization to the negative estrogen feedback was distinctively delayed in 5-day as compared to 4-day cyclic rats. (6) In short-term castrated adult male rats the implantation of estradiol, testosterone or 5α-DHT into the MPOA was not followed by reduced sensitivity to the LH-inhibiting estrogen effect.

It is proposed that the prepubertal and preovulatory increase of estrogen secretion induces desensitization to its own feedback action by inactivating a medial preoptic "feedback controller". In this way adequate gonadotropic support of final follicle maturation is guaranteed in face of a rising estrogen level in the blood.

A NEW METHOD TO PERFUSE THE RAT TESTES IN VIVO 15

E.-M. Düker, B. Wolff, W. Wuttke
Div. Clin. Exp. Endocr.,Dept. ObGyn.,Univ. Göttingen,FRG

We have recently developed an in vivo testicular perfusion method which allows us to examine the direct effects of hormones and substances on testicular function in unstressed freely-moving rats. This method has several advantages: (1) the potential importance of paracrine effects can be evaluated since the structural integrity of the testes is maintained; (2) the effects of agents can be analysed at several different times since perfusion can be carried out for several hours; and (3) the temporal relationship between intratesticular events and peripheral hormone secretion can be assessed. We have utilized this method to determine the direct effects of LHRH, of a dopamine (DA) agonist (2 Br-o-ergocryptine = CB), and a DA antagonist (sulpiride) on intratesticular testosterone (T) release. Perfusion tubing is composed of a hemodialysing fiber connected to teflon tubing via silastic tubing. The perfusion tubing was inserted into the testes and after recovery Ringer solution was perfused through the dialysis system in the testes (1 ml/h). After an initial 4 h period the substance to be tested was administered with the perfusion medium. Perfusate fractions were collected over a 15 min interval and blood samples at the end of each fraction period. Following direct intratesticular application of the substances, no effects on blood LH and prolactin levels were observed. LHRH stimulated blood LH levels resulted in a prompt rise of T concentrations in the testicular dialysates indicating a rapid diffusion of secreted T into the dialysis tubing.

When CB was administered directly into the perfusion medium (32 μg/ml) for 2 h, T concentrations in the dialysate decreased within 45 min and remained low during the entire application period. T concentrations returned to baseline upon termination of CB administration. Sulpiride at several doses had no effect on T concentrations in the dialysate.

These data demonstrate that DA may have direct effects on intratesticular T concentrations in addition to their well established effects on the hypothalamo-hypophyseal axis. We are presently testing the direct effects of several other hormones including LHRH and prolactin.

16

ADRENERGIC RECEPTORS MEDIATING STIMULATION OF CYCLIC AMP ACCUMULATION BY NOREPINEPHRINE IN HYPOTHALAMIC AND PREOPTIC AREA SLICES FROM OVARIECTOMIZED AND OVARIECTOMIZED, ESTRADIOL-PRIMED RATS

A.M. Etgen
Albert Einstein College of Medicine, Bronx, NY 10461

We have recently shown that the magnitude of norepinephrine (NE) stimulation of cyclic AMP accumulation in slices from the preoptic area (POA) and hypothalamus (HYP) of female rats varies with the endocrine state of the animals prior to sacrifice. The present experiments utilized antagonists specific for α_1, α_2, or β adrenergic receptors to: (1) identify the adrenergic receptor population(s) that mediate the cyclic AMP response to NE in POA and HYP slices, and (2) determine which receptor population(s) change in response to estradiol priming.

Slices were prepared from the POA and HYP of adult female rats that had been ovariectomized (OVX) or OVX and treated with 2 µg of estradiol benzoate (EB) 24 and 48 hr prior to sacrifice. Slices were maintained in vitro for 75 min and then incubated an additional 20 min in the presence of NE or NE plus propranolol (β antagonist), prazosin (α_1 antagonist) or yohimbine (α_2 antagonist). Control slices to assess basal cyclic AMP levels were incubated for the same total period of time with no drug additions.

In POA and HYP slices taken from OVX rats, both propranolol and yohimbine completely blocked NE stimulation of cyclic AMP accumulation. In contrast, prazosin had no effect in either the POA or HYP slices. NE-induced cyclic AMP accumulation was also abolished by yohimbine in POA and HYP slices taken from OVX, EB-treated rats. However, propranolol was only partially effective in antagonizing NE-dependent increases in cyclic AMP levels in slices from estradiol-primed rats. Moreover, prazosin partially antagonized NE stimulation of cyclic AMP content in slices from EB-treated animals. The data suggest that both α_2 and β receptors participate in NE induction of cyclic AMP accumulation in slices from OVX rats and that estradiol treatments increase the α/β receptor ratio.

17

ACUTE EFFECT OF Δ^9-TETRAHYDROCANNABINOL ON THE PULSATILE RHYTHM OF BLOOD LH IN OVARIECTOMIZED RATS

G.I. Fujimoto, D.I. Whitmoyer
Laboratory of Neuroendocrinology, Brain Research Institute and Dept. of Anatomy, UCLA School of Medicine, Los Angeles, CA 90024

A new method of collecting successive samples of rat blood at less than one-minute intervals was described by Whitmoyer (Abst. Soc. Neuroscience 10:1213, 1984). The method has enabled us to observe very rapid rises in blood LH values in the pulsatile LH rhythm characteristic of ovariectomized (OVX) animals. The average pulse interval was 21.3 ± 2.5 min with an average pulse amplitude of 6.0 ± 0.3 ng/ml. The present study employs this rapid blood-sampling technique to study the timing of effects of intravenous infusion of Δ^9-tetrahydrocannabinol (THC) on LH values and, indirectly, GnRH output during the pulsatile episodes of LH secretion in the OVX rat. In four 3-wk OVX Sprague-Dawley rats a single dose of 5 mg/kg THC (suspended in isotonic saline containing 1% sesame oil and 1% Polysorban-80) was introduced into the return line of the cannula near the animal within 50-100 min after initiation of blood collections at one-min intervals. Unless it had already started, the next LH pulse was completely suppressed, and LH steadily but not abruptly dropped to baseline levels for the duration of collections, which were continued up to 6 h. However, when 200 ng GnRH was introduced into the cannula of the THC-inhibited animal, LH values spurted within 2-3 min after injection and remained high for more than one h. This supports the finding that THC does not affect the pituitary response to GnRH but rapidly blocks the release of GnRH.

(Supported by NIH grant NS01162.)

18

PULSATILE LH SECRETION IN HYPOGONADAL WOMEN: EFFECT OF CHRONIC BROMOCRIPTINE ADMINISTRATION

M. Gambacciani, G.B. Melis, A. Cagnacci, P. Fioretti
Dept. of Obstet. Gynecol., University of Pisa, Italy

The precise role of dopaminergic system in the regulation of GnRH-gonadotropin secretion in humans is still controversial. Since pulsatile LH release is widely used as an index of endogenous GnRH secretion, we characterized LH pulse frequency in hypogonadal women, and subsequently determined the effects of dopaminergic stimulation on LH pulsatile release. Fourteen postmenopausal women (45-55 yr) and 13 short term (7-10 days) ovariectomized women (OVRW) (40-49 yr) underwent frequent blood sampling every 5 min for 4 hours before and after 15 and 30 days of bromocriptine (BCT, 3.75 mg/day) or placebo administration. LH concentrations were determined in triplicate by RIA. LH pulses were defined as nadir to peak increments that exceeded 4 times the intra-assay coefficient of variation. Overall mean LH levels were 26.4±1.7 mIU/ml in OVRW and 44.3±3.2 mIU/ml in PMW. Mean interpulse intervals (IPI) were similar in the two groups (OVRW: 57.4±4.9 min; PMW: 59.0±3.1 min). There was no significant change in mean LH IPI or pulse amplitude in either group following placebo administration. In contrast, BCT administration induced a significant ($p<0.05$) increase in mean IPI in both groups after either 15 (OVRW: 180±20.8 min; PMW: 101±9.8 min) or 30 days (OVRW: 150±30 min;PMW: 157±25.5 min) of treatment. Mean pulse amplitude was slightly but not significantly increased after BCT treatment in both groups. These results indicate that LH release is characterized by high frequency secretory pulses in hypogonadal women. Since chronic BCT administration decrease the frequency of pulsatile LH release, this study suggests that dopaminergic system may play an inhibitory role on GnRH-LH pulse generator mechanisms.

19

HYPOTHALAMIC AREAS CONTROLLING LH PULSES IN THE RAT. R.L. Goodman, Department of Physiology, West Virginia University, Morgantown,WV

While it is generally agreed that episodic LH secretion reflects the activity if a hypothalamic "GnRH pulse generator", the locale of this neural oscillator remains obscure. This study examined this question by lesioning discrete hypothalamic areas. Rats were lesioned immediately after ovariectomy on metestrus. A stainless steel electrode (0.1 mm diameter; 0.25 mm tip) was placed in the third ventricle and a radiofrequency (RF) lesion produced with a Kopf RF generator set at 20 V for 20 sec. In controls, the electrode was inserted but not activated Rats were catheterized 3 days later and LH pulses analyzed in samples (100 ul) collected every 10 min for 3 h the next day. GnRH (40 ng) was then injected iv and blood samples taken 10 and 20 min later. Rats were killed, the brains examined histologically, and rats grouped by lesion site. Lesions were at the base of the brain, extended 0.2-0.4 mm lateral to the ventricle, 0.4-0.9 mm in the AP direction, and 0.5-1.0 mm in the DV direction. When placed in the region of the anterior arcuate (AP: 6.1-5.5 Degroot atlas), bilateral lesions (n=7) decreased both LH pulse amplitude (54 ± 15 ng/ml) and frequency (1.1 ± 0.5 pulses/3h) below control (n=11) values (175 ± 18 ng/ml; 4.9 ± 0.5 pulses/3h). Unilateral lesions (n=6) decreased only pulse amplitude (103 ± 12 ng/ml;4.0 ± 0.4 pulses/3h) Bilateral lesions (n=5) just anterior (AP:6.7-6.0) also decreased pulse amplitude (105 ± 9 ng/ml), but not frequency (4.6 ± 0.5 pulses/3h). None of these lesions effected the pituitary response to GnRH. These results suggest that the region of the anterior arcuate contains axons or cell bodies integral to the GnRH pulse generator in the rat. Since lesions anterior to this area did not suppress pulse frequency, anterior input may not play a role in controlling LH pulse frequency in acutely ovariectomized rats. In contrast, such anterior input appears to be important for the maintenance of pulsatile LH secretion in chronically ovariectomized rats (Soper and Weick, Endocrinology 106: 348, 1980). There may thus be important alterations in the neural elements generating GnRH pulses with time after ovareictomy. (Supported by NIH HD15654).

A NEW MODEL FOR THE IMITATION OF PRO-ESTRUS-LIKE LH-SURGES AND CATECHOLAMINE TURNOVER FLUCTUATIONS IN OVARIECTOMIZED RATS 20

C. Hiemke, J. Hinze, A. Schmid, R. Ghraf
Institut für Physiologische Chemie, Universität Essen, Essen, F.R.G.

Ovariectomized rats are often used to study sex steroid-neurotransmitter interactions involved in the feedback regulation of gonadotropin secretion. The positive response of luteinizing hormone (LH) to a priming dose of estradiol, however, depends on the time interval between removal of the ovaries and estradiol administration. In the present investigation we have set out to establish a scheme of hormone administration to induce proestrus-like fluctuations of LH secretion and of hypothalamic catecholamine turnover in short-term as well as in long-term ovariectomized rats.

Ovariectomized Sprague-Dawley rats were injected with 20 ug estradiol benzoate (EB) on day 0, with 2.5 mg progesterone (P) on day 3 and again with EB on day 5. On day 6 blood samples were withdrawn and the turnover rates of dopamine and noradrenaline were measured in the preoptic area (POA) and the mediobasal hypothalamus (MBH).

In ovariectomized rats pretreated with EB plus P the injection of EB at noon on day 5 induced proestrus-like surges of LH in the afternoon on day 6 with maximum plasma LH levels about 17.00 h. LH-surges were observed in rats ovariectomized 1 week earlier as well as in animals ovariectomized 50 weeks earlier. The estradiol-induced stimulation of LH secretion was accompanied by time dependent fluctuations of noradrenaline turnover in the POA and MBH. The observed alterations of LH-secretion and noradrenaline turnover could be antagonised by the nonsteroidal antiestrogen monohydroxytamoxifen.

The ovariectomized rat receiving consecutive injections of EB, P and EB as described here provides a useful model for investigations on sex steroid-neurotransmitter interactions involved in the LH-surge mechanism.

NEUROCHEMICAL CHARACTERIZATION OF THE NORADRENERGIC NEUROTOXIN, 5-ADMP, IN THE RAT HYPOTHALAMUS 21

H.D. Jarry, K.J. Lookingland and K.E. Moore
Dept. of Pharmacology and Toxicology, Michigan State Univ., East Lansing, MI 48824

In regions of the hypothalamus containing incertohypothalamic dopaminergic (IHDA) neurons the concentration of norepinephrine (NE) exceeds that of DA, and this primarily reflects a higher density of NE neurons. One difficulty in studying IHDA neurons relates to this dense NE innervation, and care must be taken to ensure that neurochemical estimates of DA neuronal activity are not confounded by the presence of these NE neurons. It would, therefore, be advantageous to have a method for selectively eliminating NE input to these hypothalamic regions. Since currently available NE neurotoxins (6-hydroxydopamine, DSP4) are not very effective in destroying hypothalamic NE neurons, we examined the effects of 5-amino-2,4-dihydroxy-α-methylphenylethylamine (5-ADMP), a compound reported to selectively deplete NE in the whole mouse brain (Lin et al., Soc. Neurosci. Abst. 10: 1199, 1984), on levels of amines and their metabolites in the rat hypothalamus.

Following a single injection of 5-ADMP (100 µg/rat, icv) the concentrations of NE throughout the hypothalamus were markedly reduced by 4 h and this depletion was maintained for at least 28 days. Seven days after 5-ADMP the greatest decrease in NE occurred within periventricular regions of the hypothalamus, and this was partially prevented by pretreatment with the NE uptake inhibitor desipramine. In contrast, 5-ADMP failed to alter hypothalamic DA or dihydroxyphenylacetic acid (DOPAC) concentrations (except the median eminence), or the concentrations of 5-hydroxytryptamine (serotonin; 5HT) or 5-hydroxyindoleacetic acid (5HIAA) in any hypothalamic region. The specificity of 5-ADMP for NE neurons was lost when multiple injections (100 µg icv/rat, every 48 h x 3) of the neurotoxin were administered; this treatment did not cause a further depletion of NE but did decrease DA and 5HT concentrations in some hypothalamic regions. These results indicate that 5-ADMP is a selective neurotoxin for NE neurons and is particularly effective within the periventricular hypothalamus and should be a useful tool for determining the roles of both NE and DA neurons in these regions in the regulation of hormone release. (Supported by USPHS Grant NS15911 and a grant from The Upjohn Co.)

HORMONAL REGULATION OF THE GONADOTROPIN SUBUNIT SYNTHESIS 22

M. Jutisz, R. Counis, A. Starzec, M. Corbani
Polypeptide Hormone Laboratory, CNRS, 91190 Gif-sur-Yvette, France.

We have previously shown that in the rat, gonadectomy increases the translational capacity of mRNAs encoding gonadotropin subunits α, LHβ and FSHβ, and that injection of estradiol (in the female) or of testosterone (in the male) depresses the translational capacity of these mRNAs. This inhibitory effect of steroids can also be demonstrated in vitro using pituitary cells in culture. Hybridization experiments (Northern blots) using labeled oligodeoxynucleotide probes show that gonadal steroids act by decreasing the number of copies of mRNAs encoding LH and FSH subunits.

Using anterior pituitary cells in culture incubated in the presence of $[^{35}S]$Met, we have now obtained definite evidence that GnRH stimulates the biosynthesis of the polypeptide chains of LH subunits. The effect of GnRH is dose (0.1nM-10nM) and time dependent. It is detectable after a lag period of 1.5 h. Actinomycin D inhibits GnRH action thus suggesting that GnRH effect requires RNA synthesis. However, we have no evidence at present that GnRH acts directly on the gonadotropin subunit genes. A cAMP analogue (Br-cAMP, 1-2mM)as well as intracellular cAMP generators (6nM choleragen, 50-100µM forskolin) mimick the stimulatory action of GnRH on the incorporation of $[^{35}S]$Met into α and LHβ. The phorbol ester (TPA, 50nM) also increased the synthesis of LH subunits.

Our data demonstrate that the synthesis of pituitary gonadotropin subunits is under a dual hormonal control, by gonadal steroids and GnRH. The negative control by steroids occurs at the genomic level, while the stimulatory effect of GnRH proceeds via different mechanisms which remain to be elucidated. We have at present no evidence that either cAMP or diacylglycerol mediates GnRH effect on the synthesis of LH subunits. We postulate that protein phosphorylation plays an important role in this mechanism.

PULSATILE RELEASE OF LHRH IN THE MAMILLARY REGION OF THE HYPOTHALAMUS IN INFANT PIGS 23

S. Kanematsu, T. Hirata
Dept. of Animal Husbandry, Fac. of Agriculture, Iwate University, Morioka, 020, Japan

The present study was performed to investigate whether LHRH is released in a pattern of pulse in the hypothalamus of pigs. This would be the first demonstration on pulsatile release of LHRH in the pig.

The animals used were five littermate crossbred females and three littermate crossbred males of 21 to 46 days old pigs. Push-pull cannulae (PPC) were implanted stereotaxically in the basal hypothalamus using a rabbit head holder or modified goat head holder. The basal hypothalamus was perfused with an artificial cerebrospinal fluid at 20 µl/min. Systemic blood was collected every 10 min through a right atrial cannula simultaneously with PPC sample collection. Plasma LH and LHRH levels in the perfusate were determined by radioimmunoassay.

LHRH was not detected in the perfusates perfused in the thalamus or lateral hypothalamus. Pulsatile releasing patterns of LHRH were found in all perfusates perfused in the midline mamillary regions of the hypothalamus. LH pulses were not always accompanied by LHRH pulses. LH pulses were, however, only observed in two of eight pigs.

The results indicate that the mamillary region of the hypothalamus is involved in the pulsatile release of LHRH in the pig.

ESTROGEN MODULATION OF THE α_1-ADRENERGIC EXCITATION OF HYPOTHALAMIC PARVOCELLULAR NEURONS 24

M.J. Kelly, T.P. Condon, O.K. Ronnekleiv
Dept. of Physiology, Oregon Health Sci. U., Portland, Oregon 97201

Medial basal hypothalamic neurons control gonadotropin secretion in the guinea pig and are under the governing control of both norepineprhrine (NE) and estrogen. We have characterized the *in vitro* hypothalamic slice preparation as a model for investigating the electrical activity of arcuate-cell-poor zone (ARC-CPZ) luteinizing hormone-releasing hormone (LHRH) neurons using intracellular recording techniques (Kelly et al., Brain Res. 345:264, 1985). ARC-CPZ (LHRH) neurons in the slice remain viable for up to 12 hrs. and release LHRH into the medium in a physiological manner. ARC-CPZ neurons exhibit slow irregular firing with 12% of the cells (N=252) showing phasic bursting activity. Estradiol (E_2)(10^{-8}M) hyperpolarizes 63% of ARC-CPZ (LHRH) neurons via an increase in membrane conductance. Follicular phase and ovariectomized female guinea pigs (Group I) were compared to preovulatory and ovariectomized, estradiol benzoate (25 µg s.c.)-treated females (Group II). The latter group had serum estrogen levels greater tnan 30 pg/ml at the time of the experiment. The α_1 agonist, methoxamine (≈10 µl of 10^{-3} M pressure injected), excited 30% of the ARC-CPZ neurons in Group I (N=17). However, in Group II, 67% of the cells (N=12) were excited by the same dose of methoxamine (χ^2 Group I vs. Group II: $p<0.01$). This excitatory response was characterized by a depolarization and an increased membrane conductance, and 30% of all excited neurons exhibited phasic bursting activity with methoxamine application. A similar reponse was observed with NE, but it was not as effective as methoxamine (NE excited 15% of Group I neurons and 23% of Group II neurons). Therefore, in addition to its rapid inhibitory effects, E_2 also modulates (long term) the α_1 excitatory drive to ARC-CPZ neurons. (Supported by NIH grants HD19905, HD16793).

THE EFFECT OF SEROTONIN DEPLETERS ON PROSTAGLANDIN D_2-INDUCED LH INHIBITION IN CASTRATED MALE RATS. 25

T. Koh, Y. Nakai, F. Kinoshita, S. Tsujii, H. Takahashi, T. Usui, H. Imura
Second Division, Department of Medicine, Kyoto University, Kyoto, 606, Japan

Since prostaglandin(PG)D_2 and its receptor exist in high concentrations in the brain, especially in the hypothalamus, PGD_2 is considered to exert an important role of regulation in neurosecretion.

We reported that the intraventricular administration of PGD_2 suppressed LH secretion in castrated male rats (Endocrinology 110:2207, 1982). To elucidate the mechanism of PGD_2-induced inhibition of LH release, we examined the effect of serotonin depleters on PGD_2-induced LH suppression in castrated male rats.

Blood samples were collected every 10 min for 3h from a Silastic cannula in conscious, freely moving states and plasma LH was measured by radioimmunoassay. All animals showed elevated and pulsatile LH secretion characteristic of castrated rats after the injection of vehicle alone. Intraventricular administration of 5 µg of PGD_2 promptly blocked pulsatile LH release. This inhibitory effect of PGD_2 continued for at least 2h.

Pretreatment with p-chlorophenylalanine (PCPA, 320 mg/kg body weight ip) or 5,6-dihydroxytryptamine (5,6-DHT, 50 µg icv), a well-known serotonin depleter of the brain, had few effects on pulsatile LH release in castrated male rats. However, the pretreatment with the serotonin depleter, either PCPA or 5,6-DHT, completely blocked the inhibitory effect of PGD_2 on LH secretion.

These results suggest that a possible involvement of serotonin in PGD_2-induced inhibition of LH release in castrated male rats.

DOSE-DEPENDENT SUPPRESSION BY LHRH OF THE POSITIVE EFFECT OF ESTRADIOL ON THE PITUITARY GLAND 25a

T.R. Koiter, H. Moes, G.A. Schuiling
Dept. of Obstetrics & Gynecology, University of Groningen, The Netherlands

In the present study the effects of combined treatment with estradiol and LHRH on the pituitary gland were studied. Ovariectomized rats were during 6 days pretreated with LHRH, which hormone was continuously administered by way of sc implanted osmotic minipumps at the rate of either 25,50,100,250 or 500 ng/h, and with estradiolbenzoate (EB;3 ug/sc injection) on days 3,5 and 6. Subsequently the pituitary LH secretion was assessed using a superfusion system. First the pituitary glands were superfused with TC 199 medium containing no LHRH to assess the autonomous secretion of LH, and subsequently with medium containing LHRH at the maximally stimulating concentration of 1 ug/ml. LHRH pretreatment dose-dependently decreased the autonomous and the LHRH-stimulated secretion of LH. This decrease was associated with a dose-dependent depletion of the LH stores by LHRH. EB did not affect by itself the pituitary LH content, but potentiated the depleting effect of LHRH. EB increased the LHRH-stimulated secretion of LH (positive effect of EB) and this positive effect of EB was decreased by LHRH in a dose-dependent way. When LHRH had been infused at a rate higher than 100 ng/h (which established an LHRH plasma concentration of 63 pg/ml) the effect of EB became inhibitory. This was mainly due to the very low pituitary LH content: relative to the pituitary content the effect of EB on the LHRH-stimulated secretion of LH varied between positive (LHRH infusion rates of 0,25,50 and 100 ng/h) and zero (250,500 ng LHRH/h). The positive effect of EB on the autonomous secretion of LH was not depressed by LHRH. It is concluded that LHRH and estradiol influence each other's effect on the pituitary gland at concentrations which are within the "physiological" range.

EFFECT OF TRADITIONAL HERBAL MEDICINE ON HYPOTHALAMIC-PITUITARY-OVARIAN FUNCTION IN WOMEN WITH OVARIAN INSUFFICIENCY 26

T. Koyama, M. Ichimura, M. Ohara, Y. Kido, M. Saito
Department of Obstetrics and Gynecology, Tokyo Medical and Dental University, Tokyo, 113, Japan

Recently oriental herbal medicine has been widely used for women with infertility and climacteric symptoms in clinical gynecology in Japan. In this study, effects of most popular herbal medicine for women with ovarian insufficiency, Toki-Syakuyaku-San (TSS, Tsumura No 23, Tsumura Juntendo Co., Tokyo) and Unkei-to (UKT, Tsumura No 106), on hypothalamic-pituitary-ovarian function were endocrinologically investigated. Twenty-one women with ovarian insufficiency, 16 of whom wished to have children, were treated with TSS (7.5 g/day, per os) for 10 to 16 weeks and next were treated with UKT (7.5 g/day, per os) for 8 to 16 weeks. In some cases premarine test and LH-RH · TRH test were performed for assessment of hypothalamic-pituitary function before and after administration of TSS and/or UKT. During treated period, blood was taken every two week for determination of serum LH, FSH, prolactin, E_2,progesterone (P) and testosterone with BBT record. Concerning premarine test tendency of betterment of LH response was observed with TSS treatment (48% to 62% of positive response) and UKT (55% to 67%). On LH-RH · TRH test tendency of betterment of response was observed in amenorrheic women. Two ovulatory cycles were observed with TSS treatment and one ovulatory cycle was observed with UKT in 7 amenorrheic women. Four ovulatory cycles were obtained during 12 treated cycles with TSS and 4 ovulatory cycles during 14 treated cycles with UKT in 4 anovulatory women. In 10 women with luteal phase dysfunction normal midluteal P level was obtained in 20 cycles during 38 TSS treated cycles and in 19 cycles during 45 UKT treated cycles , respectively. Four pregnancies were observed during TSS treatment and one pregnancy during UKT treatment. These results infer that TSS and UKT mainly may exert their effects on hypothalamic-pituitary area and secondary may exert on ovary ; however, in part, direct effect on ovary may not be excluded.

THE EFFECT OF BARBITURATES ON PITUITARY SENSITIVITY TO LHRH IN THE OVARIECTOMIZED RAT 27

C.B. Lambalk, J.A.M.J. van Dieten, J. de Koning, J. Schoemaker* & G.P. van Rees
Dept. of Pharmacology of the University of Leiden, P.O. Box 9503, 2300 RA Leiden, The Netherlands and *Dept. of Obstet./Gynaecology, Academic Hospital of the Vrije Universiteit, P.O. Box 7095, 1007 MB Amsterdam, The Netherlands.

Recent experiments in ovariectomized (OVX) rats have shown that the pituitary is refractory to LHRH for a short period after an LHRH pulse. The duration of this period depends on the dose.

It is postulated that even under physiological conditions the pituitary is always refractory to endogenous LHRH in some degree.

When the action of endogenous LHRH was suppressed in vivo by anti-LHRH or an antagonist, an enhanced response was found after administration of an agonist or LHRH itself in vitro.

Phenobarbital presumably suppresses LH release by blocking endogenous pulsatile LHRH.

In view of earlier findings it can therefore be expected that under phenobarbital an enhancement of the pituitary LH response to exogenous LHRH pulses develops.

In this experiment we show that in OVX rats the LH response to exogenously administered LHRH pulses (1.25 or 5.0 ng/100 g body weight) is increased when given 1 h after an intraperitoneal injection of 80 mg/kg phenobarbital in comparison with the response in the absence of phenobarbital. In both situations there was a relationship between the LH response and the pulse dosage. Phenobarbital has no direct stimulating effects on pituitary LH release.

We assume that the increased response is the result of the removal of endogenous LHRH by phenobarbital, leading to the recovery of the pituitary from a certain degree of refractoriness.

THE EFFECTS OF HIGHLY SPECIFIC OPIATE RECEPTOR AGONISTS ON LH AND PROLACTIN SECRETION IN RATS. 28

C.A. Leadem and S. Johnson, Department of Anatomy, University of Arizona, Tucson, AZ

With the recent development of highly specific ligands for the mu, delta and kappa receptors it was of interest to define the effects of activation of each of these receptor types on LH and prolactin(PRL) secretion. The agonists were: DAGO for mu receptors, DPDPE for delta receptors and U50,488H for kappa receptors. Each of these agonists exhibits at least a 100-fold preference for binding to its receptor versus other opiate receptors. The compounds were infused (10 µl/h) at various concentrations into the third cerebroventricle of unanesthetized, ovariectomized rats (n=5-20/group) while blood samples (50 µl/5 min) were continually withdrawn through a jugular cannula. Blood withdrawal was begun 30 min prior to initiating drug infusion so as to estimate baseline hormone titers; drugs were then infused for two additional hours. PRL and LH were measured in the same sample by radioimmunoassay. For each group, post-infusion samples were compared to the same animal's mean pre-infusion hormone levels by paired t-test. The mu agonist, DAGO, at both 1 and 10 µg/h caused a significant suppression of LH secretion and a significant stimulation of PRL release. DPDPE, the delta agonist, had no effect on either hormone at 1 µg/h but inhibited LH secretion at 10 µg/h. There was still no effect of this high dose of DPDPE on PRL release. The kappa agonist, U50,488H, had no effect on either hormone at 10 µg/h but at 100 µg/h produced a significant suppression of LH release and a highly variable, non-significant increase in PRL. Co-infusion of 100 µg/h of naloxone with the high dose of each of the agonists completely blocked the responses of both hormones to each of the agonists with one exception: the highly variable stimulation of PRL by U50,488H was not affected, thus indicating a non-specific effect of U50,488H on PRL secretion. These results demonstrate that: 1) activation of the mu receptors produces an inhibition of LH secretion and a stimulation of PRL release; 2) activation of the delta or kappa receptors produces an inhibition of LH secretion but has no effect on PRL release. (Supported by PHS S07 RR05675 and NIH Grant HD 19965)

HYPOTHALAMIC FACTOR THAT INHIBITS LH SECRETION: RELATIONSHIP WITH GnRH (1-5). 29

J. Leal, M. De la Lastra
Laboratorio Endocrinología, Facultad Ciencias Biológicas Pontificia Universidad Católica de Chile. Casilla 114-D. Santiago, Chile.

A gonadotropin inhibitory activity has been obtained with different extraction procedures from rat and human hypothalami. We report here the obtention from cow's median eminence (ME) of a peptidic material, soluble in acetic acid 0.5 M and methanol, which inhibits LH, but not FSH release stimulated with 200 ng GnRH in immature male rats. The inhibitory dose was equivalent to 0.33 - 1 median eminence and higher doses were not effective.

The inhibitory material cross reacts with a monoclonal antibody against GnRH and has an estimated molecular weight of approcimately 750 daltons. These characteristics suggest that it could be a fragment cleaved from GnRH by the endopeptidase that occurs in hypothalamus. The principal product of this enzymatic process is GnRH (1-5) which has a molecular weight of 739 daltons, similar to that estimated for the natural inhibitory material. On these grounds we resolved to assay the sequence GnRH (1-5) supply by Dr. J. Rivier, La Jolla, CA, on gonadotropin release stimulated with 200 ng GnRH in immature male rats and upon ovulation induced with GnRH or LH. The release of LH, but not FSH, was significantly inhibited with 50 and 100 ng of GnRH (1-5), but not with higher doses. No effect was observed upon basal, non estimulated levels of LH. Ovulation induced with 200 ng of GnRH in chlorpromazine treated proestrous rats was significantly inhibited by 50 ng but not with 450 ng of GnRH (1-5). Ovulation induced with LH (3ug/100g bw) in hypophysectomized proestrous rats was not modified by 50 ng of GnRH (1-5).

On the basis of these results we propose that GnRH (1-5) is the LH-release inhibitory material that occurs in cow's median eminence and we suggest a possible role of this peptide in gonadotropin regulation at adenohypophiseal level.

This study was supported by Grant RF 83016; DIUC 71/84 and DIUC 69/86, and CONICYT 1186/85.

INHIBITION OF LH AND PRL BY Δ^9-TETRAHYDROCANNABINOL IN MEDIAL BASAL HYPOTHALAMIC DEAFFERENTATED OVARIECTOMIZED RATS. 30

L.L.Murphy, C.D.Thomas and L.Tyrey, Dept. of Obstetrics and Gynecology, Duke University, Durham, NC 27710

The inhibition of luteinizing hormone(LH) and prolactin(Prl) by Δ^9-tetrahydrocannabinol(THC), the major psychoactive constituent in marihuana, is well documented. The site at which THC acts to inhibit these hormones is unclear although a supra-pituitary site of THC action is implicated. In the present study, medial basal hypothalamic(MBH)-deafferentated female rats were used to investigate the MBH as a potential site of THC inhibitory action. Following MBH deafferentation, rats were acyclic with predominantly leukocytic vaginal smears. Sham-cut rats (knife inserted but not rotated) continued to exhibit regular 4-day vaginal smear patterns. Rats were ovariectomized approximately 3 wk after brain surgery and were utilized 4-6 wk later. Serial blood samples were taken via intra-atrial cannulae every 10 m for 60 m before and after administration of THC (0.5 or 1.0 mg/kg bw). After treatment with THC, serum LH was reduced to 50-60% of the pretreatment mean within 20 m ($p<0.05$). With 0.5 mg THC/kg bw, serum LH remained suppressed at 30 m ($p<0.01$) in sham-cut rats, but not in rats with MBH cuts. With 1.0 mg THC/kg bw, serum LH in sham-cut rats remained suppressed for the duration of the sampling period(30% of pretreatment by 60 m). In contrast, serum LH increased after 30 m in MBH-cut rats and returned to the pretreatment level by 60 m. In both sham- and MBH-cut rats, THC treatment suppressed serum Prl within 20 m ($p<0.05$). At 20 m serum Prl was reduced to 60-80% of the pretreatment level by 0.5 mg THC/kg bw and 50-55% of pretreatment by 1.0 mg THC/kg bw. Serum Prl remained suppressed for the duration of the sampling period in all groups. An earlier study using rats with small MBH islands failed to detect Prl suppression after THC treatment. With larger MBH islands, extending from the retrochiasmatic plane to the premammillary region, THC-induced inhibition of both LH and Prl was readily apparent. These data suggest that THC inhibits LH and Prl secretion by actions within the MBH, although differences in the durations of LH suppression between sham and MBH-cut rats suggest that THC also may act through extra-hypothalamic sites. (Supported by NIDA #DA 02006).

USE OF POTENT LHRH ANALOGS IN THE CONTROL OF FERTILITY AND TREATMENT OF ENDOMETRIOSIS 31

R.M.G. Nair, G.K. Nambiar, M.A. Barnes, R.S. Mathur, M.R. Neff, G. Holtz, R.E. McIntosh
VA Medical Center & Depts. of Medicine and Obstetrics and Gynecology, Charleston, SC, School of Sciences & Technology, Savannah, GA, Mount Sinai Medical Center, Milwaukee, WI, and The Fertility Clinic, Seattle, WA

A superactive agonist (S1), His-2Me-DAla-6,DesGly-10 LHRHethylamide and an antagonist (S2) D-p-Glu-D-Phe-D-Trp-Ser-D-Tyr-D-Trp-D-Leu-Arg-Pro-Gly-NH2 were chronically administered in groups of male rats, hamsters, and rabbits (2 µg/kg BW, IM) for 3 months. Decreased testicular weights were observed at 4 wk post-treatment with S1 or S2, in the rats and hamsters. A decrease in the number of germinal cells and disruption in the cellular association occurred. Gradual decrease in the plasma concentration of LH, FSH, and testosterone with degenerative changes in the sertoli cells and seminiferous tubules followed by disruption of spermatogenesis, resulted for both treatment groups. Sperm/gram cauda of the hamsters or sperm counts in the semen from rabbits after prolonged treatment were reduced by 95%. During a recovery period of 8 weeks following the treatment, the sperm count reached normal limits.

S1 was used intranasally for the treatment of endometriosis and uterine leiomyoma (IND 20,729), by two clinical groups. The treatment consisted of the administration of 100 µg of S1, t.i.d., intranasally using a metered dropper, beginning on day 3-5 of the menstrual cycle and continuing for a minimum of 3 months. Response to treatment was monitored by serial estradiol, LH and FSH measurements and also ultrasonography or laparoscopy. The E2 and gonadotropin levels gradually decreased after an initial acute rise during the beginning of the therapy. Patients experienced estrogen withdrawal bleeding during the first month of therapy but subsequently became amenorrheic. Hot flushing was the only side effect suffered. Clinically significant regression was obtained in the treatment group, although the E2 concentrations were not as low as castrate levels. Further work is in progress.

These studies indicate the efficacy of LHRH analogs as very valuable therapeutic or contraceptive agents.

OPIOID PEPTIDE INHIBITION OF THE HYPOTHALAMIC-PITUITARY AXIS IN THE RABBIT 32

K.M. Orstead and H.G. Spies
Oregon Primate Research Center, Beaverton, Oregon 97006

Indirect evidence suggests that the endogenous opioid peptides (EOPs), in the appropriate ovarian steroid milieu, inhibit hypothalamic gonadotropin-releasing hormone (GnRH) release. This study compared the simultaneous release of GnRH from the mediobasal hypothalamus (MBH), and luteinizing hormone (LH) and follicle-stimulating hormone (FSH) from the pituitary in intact (INT) and ovariectomized (OVX) does during either intravenous (IV) infusion or intrahypothalamic perfusion of the opiate receptor antagonist naloxone (NAL). All does were fitted with a push-pull perfusion (PPP) cannula directed into the MBH and subsequently subjected to PPP at a flow rate of 20 µl/min for 6 h to measure hypothalamic GnRH release. GnRH in PPP samples and LH and FSH in plasma samples collected at 10-min intervals were measured by specific RIAs. In experiment I, INT (n=3) and OVX (n=4) does received saline (IV) for 4 h, followed by 2 h of NAL (10 µg/min/kg, IV) during PPP. In experiment II, INT (n=3) and OVX (n=3) does received NAL that was added directly to the PPP medium at a rate of 0.2 µg/min for 2 h during the 6 h of MBH perfusion. In OVX does, either IV infusion or intrahypothalamic perfusion of NAL stimulated prompt, parallel increases in both GnRH and LH release. In these does, mean basal GnRH levels increased from 0.24 to 0.81 pg/10 min ($p < 0.001$) during the first h of IV NAL infusion. Mean basal GnRH release in OVX does also increased from 0.40 to 2.38 pg/10 min ($p < 0.025$) during the first h of intrahypothalamic NAL perfusion. In contrast, either route of NAL administration tended to augment both GnRH and LH release in INT does, but these increases were not significant. NAL also did not alter FSH secretion in any group. We have concluded that: 1) the EOPs inhibit the release of hypothalamic GnRH and thus pituitary LH; and 2) the more robust responses of GnRH and LH release to NAL administration in OVX vs. INT animals suggest that ovarian steroids influence the inhibition by EOPs of GnRH release. Furthermore, the failure of NAL to alter FSH secretion suggests, under these circumstances, a divergence in the hypothalamic regulation of pituitary LH and FSH secretion. Supported by NIH grants HD-07133, HD-18185, HD-16631 and RR-00163.

THE EFFECT OF Δ^9-TETRAHYDROCANNABINOL ON SOMATOSTATIN AND LH-RH RELEASE FROM RAT MEDIAN EMINENCE "IN VITRO". 33

V. Rettori, C. Aguila, S. Dalterio* and S.M. McCann. Dept of Physiology, Univ Tx Hlth Sci Ctr at Dallas, Texas 75235 and *Dept of Pharmacology UTHSC at San Antonio, Texas 78284

It has been demonstrated that Δ^9-tetrahydrocannabinol (THC), the principal psychoactive component of marihuana, inhibits the secretion of LH and GH *in vivo* in the rat. In the present study the direct effect of THC on somatostatin (SRIF) and LH-RH release by median eminence (ME) fragments from adult male (Sprague-Dawley) rats incubated *in vitro* was investigated. ME and the proximal stump of the pituitary stalk were dissected free under a stereoscopic microscope. After 30 minutes of preincubation in Krebs-Ringer bicarbonate glucose buffer (KRBG), pH 7.4 at 37°C in an atmosphere of 95% O_2-5% CO_2, doses ranging from 10^{-11} to 10^{-8}M of THC were added to fresh KRBG and the tissues were incubated for an additional 30 minutes. The media were assayed by RIA for SRIF using highly specific antisera for somatostatin (R-110) and LH-RH ($R_{11}B_{73}$). There was a signifianct dose-related increase in SRIF release with concentrations of 10^{-9}M and 10^{-8}M THC. LH-RH release was not significantly affected by any of the THC concentrations tested. It appears that the lowering of GH in serum after THC administration may result from its stimulatory action on SRIF release from the ME. Although an effect of THC on LH-RH release was not observed in the present experimental conditions, a central neuroendocrine mechanism inducing a reduction in serum LH is likely since plasma LH decreased following intraventricular THC in earlier experiments in the face of normal pituitary responsiveness. It is possible that THC inhibits LHRH release *in vivo* by an action on the cell bodies of the LHRH neurons which would not be included in the incubation. Alternatively, THC might block stimulated LHRH release from the fragments *in vitro*. (Supported by PHS grants AM 10073 and HD 09988).

PROCESSING OF PREPRO-LUTEINIZING HORMONE-RELEASING HORMONE IN THE HYPOTHALAMUS 34

O.K. Ronnekleiv, J. Adelman, W.E. Ellinwood, M.J. Kelly
Dept. Physiology and IABR, Oregon Health Sciences U. Portland, Oregon

Recently, it has been demonstrated that mammalian luteinizing hormone-releasing hormone (LHRH) is synthesized from a larger polypeptide, preproLHRH (Seeberg and Adelman, Nature 311:666, 1984). The processing of the preproLHRH to the mature decapeptide has been suggested to occur as the precursor is transported down the axon to the terminal (King and Anthony, Peptides 4:963-70, 1983). However, we developed an antiserum to LHRH (EL-14) which appeared to recognize the mature decapeptide and found that the antiserum immunocytochemically stained LHRH cell bodies and fibers in the rat, guinea pig and monkey hypothalamus (Ellinwood et al., Peptides 6:45, 1985). Presently, we have further characterized the EL-14 antiserum by determining the ability of up to 10 µg of rat brain preproLHRH and up to 1 ng of a synthetic peptide consisting of amino acids 6-16 of preproLHRH to inhibit the binding of [^{125}I]LHRH to synthetic LHRH under RIA conditions. For immunocytochemical specificity testing, 1 ml of the EL-14 antiserum, diluted 1:4000, was preabsorbed with 1 to 25 µg of the preproLHRH or 1 to 10 µg of the 6-16 fragment. As determined by RIA, the EL-14 antiserum bound 25 - 30 % of the [I^{125}]LHRH at a final dilution of 1:630,000. preproLHRH or the 6-16 fragment exhibited no signifcant cross reactivity in the RIA (less than 0.01 %). Moreover, we were unable to block the staining of LHRH cells or fibers through preabsorption of the EL-14 antiserum with the preproLHRH or the 6-16 fragment. Preabsorption of the antiserum with 1 µg/ml of LHRH prevented all immunoreactive staining in the rat, guinea pig and monkey hypothalamus. This data suggests that the precursor is being processed to the mature decapeptide in the cell body of these species. However, the extent of this processing in the cell soma, and regional and species differences needs to be determined. (Supported by NIH grants HD19905, HD16793)

GONADAL MODULATION OF NEUROPEPTIDE Y RELEASE FROM THE MEDIOBASAL HYPOTHALAMUS (MBH) IN VITRO 35

A. Sahu, W.R. Crowley, T.L. O'Donohue, P.S. Kalra, S.P. Kalra
Dept. OB-Gyn, Univ. Fla. Col. Med., Gainesville, FL 32610 and Dept. Pharmacol., Univ. Tenn., Memphis, TN

Neuropeptide Y (NPY) is present in high concentrations in the rat hypothalamus. Intracerebroventricular injection of NPY modifies LH secretion, the response is dependent on the steroid background. To study further the role of steroids in regulation of NPY secretion, we have studied the in vitro NPY release from the MBH of intact (sham control) and castrated (20 days) male rats. Five MBH/chamber were incubated in 0.5 ml Krebs-Ringer bicarbonate (KRB); KRB was changed at 15 min intervals. In the first experiment, after a preincubation period of 60 min (0 time), the MBH were exposed for 15 min to a pulse of 23 mM followed 30 min later with 45 mM KCl. NPY concentration in the medium was measured by a specific RIA. Whereas 23 mM KCl was ineffective, 45 mM KCl evoked a 4-8 fold higher release of NPY from the MBH of intact and castrated rats. In the second experiment, MBH were exposed for 15 min to two pulses of 45 mM KCl 30 min apart. NPY released in response to the first K^+ pulse was significantly smaller from the MBH of castrated than intact rats ($p < 0.05$). In the third experiment, NPY release in vitro was also significantly lower from the MBH of castrated rats. In an additional experiment the MBH were exposed to two 15 min pulses, 30 min apart, of 0.568 and 56.8 µmole prostaglandin E_2 (PGE_2). Unlike K^+, PGE_2 failed to stimulate NPY release from the MBH of either intact or castrated rats. These studies show that (1) KCl stimulates NPY release from the MBH in vitro, (2) NPY response to K^+ is significantly lower from the MBH of castrated than intact males, thereby suggesting that testicular secretions may modulate NPY release and (3) since PGE_2 failed to stimulate NPY release in vitro, intracellular processes in NPY release may not involve PGE_2 mediation. (Supported by NIH HD 08634, 11362).

PULSATILE RELEASE OF HYPOTHALAMIC LHRH INTO PITUITARY PORTAL BLOOD OF OVARIECTOMIZED RATS: EVIDENCE FOR AN AUTOFEEDBACK MECHANISM 36

D.K. Sarkar
University of California, San Diego, La Jolla, CA-92093.

The secretory profile of hypothalamic LHRH and the possible existence of an autofeedback mechanism controlling LHRH release were determined in ovariectomized rats.

The profile of LHRH release was studied by measuring the concentration of LHRH in pituitary portal blood samples collected every 10 min from ovariectomized rats. Pituitary portal blood samples were collected in rats using an anesthetic consisting of alphaxalone and alphadolone acetate. This anesthetic had no significant effect on the secretion of pituitary LH in ovariectomized rats; LH release was pulsatile in nature and showed 4-5 peaks during 3 h period. Under this anesthesia, LHRH was also released into pituitary portal blood in a pulsatile manner with 4-5 peaks during 3 h collection period.

The effect of an LHRH agonist analog with or without an LHRH antagonist analog on the endogenous release of LHRH was studied to determine the possible autofeedback regulation of LHRH release. Both of these analogs had no significant cross reaction in RIA of LHRH. The LHRH agonist significantly reduced the pulse amplitude of endogenous LHRH secretion. This inhibitory action of the LHRH agonist was blocked by the LHRH antagonist.

These results suggest that the hypothalamic secretion of LHRH is pulsatile in nature in ovariectomized rats and that LHRH may modulate its own release through an autofeedback mechanism.

This study was supported by NIH AG-05453.

PATHOLOGIC EFFECTS OF ESTRADIOL ON THE HYPOTHALAMIC ARCUATE NUCLEUS 37

H.M. Schipper, J.R. Brawer
McGill University, Montreal, Canada

The pathologic effects of sex steroids on the hypothalmic arcuate nucleus of adult rats were examined using numbers of reactive microglia and astrocytic granules as quantitative indices of neuropathology.

Microglial and astrocytic reactions were observed in adult female rats entering a state of "persistent estrus" following a single injection of 2 mg estradiol valerate (EV) or exposure to continuous illumination. Lower doses of EV failed to elicit both the persistent estrus state and significant glial responses. In EV-treated animals, a hypothalamic lesion could be prevented by prior ovariectomy or by pituitary-ovarian suppression with medroxyprogesterone acetate indicating that an ovarian factor is responsible for the neuropathological changes. This ovarian product is probably estradiol since dose-related enhancement of glial reactivity occurs in male rats treated with multiple injections of EV.

Arcuate pathology developed spontaneously in "senile persistent estrus" female and aging male rats. In females, but not in males, early gonadectomy suppressed age-related arcuate glial reactivity. Conceivably, estrogen withdrawal or EV-treatment respectively retards or accelerates histologic aging of the female gonadotropic hypothalamus.

Testosterone treatment occasionally elicited mild arcuate glial responses, possibly through prior aromatization to estradiol. In contrast, 5α-dihydrotestosterone (a non-aromatizable androgen) appeared to suppress astrocytic granule counts below control values.

The EV-induced persistent estrus rat may serve as a useful model for Clover disease of the ewe and the human polycystic ovarian syndrome.

CHOLECYSTOKININ AND REPRODUTION: CASTRATION ALTERS CCK LEVELS WITHIN CELLS OF THREE SEXUALLY DIMORPHIC NUCLEI. 38

R.B. Simerly and L.W. Swanson, Howard Hughes Medical Institute and The Salk Institute, La Jolla, California, USA.

Three sexually dimorphic cell groups, the central part of the medial preoptic nucleus(MPNc), the encapsulated part of the bed nucleus of the stria terminalis(BSTe), and the posterodorsal part of the medial nucleus of the amygdala(MeAp), contain high densities of steroid concentrating cells and are thought to play important roles in the control of reproductive behavior and physiology. Cholecystokinin(CCK) has also been implicated in these functions and particularly high densities of CCK- immunoreactive cells are concentrated in these regions. In addition, CCK levels in specific parts of the forebrain appear to be sensitive to circulating gonadal steroids in the adult (Micevych et al.,'85; Frankfurt et al.,'85).

In order to examine the sensitivity of CCK cells in the MPNc, BSTe, and MeAp to the effects of differential levels of circulating gonadal steroids, we employed an indirect immunohistochemical method using an antiserum directed toward CCK-8. Two groups of male Sprague-Dawley rats were gonadectomized at 60 days of age, and one group each was sacrificed at 3 days and 14 days after gonadectomy. Each animal received 50-70ug of colchicine in the lateral ventricle 3 days prior to being sacrificed along with an intact, colchicine-treated male rat. Sections through the forebrain of all animals were processed for indirect immunohistochemistry as described elsewhere (Simerly et al. '86). Although CCK-8 staining was not significantly diminished in the MeAp at 3 days after gonadectomy, fewer cells were stained in the BSTe, and CCK-immunoreactivity was barely visible in the MPNc. In contrast, CCK-staining in cells within each region was nearly eliminated in animals sacrificed 2 weeks after gonadectomy. The distribution of CCK-immunoreactive cells in each region was also examined in female rats. The distribution of CCK-stained cells in the MPNc and BSTe was found to be similar to that of males, although fewer immunoreactive cells were found in both regions in females in accordance with the smaller size of each cell group in animals of this sex. Notably, virtually no CCK-stained cells were found within the MeAp of females, although a few stained cells were found in the anterior part of the medial amygdaloid nucleus. These findings suggest that CCK levels within cells of each of the sexually dimorphic cell groups examined here are regulated by circulating gonadal steroids, and may be related to hormonal modulation of the reproductive functions in which these cell groups participate.

Supported by NIH grants AM26741, NS16686, NS07573.

QUANTITY, IN SITU ACTIVITY, AND PHOSPHORYLATION OF TYROSINE HYDROXYLASE IN THE MEDIAN EMINENCE AS A FUNCTION OF ESTROGEN AND PROGESTERONE 40

P.S. Wang and J.C. Porter
University of Texas Health Science Center, Dallas, Texas 75235

The effect of estradiol benzoate (EB) and/or progesterone (P) on the quantity, in situ activity, and phosphorylation of tyrosine hydroxylase (TH) in the median eminence (ME) was investigated in long-term ovariectomized rats. The in situ activity of TH was evaluated from the rate of accumulation of dihydroxyphenylalanine (DOPA) in the ME of animals treated with NSD 1015, a DOPA decarboxylase inhibitor. TH was quantified by means of an immunoblot assay using purified rat TH as the standard. Phosphorylation of TH in the ME was evaluated by quantifying ^{32}P-labelled TH. ^{32}P-labelled TH was purified by immunoprecipitation and polyacrylamide gel electrophoresis and quantified by radioautography and densitometry. The animals were treated for 1, 2, or 3 days with EB (25 µg/kg BW per day), P (5 mg/kg BW per day), or both EB and P.

The effects of these treatments of ovariectomized rats with EB and/or P on the quantity of TH in the ME are shown in Table 1.

TABLE 1. TH in the ME.

Days of Treatment	TREATMENT: Solvent Vehicle	EB	P	EB + P
1	.23 ± .011(6)*	.21 ± .005(6)	.17 ± .007(6)	.14 ± .015(6)
2	.22 ± .011(6)	.21 ± .010(6)	.17 ± .011(6)	.19 ± .009(6)
3	.24 ± .020(6)	.22 ± .020(6)	.13 ± .014(6)	.13 ± .010(6)

*Values are presented as pmoles TH per ME (Mean and SE). Number of animals is shown in parentheses.

The in situ activity of TH in the ME of ovariectomized rats treated with EB and/or P is shown in Table 2.

TABLE 2. In situ activity of TH in the ME.

Days of Treatment	TREATMENT: Solvent Vehicle	EB	P	EB + P
1	29 ± 3.6(6)*	40 ± 3.4(6)	42 ± 3.2(6)	66 ± 11.8(6)
2	34 ± 2.2(6)	39 ± 3.6(6)	39 ± 4.5(6)	74 ± 6.8(6)
3	26 ± 4.7(6)	31 ± 1.0(6)	52 ± 6.6(6)	114 ± 13.5(6)

*Values are presented as moles DOPA/hr X mole TH.

When in vitro phosphorylation of TH in the ME was evaluated in the presence of .1 mM veratridine (a condition known to stimulate phosphorylation of TH in the ME), it was found that the incorporation of ^{32}P into TH in the ME of rats treated with EB + P was significantly greater ($P < .05$) than that into TH in the ME of vehicle-treated animals.

These data support the view that treatment with both EB and P results in an increase in the in situ activity of TH in the ME. The increase in the in situ activity of TH in the ME may in part be the result of increased capacity of the ME to phosphorylate TH.

INTRAVENTRICULAR INJECTION OF OVINE FSH SUPPRESSES LH AND TO A LESSER EXTENT FSH RELEASE IN OVARIECTOMIZED RATS. 41

W.H. Yu and S.M. McCann
Dept. of Physiol., University of Texas Health Science Center, Dallas, Texas, 75235.

To test for possible feedback control of FSH to alter its own release and that of LH within the CNS, conscious ovariectomized rats were injected in the 3rd ventricle (icv) with ovine (o) FSH or 0.9% NaCl (3 µl). Blood samples were collected from jugular cannulae before and after icv injection. Synthetic LHRH (25 ng/100 g B.W.) was administered iv to test for pituitary sensitivity at the end of the experiment. Plasma concentrations of FSH and LH were measured by specific RIAs. Plasma LH was significantly lowered by icv injection of ovine FSH with all doses (0.5 µg and higher) ($p<0.001$). FSH suppressed LH release within 10 min; the maximal effect occurred within 3 h and was maintained for 6 h. With higher doses of oFSH (8 and 20 µg), plasma levels of FSH declined to minimal values at 2-3 hours after injection and then rebounded to elevated levels during the period from 8 to 12 hours. There was minimal cross-reactivity between oFSH and antisera against rat FSH but cross-reactivity between oFSH and the antiserum against oLH used for RIA was about 30%. Consequently the decreased levels of LH after icv injection of oFSH could not be caused by leakage of ovine FSH into the circulatory system. The suppression of LH release by FSH was hypothalamic since responsiveness to LHRH was unimpaired. The biphasic effect on plasma FSH indicates the existence of a short-lived negative short-loop feedback of FSH on its own release. The late elevation may be the result of removal of this inhibition, accompanied by enhanced responsiveness of the gonadotropes to renewed stimulation by FSH-releasing factor. (Supported by HD 09988 and AM 10073).

EFFECTS OF HORMONAL TREATMENT ON HYPOTHALAMIC LHRH CONTENT. 42

M. Zanisi, E. Messi, M. Motta
Department of Endocrinology, University of Milano, Italy.

Gonadotropin secretion is controlled by a variety of hormonal modulators that may also act at hypothalamic level. The possible involvement of some of these modulators on the hypothalamic stores of LHRH has been investigated. Role of androgens. Testosterone (T) is known to exert some of its effects after aromatization to estradiol. Long-term treatment of castrated male rats with T is able to increase the low intrahypothalamic levels of LHRH induced by castration, a phenomenon not inhibited by the simultaneous administration of a potent antiestrogen (tamoxifen). In keeping with these results estradiol injected in low doses to castrated male rats does not influence intrahypothalamic LHRH stores. Role of LHRH. Long-term treatment with LHRH analogs is known to inhibit gonadal function. The possibility that these compounds may also influence hypothalamic LHRH stores has been tested by treating either normal or castrated male rats with a biodegradable depot preparation of an LHRH analog either alone or in association with silastic implants of T. In normal male rats the analog significantly reduces the intrahypothalamic LHRH stores, while T is ineffective; when the two hormones are given in association, T is able to overcome the inhibitory effect of the analog given alone. Conversely, in castrated male rats, the LHRH analog does not modify the reduced levels of LHRH induced by orchidectomy. As expected, T increases LHRH levels; when the analog is given in association with T, the facilitatory effect of the steroid is still evident. These data suggest that in the male: 1) the effect of T on the intrahypothalamic stores of LHRH is exerted by the steroid as such; 2) LHRH analog has a different effect depending on the presence or absence of the testes; 3) T seems to be the main controller of the LHRH hypothalamic stores. (Supported by C.N.R. grants no. 85.00679.56 and 85.00715.56).

THE POSSIBLE ROLE OF CALMODULIN IN THE RELEASE OF SRIF INDUCED BY GRF. 43

M.C. Aguila and S.M. McCann
Department of Physiology, Univ of TX Hlth Sci Center at Dallas, Texas 75235.

The present in vitro experiments were performed to examine the possible role of calcium and calmodulin on growth hormone-releasing factor (GRF) induced somatostatin (SRIF) release from the median eminence (ME). Adult male rats were used as tissue donors. The ME's were first preincubated in 0.4 ml of Krebs Ringer bicarbonate glucose (KRBG) buffer (pH 7.4) containing bacitracin at 37°C in an atmosphere of 95% O_2, 5% CO_2 with constant shaking for 30 minutes. When the calcium concentrations were altered, the altered medium was used during the preincubation and incubation periods. After preincubation, the medium was discarded and replaced by medium containing the different substances to be tested (GRF, EGTA and calmodulin inhibitors).

The stimulation of SRIF release induced by 10^{-10}M GRF was not inhibited by omission of extracellular calcium or omission of Ca^{++} plus chelation of residual extracellular calcium by 10^{-4}M EGTA which suggests that the GRF effect on SRIF release from the ME is independent of extracellular calcium. Two calmodulin inhibitors were employed to examine the possible influence of calmodulin on GRF-induced SRIF release. Both Trifluopromazine (1 µM) and Trifluoperazine (1 µM) had an inhibitory effect on the stimulation of SRIF release induced by GRF and failed to alter resting release. Thus, the inhibitory effect of calmodulin inhibitors on GRF-induced SRIF release, suggests that calmodulin may be involved in this process. Examination of the mechanism by which GRF may mobilize intraterminal calcium in the ME warrants further investigation. (Supported by AM grant # 10073).

ANGIOTENSIN II (A_{II}) ACTS ON ANTERIOR PITUITARY (AP) CELLS TO INCREASE INTRACELLULAR FREE CALCIUM [Ca++]i AND STIMULATE PROLACTIN RELEASE

44

J.M. Anderson, M.J. Cronin
University of Virginia, Charlottesville, Virginia 22908

A_{II} and dopamine (DA) are stimulatory and inhibitory hormones affecting the AP lactotroph. A_{II} receptor activation releases into AP cells inositol trisphosphate, an agent that increases [Ca++]i in other cell types, whereas DA activity is correlated with reduced AP [Ca++]i. Because it is unknown whether A_{II} action in AP is associated with an elevation of [Ca++]i, we used the [Ca++]i indicator fura-2 to monitor any such response. DA provided an inhibitory control. Dispersed rat AP cells were loaded with fura-2 and then monitored fluorometricaly. A_{II} (10 nM) induced a spike of [Ca++]I that peaked within 15 sec at 33 $\pm$ 7% (n=4) above baseline. DA (1 uM) immediately reduced this plateau level of [Ca++]i, reaching a minimum within 40 sec. As a positive control, DA (100 nM) also attenuated basal [Ca++]i, confirming an earlier report (FEBS Lett 159: 79, 1983). It is also possible that A_{II} acts as a secretagogue only on a subset of lactotrophs, rather than on the entire lactotroph population, or that some lactotrophs are particularly sensitive to A_{II}. To address this andto further characterize the A_{II} effect on prolactin release, we applied the reverse hemolytic plaque assay. When challenged with the Ca++ channel blocker D600 (1 uM), A_{II}-stimulated prolactin release was inhibited, indicating a dependence on extracellular Ca++. DA (1 uM) also attenuated A_{II}-stimulated prolactin release. The plaque areas were then plotted as frequency-area histograms to assess secretory trends. Preliminary studies indicate that A_{II}-responsive subpopulations of lactotrophs exist. We conclude that AP cells respond to A_{II} by increasing [Ca++]i and prolactin release.
(Supported by FIDIA, Italy & RCDA 1K04NS00601)

ACTH RELEASE IN RESPONSE TO CRF, FORSKOLIN, MAITOTOXIN, PHORBOL ESTER AND ATRIAL NATRIURETIC FACTOR (ANF).

45

A.J.Baertschi, T. Yasumoto, R. Pence, M.J. Cronin
University of Virginia, Charlottesville VA 22908
Tohoku University, Sendai 980 Japan

The role of ANF in corticotroph function was examined on dispersed, cultured anterior pituitary cells of rats, because (1) ACTH secretion is inversely related to atrial stretch; (2) ANF immunoreactivity has been detected in the median eminence (Neuroscience 16:521, 1985); and (3) ANF weakly binds to anterior pituitary cells (Peptides 5: 1167, 1984) and inhibits basal and CRF-stimulated adenylate cyclase activity (Life Sci 36: 1873, 1985). CRF (10nM), forskolin (3 µM; a catalytic adenylate cyclase stimulator), and phorbol dibutyrate (PDB, 100nM; a protein kinase C activator) significantly enhanced ACTH release within 15 min by 2.5-fold, 1.8-fold and 4.9-fold, respectively, confirming previous observations. Both CRF and forskolin, but not PDB, increased cellular cAMP levels. Maitotoxin, shown elsewhere to activate native Calcium channels, enhanced ACTH secretion (ng/mg protein/15min) from 4.81+-0.58 (vehicle) to 8.47+-0.8 (maitotoxin, 3ng/ml) and 9.96+-1.25 (maitotoxin, 10ng/ml). ANF (30-100nM) had no effect on basal cAMP levels, but significantly increased basal ACTH release by 2.2-fold (average of 2 independent 2-3h experiments). ANF had no effect on ACTH secretion induced by 3µM forskolin, 100nM PDB, and 30ng/ml maitotoxin, weak or non significant stimulatory effects on the 10nM CRF-evoked increase in cellular cAMP levels and ACTH secretion, and no effect on cellular cAMP levels stimulated by 10nM GRF or 30nM TRH. In conclusion, high levels of ANF have weak or non significant effects on basal or TRH, GRF and CRF-stimulated cAMP levels in the anterior pituitary gland, no effect on ACTH release evoked by activators of protein kinase C, Ca-channels or adenylate cyclase, and only moderate effects on basal release of ACTH. In view of these findings, other roles of ANF in pituitary function (e.g. vascular) should also be examined. (Supported by RCDA 1K04NS00601, CIT BIO-85-025, NIH HL31133.)

INTERACTIONS BETWEEN STIMULATORY AND INHIBITORY NEUROHORMONES ON RAT ANTERIOR PITUITARY ADENYLATE CYCLASE ACTIVITY.

46

P. Bertrand, J. Epelbaum, C. Kordon and A. Enjalbert,
U. 159 INSERM, U. de Neuroendocrinologie, 2ter rue d'Alésia, 75014 PARIS, France.

Cyclic AMP (cAMP) is involved in the mechanism of action of various hypothalamic neurohormones each of them acting on several pituitary cell types. In the present work we characterized the interactions between the effect of some stimulatory (VIP, CRF, GRF) and inhibitory (dopamine, SRIF, angiotensin II) neurohormones on adenylate cyclase activity of anterior pituitary membrane preparations. In an heterogeneous cell population non additivity of the effects of two neurohormones indicates that corresponding receptors coupled to adenylate are localized on the same cell type, since it is generally accepted that there is a single pool of adenylate cyclase in a single cell. In male rats, VIP, CRF and GRF stimulated basal adenylate cyclase activity by 349 %, 228 % and 710 % with an apparent affinity of K_D = 4.0 10^{-8}, 1.2 10^{-7}, 1.6 10^{-8} M respectively. Amplitude of these effects were twice lower in female pituitary membranes without changes in the apparent affinities. On the contrary, dopamine SRIF and angiotensin II inhibited basal adenylate cyclase of 47 %, 25 % and 23 % in males with apparent affinities of 10^{-6}, 10^{-7}, 2.10^{-9} M and 45, 20, 38 % in female. The effects of the three stimulatory neurohormones were strictly additive. In the case of inhibitory factors, the effects of dopamine and angiotensin II were not additive, while somatostatin effect was partially additive with dopamine or angiotensin effects. Finally, a selective interaction resulting in higher effects of inhibitors on stimulated than on basal adenylate cyclase activity was only observed between VIP and dopamine, VIP and angiotensin II and GRF and somatostatin. In summary our results demonstrate that VIP, DA, AII and some SRIF receptors coupled to adenylate cyclase are localized on the same cell (lactotrophs) type while SRIF and GRF receptors are localized on another (somatotrophs) and CRF receptors on a third type (lactotrophs).

SECRETION OF GROWTH HORMONE BY 5,6-EPOXYEICOSATRIENOIC ACID IN NORMAL RAT PITUITARY CELLS

47

J.R. Cashman, D. Grandsaert, R.I. Weiner
University of California San Francisco, San Francisco, California

Growth hormone profoundly influences development, differentiation, and metabolism. The regulation of growth hormone (GH) secretion is primarily under the control of peptide hypothalamic GH-releasing factor and a GH-release-inhibiting factor (somatostatin). Thyroid and glucocorticoid hormones stimulate GH synthesis in cultured rat pituitary cells probably by regulating specific mRNAs. GH can also be released from somatotrophs by prostaglandin E_2 (PGE_2). In addition to the prostaglandin pathway, two other arachidonate metabolic pathways (i.e., lipoxygenase and epoxygenase) may also participate in the mediation of GH release. The epoxide metabolite of arachidonic acid: 5,6-epoxyeicosatrienoic acid, 5,6-EET, stimulates the release of GH from normal rat pituitary cells.

Normal female rat anterior pituitary cells were isolated, dispersed and grown for 24 hours in wells coated with corneal extracellular matrix. Cells were determined to be viable before and after challenge experiments by observing the exclusion of trypan blue dye. GH was quantitated from each sample with a double antibody radioimmunoassay.

GH secretion was greatly stimulated in a time and dose dependent fashion by 5,6-EET. GH release from normal rat pituitary cells reached apparent maximal values at 50 µM 5,6-EET. Employing 50 µM 5,6-EET, a time course study revealed an apparent maximal response after only 10 minutes. In both cases 5,6-EET produced a 13-17 fold increase in GH release compared to basal levels.

These data suggest that (1) Cytochrome P-450 epoxygenase may provide a mediator for GH release and (2) that 5,6-EET may be one of the most potent intracellular mediators for GH release known. We are currently investigating the molecular mechanism for this remarkable process.

INOSITOL PHOSPHATES, DIACYLGLYCEROL, AND ARACHIDONIC ACID IN GnRH ACTION 48

J.P. Chang, R.O. Morgan, K.J. Catt
Endo. & Reprod. Res. Branch, NICHD, Bethesda, Maryland.

GnRH-stimulated LH release is accompanied by rapid increases (within 15 sec) of 50-100 nM in intracellular $[Ca^{2+}]$, and the LH response is mediated by Ca^{2+}-dependent mechanisms that involve both arachidonic acid (AA) and protein kinase C (PKC) pathways. In dispersed rat anterior pituitary cells prelabelled to equilibrium with $[^3H]$-inositol, GnRH treatment caused increases in levels of inositol-1,4,5-tris- (IP_3), inositol-1,4-di-, and inositol-4-mono-phosphate (I-4-P) within 15 sec. The GnRH-induced increases in inositol phosphates were reversed by the addition of a GnRH antagonist. GnRH also elevated diacylglycerol (DG) levels in $[^{14}C]$-glycerol or $[^{14}C]$-AA prelabelled gonadotropes within 15 sec. Although the initial elevation of IP_3 was not uniformly maintained in all cell preparations, marked and prolonged increases in I-4-P, a specific metabolite of IP_3, were consistently observed during continuous GnRH action. These results indicate that GnRH-induced phosphatidyl-4,5-bisphosphate (PIP_2) hydrolysis is not only rapid, but is also sustained throughout the duration of GnRH action. IP_3 acts on intracellular receptor sites to mobilize stored Ca^{2+}. DG is a known activator of PKC as well as a source of AA, which, like IP_3, may also regulate Ca^{2+} metabolism. The LH response to AA in a pituitary cell column perifusion system resembled the initial, rapid phase of LH release induced by GnRH, whereas the response to synthetic DG or phorbol ester coincided with only the second phase of the GnRH-stimulated LH secretion. Pretreatment with nordihydroguaiaretic acid (NDGA, inhibitor of AA metabolism) and retinal (inhibitor of PKC activation) reduced the first and second phases of the LH response to GnRH, respectively, and exposure to both NDGA and retinal completely abolished the LH response. These results suggest that phospholipase C-dependent hydrolysis of PIP_2 is a primary event in GnRH action. The resulting products, IP_3, DG, and AA, represent intracellular signals that mediate components of the secretory response to the releasing peptide. IP_3 and AA may participate in the early LH response, while the DG-activated PKC probably mediates the prolonged phase of GnRH-induced LH release.

LEUKOTRIENES C4 AND D4 ARE POTENT STIMULATORS OF LHRH RELEASE IN VITRO. 49

K. Gerozissis, C. Rougeot, F. Dray
INSERM U. 207 - Institut Pasteur, URIA, 75015 Paris.

Prostaglandin E2 (PGE2), 12-hydroxyeicosatetraenoic acid (12-HETE) and leukotrienes C4 and D4 are produced by the rat hypothalamus predominantly in the median eminence (ME). PGE2 and 12-HETE were shown to stimulate the release of LHRH by the ME (1). Furthermore LTC4 has recently been shown to act directly on the hypophysis increasing LH secretion at concentrations as low as 10^{-14} M (2). Therefore we have investigated the effect of leukotrienes on LHRH release from rat ME using a large spectrum of concentrations (10^{-6} to 10^{-20} M).

Two MEs/tube were incubated for 30 min at 37°C in 0.4 ml Krebs Ringer bicarbonate glucose buffer, pH 7.4 containing 2.3×10^{-5} M bacitracin and 5×10^{-5} M ascorbic acid. LHRH, somatostatin (SRIF) and rat Growth Hormone Releasing Factor (GRF) were radioimmunoassayed in the supernantants. LTC4 significantly stimulated LHRH release (two fold), showing a bimodal pattern of action, with two equipotent maxima observed at 10^{-8} and 10^{-16} M. At 10^{-10} and 10^{-20} M LTC4 did not alter basal LHRH release.

LTD4 also stimulated LHRH release but with a different dose-response curve. The maximum (two fold) was obtained at 10^{-8}, 10^{-10} M and no effect was observed at lower concentrations. LTE4 had no significant effect on LHRH release at 10^{-8} and 10^{-16} M. LTB4 stimulated significantly LHRH release only at 10^{-6} M. 80% of $[^3H]$ LTC4, incubated with ME under the same conditions, was found unaltered, after HPLC analysis. LTC4-induced LHRH release was selective, since no significant change of SRIF and GRF release was observed.

These results strengthen the hypothesis for a biological role of the peptidoleukotrienes on the regulation of LH secretion, suggesting, particularly for LTC4, a dual effect at both the hypothalamic and hypophyseal levels.

1. Gerozissis et al, Neuroendocrinology (1985) 40:272
2. Hulting et al, Proc. Natl. Acad. Sci. (1985) 82:3834

PITUITARY CYCLIC AMP RESPONSE TO CRF ADMINISTRATION IN VIVO 50

G.J. Kant, M.A. Oleshansky, D.D. Walczak, E.H. Mougey, and J.L. Meyerhoff
Dept Medical Neurosciences, Walter Reed Army Institute of Research, Washington DC 20307

The hypothalamic peptide, corticotropin releasing factor (CRF), isolated and characterized by Vale and colleagues in 1981 has been shown to be a potent secretagogue of ACTH and related pituitary hormones both in vivo and in vitro. The in vitro CRF-stimulated release of ACTH is parallelled by concomitant increases in pituitary adenylate cyclase activity and levels of cyclic AMP. Thus it has been suggested that cyclic AMP is involved in the release or synthesis of pituitary hormones regulated by CRF.

The present study was conducted to assess the response of pituitary cyclic AMP in vivo to CRF administration. Rats were anaesthetized and implanted with indwelling jugular catheters 3 days prior to CRF administration. In the first experiment, rats were pretreated with either normal sera or specific CRF antisera. Six min later, rats were given a second iv injection of either CRF (5ug) or vehicle. Rats were killed by decapitation 15 min following the second injection. Plasma was assayed for ACTH and pituitaries were assayed for cyclic AMP by radioimmunoassays.

CRF administration markedly increased levels of pituitary cyclic AMP (7 fold) in normal sera pretreated rats. In CRF antisera pretreated rats, the increase in pituitary cyclic AMP following CRF was attenuated (2 fold increase). CRF also increased plasma ACTH levels and antisera pretreatment lowered basal and CRF-stimulated ACTH levels.

In a second experiment, CRF was administered to separate groups of animals maintained on reverse lighting regimens. Animals were not pretreated with antisera in this experiment. CRF was adminstered at lights "on" for one group of rats and at lights "off" for the other group. Both pituitary cyclic AMP and plasma ACTH responses to CRF (5ug) were much larger at lights "on" than at lights "off".

Taken together these experiments demonstrate similar responses of pituitary cyclic AMP synthesis and ACTH release to administration of CRF in vivo and support the hypothesis that cyclic AMP is involved in the release of ACTH.

SOMATOSTATIN RECEPTORS ON GH, TSH AND PRL CELLS : PHARMACOLOGICAL CHARACTERIZATION OF 125I NTyr SRIF BINDING SITES AND COUPLING TO ADENYLATE CYCLASE. 51

S. Krantic, P. Bertrand, C. Shu, A. Enjalbert, C. Kordon and J. Epelbaum
U. 159 INSERM, 2 ter rue d'Alésia, 75014 Paris, France.

Somatostatin (SRIF) can inhibit GH, TSH and PRL secretion from anterior pituitary cells in culture. In the present work, we characterized the pharmacological properties of SRIF receptors localized on the three target cells of the neurohormone and we further defined their coupling with adenylate cyclase. We checked the ability of 14 structural agonists of SRIF to displace 125I NTyr SRIF binding from pituitary cell membranes and their potency to inhibit adenylate cyclase activity and we measured the effect of those analogs on basal or GRF stimulated GH secretion and on TRH stimulated TSH and PRL secretion. There was a very good correlation (r = 0.98) between the displacement of 125I NTyr SRIF and the inhibition of adenylate cyclase activity by the analogs. The effects of analogs on the three hormones tested also followed the same order of potency. Furthermore pretreatment of the cells with pertussis toxin (10 ug/ml for 24 h) which blocks negative receptor cyclase coupling through guanine nucleotide dependent transducing protein (Ni) blocked somatostatin inhibition of PRL as well as of GH secretion.

We conclude from our data that SRIF binding sites located on three target cell types of the anterior pituitary represent a unique class of receptors, all negatively coupled with adenylate cyclase.

ROLE OF Na^+ AND Ca^{2+} IN DOPAMINE INHIBITION OF STIMULATED PROLACTIN RELEASE BY 7315a AND MtTW15 RAT PITUITARY TUMORS 52

J. Lafond, C. Bouvier, R. Collu
Research Unit on Reproductive and Developmental Biology, Pediatric Research Center, Hôpital Ste-Justine and University of Montreal, Montreal, Canada, H3T 1C5

The secretion of prolactin (PRL) by normal cells is under a tonic inhibitory control exerted by dopamine (DA) through specific receptors. We have recently demonstrated that Na^+ is essential for DA inhibition of baseline pituitary PRL release (Endocrinology 114: 1302, 1984) and that Ca^{2+} is probably the main second messenger involved both in stimulated and inhibited PRL release (Proc Endocr Soc, 1986, abstract 497). Recently, we have performed several in vitro experiments with cells obtained from 7315a and MtTW15 tumors that possess high affinity DA receptors but are resistant to dopaminergic inhibition of PRL release. The cells were enzymatically dispersed and subsequently plated in multi well dishes and cultured for 4 days in DMEM medium. On the fifth day, the cells were washed and then incubated for 30 min in simili-DMEM media with or without Na^+ and in the presence of BAY K 8644, A23187, TRH, Nifedipine or DA alone or in various combinations. PRL release by the cells was determined by RIA under basal and experimental conditions. With both types of tumoral cells, DA and Nifedipine were completely incapable of inducing an inhibition of basal PRL release in the presence or in the absence of Na^+. BAY K 8644, A23187 and TRH stimulated PRL release with or without Na^+ but the stimulatory effects of BAY K 8644 and A23187 were enhanced in the absence of Na^+. PRL release by 7315a cells when stimulated by BAY K 8644, A23187 or TRH could be inhibited by DA with or without Na^+, while DA was incapable of inhibiting PRL release by MtTW15 cells stimulated by BAY K 8644 or A23187. These data suggest the existence of a difference between 7315a and MtTW15 mechanisms of resistance to DA inhibitory action and their location at two different cellular sites.

SUPPRESSION OF TRH-INDUCED $^{45}Ca^{2+}$ FLUX IN 7315a TUMOR CELLS 53

I.S. Login, A.M. Judd, W.D. Jarvis, R.M. MacLeod
University of Virginia School of Medicine, Charlottesville, Virginia 22908

7315a prolactin-secreting tumor cells appear to have a defect in Ca^{2+} handling systems: basal prolactin release is low compared with normal cells, dopamine inhibits prolactin release only when Ca^{2+} mobilization is augmented, and D-600 does not block uptake of $^{45}Ca^{2+}$. Ca^{2+}-dependent TRH-evoked prolactin release is also markedly suppressed in 7315a cells. In this study, we compared TRH-induced $^{45}Ca^{2+}$ flux in normal pituitary and 7315a tumor cells. After 2-4 days in culture, cells of the female rat anterior pituitary or of the 7315a tumor were prelabeled in 1.5 mM $^{45}CaCl_2$ (2.5 hr) and perifused at 37°C with unlabeled media. After a 45 min washout, 1-min fractions (0.54 ml/min) were collected to monitor simultaneously fractional $^{45}Ca^{2+}$ efflux and prolactin release. The integrated response of each parameter to a 2-min pulse of TRH was determined. In 2-7 columns each, for 0 (control), 0.1, 1, 10 and 100 nM TRH, integrated fractional efflux (X 10^4) in normal cells was (mean $\pm$ SE) 5 ± 6, 23 ± 3, 213 ± 82, 389 ± 79 and 653 ± 59, respectively; whereas in 7315a cells for 0, 1, 10, 100 and 1000 nM TRH, the values were $-.8 \pm 7$, 27 ± 9, 87 ± 11, 164 ± 27 and 123 ± 20, respectively. Prolactin responses showed a similarly striking dose-dependent difference between the normal and 7315a cells. At 10 nM TRH, inositol trisphosphate production (mobilizing intracellular Ca^{2+}) was only 25% less in 7315a cells than in normal cells, versus a 4.5-fold reduction in Ca^{2+} mobilization. Thus 7315a cells have been directly shown to have an abnormality of Ca^{2+} kinetics. These tumor cells have evolved into a state of essentially autonomous secretion apparently because calcium exchange or storage is so low that physiologically, the basal secretory rate can be neither suppressed nor stimulated. In effect, stimulus and secretion mechanisms seem to have become uncoupled through an alteration in calcium ion kinetics. This concept may have relevance for selected patients with prolactinomas refractory to medical therapy.

THYROLIBERIN (TRH) RELEASE IS DEPENDENT ON EXTRACELLULAR Ca+ AND PARTIALLY MEDIATED BY AN ACTIVATION OF PROTEIN KINASE C IN HYPOTHALAMIC CELLS GROWN IN SFM. 54

C. Loudes, A. Faivre-Bauman, A. Barret and A. Tixier-Vidal
UA_CNRS 1115, Collège de France, Paris (FRANCE)

Hypothalamic cell cultures were initated from fetal mouse hypothalamus on the 16th day of gestation, and grown in a serum-free defined medium which allows neuronal maturation up to complete synaptogenesis after 10-12 days in vitro (FAIVRE-BAUMAN et al, 1984). At that stage, Thyroliberin (TRH) neurons express release capacities in response to K^+ depolarization in the presence of extracellular Ca^{++} (LOUDES et al, 1983). This is correlated with acute synaptic vesicles depletion (TIXIER-VIDAL et al, 1986).

Several neurotransmitters were tested as effectors of TRH release in the absence or in the presence of K^+. None of the following ones were efficient: Serotonine, Histamine, Nor-Adrenaline, Somatostatine or GABA. In contrast, Dopamine in presence of 60 mM K^+ elicited, in a dose dependent manner, a higher TRH release than depolarization alone (up to 600% of the basal release). This was blocked by Fluophenazine, while sulpiride, an effector of D2 type receptors, had no effect.

The possible involvement of protein kinase C activation was investigated, using di-acylglycerol(DAG) or phorbol esters. DAG provoked TRH release, with a dose-response curve, but its effect was not so constantly observed than that of TPA. Kinetic studies show that TPA effect reaches a plateau after 30 min. and is maximum at 10^{-7}M. At this concentration, the TRH response remains however lower than in presence of 60 mM K^+. In absence of extracellular Ca^{++}, or in presence of cobalt, TPA effect on TRH release is reduced by about 1/3 . Inactive analogs of TPA, such as 12-13 dodecanoate 4-ß phorbol, had no effect on TRH release. Dopamine added together with TPA could not increase the response more than TPA alone.

From these results, we may conclude that the stimulation of TRH release is mediated by an activation both of voltage-dependent Ca^{++} channel, and of protein kinase C. Since Dopamine amplifies the effect of high K^+ response but not that of TPA, it is suggested that DA might induce a breakdown of phosphatidylinositol, which is presently under investigation.

THE DESENSITIZATION PHASE OF GnRH STIMULATED LH RELEASE FROM SHEEP PITUITARY CELLS IN PERIFUSION 55

R.P. McIntosh, J.E.A. McIntosh, L. Starling, W.R. Smith*
Wellington Clinical School of Medicine, University of Otago at Wellington, New Zealand and *University of Guelph, Ontario, Canada.

The diminished release of LH from sheep pituitary cells upon continued stimulation by GnRH ("desensitization") can readily be interpreted by a simple model involving a limited availability of an essential component in the mechanism of release. Recovery of sensitivity of cells after pulsatile or continuous GnRH stimulation would then be controlled by the rate of regeneration of the essential component which would account for the dependency of response on the frequency of pulsatile stimulation. However, this model leaves unexplained our observation that cells desensitized to a maximally stimulating concentration of GnRH can produce a further release of LH to even higher levels of GnRH ("supramaximal stimulation"). A model including a shift in dose response curve which reduces sensitivity of the cells to GnRH after the initial receptor occupancy would account for this.

Using a multiple column, computer-controlled perifusion apparatus we have quantitatively characterized the dynamics of these desensitization related events, investigated some possible factors controlling them and tested predictions from both models.

The rate of appearance and size of the supramaximal response depends on the rate at which desensitization is occurring and takes about 40 min to become maximal. Neither the supramaximal response, nor the rate of appearance of and recovery from desensitization, are altered by substances modifying the cytoskeleton. The greatly increased rate of LH release immediately upon stimulation with phorbol esters, and the reduced rate of desensitization in comparison with responses to GnRH, indicate that availability of secretory granules and mechanistic events after stimulation of protein kinase C are unlikely to be limiting to cell responses. The presence of Li^+ causes a reduced rate of desensitization to GnRH and diminished supramaximal response. The relative desensitized response levels of LH using different concentrations of applied GnRH support predictions from neither model.

This signalling system has been shown to have characteristics of high responsiveness to increases at low levels of stimulation, lower responses to increases at high levels, and very low responses to any constant stimulation. While both models (limiting rate of regeneration of an essential component in the release mechanism and a shift in dose response characteristics after initial binding of agonist to receptor) explain most of these characteristics of the dynamic release of LH on stimulation with GnRH, further refinements are necessary.

SOMATOSTATINERGIC INHIBITION OF HYPOTHALAMIC AND ANTERIOR PITUITARY ADENYLATE CYCLASE ACTIVITY 56

G. Schettini, T. Florio, O. Meucci, E. Landolfi, M. Grimaldi, G. Magri
Dept Pharmacol, II Medical School, 80131 Naples, ITALY

Somatostatin (SRIF)-like immunoreactivity has been identified in the hypothalamus, and SRIF receptors have been characterized at pituitary level. SRIF role in the regulation of anterior pituitary (AP) hormone secretion has been extensively studied, while the postreceptor mechanisms of its hypothalamic and AP action have not been fully characterized.

Here we report the SRIF inhibition of basal and stimulated adenylate cyclase (AC) activity in hypothalamic and AP membrane preparations. SRIF (1-100 uM) inhibits basal and 1 uM VIP stimulated hypothalamic AC activity, an effect shared also by the SRIF analogue SMS 201-995. GRF, which has been identified by immunocytochemistry at hypothalamic level, did not modified either basal or SRIF inhibited hypothalamic AC activity.

The studies conducted on AP membrane preparations showed that SRIF (1-100 uM) inhbited basal AC activity. Its inhibitory effect was also shown in presence of GRF (1-100 nM). Indeed SRIF inhibited in a non competitive manner GRF-stimulated anterior pituitary AC activity, increasing its effectiveness with the higher GRF concentrations. Forskolin stimulation of anterior pituitary AC activity was also inhibited by SRIF in a non competitive manner, an effect reverted by pretreatment of AP cells with pertussis toxin, that uncouples inhibitory receptors from AC catalytic subunit.

These results show that hypothalamic SRIF receptors are coupled with AC enzyme in an inhibitory fashion. Similarly anterior pituitary SRIF receptor stimulation inhibits basal, GRF or forskolin enhanced AC activity, likely interacting with the inhibitory regulatory subunit. (Supported by a grant from the Italian MPI 60%)

ADENOSINE MODULATION OF ANTERIOR PITUITARY ADENYLATE CYCLASE ACTIVITY 57

G. Schettini, E. Landolfi, O. Meucci, T. Florio
Dept Pharmacol, II Medical School, 80131 Naples, ITALY

Adenosine (ADO) modulates hormonal secretion and adenylate cyclase (AC) activity in several tissues. Two adenosine-reactive sites coupled with AC have been identified: the extracellular R and the intracellular P site. The R site requires the integrity of the ribose ring and expresses two receptor subtypes, A1/Ri (high affinity inhibitory receptor) and A2/Ra (low affinity stimulatory receptor). The P site requires an intact purine ring and mediates inhibition only.

We report here the effect of ADO and its analogs N6-phenylisopropyladenosine (PIA), 2-chloroadenosine (2-Cl ADO), on basal and stimulated anterior pituitary AC activity. The experiments were performed on membrane preparations using 10 uM RO 20-1724, a phosphodiesterase inhibitor which does not block ADO receptors. ADO (1 to 100 uM) dose dependently inhibited basal AC activity (maximum -40%). PIA (3 to 300 uM) and 2-ClADO (100 nM to 30 uM) showed a bifasic pattern of response, being inhibitory at low, but stimulatory at high micromolar concentrations. The effects of PIA (inhibition -15%; stimulation +38%) were more pronounced than 2-ClADO (-7%; +15%). In stimulated conditions, ADO reduced both 100 nM GRF (-35%) and 1 uM VIP (-30%) activation of AC. PIA potentiated 10 uM DA inhibition of AC activity. At lower concetrations PIA inhibited 1 uM VIP stimulation of AC, while the highest PIA concentration showed no addictive stimulatory effect with VIP on AC activity.

These results show the presence on anterior pituitary cells of both types of ADO receptors, R and P, and their coupling with AC activity. Moreover the R site appears to be expressed in both receptor subtypes, as shown by the AC bifasic response to PIA and 2-ClADO. It is suggestive that these receptors may be involved in the regulation of anterior pituitary hormone release.

GROWTH INHIBITION OF PITUITARY TUMOR CELLS BY GM_1, PHORBOL ESTER, FORSKOLIN, AND BUTYRATE. 58

M.A. Sortino, S.T. Summers, R. Steward, A. Fedson, M.J. Cronin
University of Virginia, Charlottesville, Virginia 22908

Identification of cellular mechanisms that have the potential to regulate cell division is essential to fully understand tumor biology, growth and differentiation. We tested several agents known to affect specific processes for their effects on 235-1 cell growth. This rat cell line was derived from the prolactin-secreting 7315a pituitary tumor (ACTA Endocrinol 106: 459, 1984) and was grown in RPMI-1640 medium supplimented with 7.5% horse and 2.5% fetal calf serum. Cells were added at 50,000/2 cm^2 well and had a 50% plating efficiency. The following agents were tested: ganglioside GM_1 [associated with oncogenic transformation], phorbol myristate acetate [PMA, a direct stimulator of protein kinase C], forskolin [a direct stimulator of catalytic adenylate cyclase], and butyrate [a stimulus for G1 arrest]. These agents were added to 235-1 cells a day after passaging, and then renewed daily except for GM_1, which was added only once. Neither 0.01% ethanol vehicle nor the protein kinase C inactive 4-alpha-didecanoate affected 235-1 cell number. In contrast, all of the test agents significantly reduced cell number as follows: 100 uM GM_1 (-64 $\pm$ 3% at 3 days); 100 nM PMA (-48 $\pm$ 4% at 3 days & -32 $\pm$ 9% at 5 days); 10 uM forskolin (-42 $\pm$ 6% at 5 days) PMA + forskolin (-85 $\pm$ 1% at 5 days); 1 mM butyrate (-88 $\pm$ 3% at 5 days). It was of interest that the combination of PMA (100 nM) and forskolin (10 uM) induced a profound increase in the size and number of processes of the cells. These data provide an entré for more detailed assessment of the molecular requirements for growth and differentiation in 235-1 pituitary tumor cells.

(Supported by FIDIA, Italy, RCDA 1KO4NS00601 & MSTP GM 07267)

PROTEIN KINASE C ENHANCES GROWTH HORMONE RELEASING FACTOR (GRF) AND CORTICOTROPIN RELEASING FACTOR (CRF) STIMULATED CYCLIC AMP (cAMP) PRODUCTION IN ANTERIOR PITUITARY (AP) CELLS 59

S.T. Summers, A.J. Baertschi, J.R. Zysk, M.J. Cronin
University of Virginia, Charlottesville, Virginia 22908

Influences of protein kinase C on cAMP production have been observed in a number of tissues, including the AP. We have characterized the ability of activators of protein kinase C (phorbol esters, teleocidin) to augment GRF- and CRF-stimulated cAMP accumulation in dispersed and cultured AP cells.

The time course of phorbol myristate acetate (PMA) potentiation of GRF-induced cAMP accumulation is rapid; after 60 sec, coincubation with GRF (100 nM) + PMA (100 nM) produced significantly higher cAMP levels than incubation with GRF alone. Cells exposed to GRF + PMA continue to display increased cAMP content up to 2 hr; longer incubations with GRF + PMA result in lower cAMP levels than GRF alone. The mean ED_{50}'s from independent studies were 9 nM for PMA, 4 nM for phorbol dibutyrate, and 7 ng/ml for teleocidin, a stimulator of protein kinase C without a phorbol structure. These concentrations are consistant with the binding and activity constants of protein kinase C. The PMA-induced increase in GRF responsiveness appears to be due solely to an increased efficacy because the GRF potency was not altered. The ability of somatostatin to reduce GRF-stimulated cAMP levels was not abolished by cotreatment with PMA.

Stimulation of protein kinase C also rapidly enhances CRF-initiated cAMP accumulation. This potentiation is greater than with GRF, reaching an elevation of 900% of CRF alone at 15 min versus only 200% with GRF. The mean ED_{50}'s were 10 nM for PMA, 4 nM for phorbol dibutyrate, and 5 ng/ml for teleocidin, while 4-alpha-PMA, which is inactive at protein kinase C, was without effect. We conclude that protein kinase C can determine the efficiency with which GRF and CRF receptors generate a cAMP signal in AP cells.

(Supported by AM32632, AM 22125, 1KO4NS00601, HL31133 & FIDIA, Italy)

CHARACTERIZATION OF PGE2 RECEPTORS IN PORCINE AND MURINE ANTERIOR PITUITARIES. 60

C.Tiberghien, V. Fafeur, A. Wisner-Provost, M.C. Bommelaer, F. Haour, F. Dray.
INSERM U. 207 - Institut Pasteur, URIA, 75015 Paris

Specific PGE_2 binding sites have been previously demonstrated in rat anterior pituitary (1). These data have been confirmed and developped using porcine pituitary membranes and rat pituitary cell preparations.

The binding of $[^3H]$ PGE_2 was achieved in PBS for two hours at 22°C. This binding was saturable and partially reversible with excess cold. Among the ions tested, Ca^{++}, Cu^{++}, Mg^{++}, a significant increase of the specific binding to pituitary membranes was found with Mg^{++} ion only.

Saturation experiments followed by Scatchard analysis of the binding data indicate the presence of two classes of binding sites. The KD of the high affinity binding sites was 1.5 nM (n1 in the order of 5 fmol/mg protein). The KD of the lower affinity sites was 25 nM (n2 in the order of 25 fmol/mg protein). The affinity of both classes of sites were in the same order in the presence of Mg^{++} (10 mM). The specificity of the binding was investigated using various analogues in competitive experiments. The order of potency was PGE2 $\geqslant$ PGE1 > 11 epi PGE2 > 13-14 DH PGE2 > 8 iso PGE2. The biological activity of these analogues was measured by their capacity to induce GH release in isolated rat pituitary cells in perifusion (10^{-6} M). The biological activity was highly correlated with the binding capacity (r=0.8). Both very weak competitive effect and biological activity were observed with 15 keto PGE2, 5 trans PGE2, PGB2, PGD2, PGF2α and 15 epi PGE2 . The average number of sites was 1000 sites/cell (ligand 2 nM) when measured on a cells population obtained from rat anterior pituitary following a Percoll gradient.

These results demonstrate the presence of high affinity and low capacity PGE2 receptors in the pituitary cells. This fact, correlated with the recent finding that GRF induced PGE2 release (2), suggests that PGE2 is among the physiological regulators of the somatotroph cells.

1. Malet et al, Brain Research 236, 227, 1982
2. Fafeur et al, BBRC 126, (2) 725, 1985

CHEMICAL CROSSLINKING OF A GROWTH HORMONE RELEASING FACTOR BINDING SITE IN ANTERIOR PITUITARY CELLS 61

J.R. Zysk, M.O. Thorner, J.M. Anderson and M.J. Cronin
University of Virginia, Charlottesville, Virginia 22908

Growth hormone-releasing factor (GRF) stimulates the secretion of growth hormone (GH) from the anterior pituitary (AP) somatotroph and is closely coupled to the cyclic AMP generating system. However, little is known concerning the nature of the GRF receptor itself. Therefore, we undertook a study of the GRF receptor by chemically coupling ^{125}I-His^{1}Nleu^{27} hGRF (132) (GRF analog) to cultured rat anterior pituitary cells with the protein crosslinker disuccinimidyl suberate (DSS, 0.1 mM). Cells were maintained in 24 well plates and allowed to bind the labeled ligand in the absence or presence of unlabeled peptide hormones prior to the addition of DSS. After stopping the reaction, whole cell extracts were prepared from the crosslinked cells and then subjected to SDS polyacrylamide gel electrophoresis followed by autoradiography of the dried gels. After binding for 20 min at 22°, the analog was found to crosslink to protein bands of 72, 50 and 26 kilodaltons (kd). The 72 kd band was found to be serum albumin (which was used as a carrier in the initial studies). The 50 kd band diminished to equal extents when cells were labeled in the presence of excess unlabeled (luM) analog, human GRF or vasoactive intestinal peptide (VIP). This band may be similar or identical to the 50 kd receptor for VIP described in other tissues. The 26 kd band was diminished in the presence of excess unlabeled analog and GRF but not VIP. Thus, the best candidate for the putative GRF receptor (or subunit) appears to be the 26 kd band. The GRF analog (1-100 nM) increased cellular cyclic AMP levels to an extent comparable to human GRF. The analog also induced GH secretion in anterior pituitary cells when tested by the reverse hemolytic plaque assay. These results suggest an approximate molecular weight of 26 kd for the GRFspecific binding site and indicate that his^1-Nleu^{27} binds to both GRF and VIP-preferring sites in the anterior pituitary cells. Supported by AM32632, AM22125, RCDA 1K04NS00601.

DUAL EFFECT OF GABA ON TRH-INDUCED TSH RELEASE FROM PERIFUSED RAT PITUITARIES. 62

H. Astier, J.P. Roussel, L. Tapia-Arancibia
Lab. Neuroendocrinology, University of Montpellier II, 34060 Montpellier, France.

The presence of GABA in hypophysial portal blood at concentrations higher than in systemic blood (RACAGNI et al. 1982, Life Sci. 31, 823) and of high affinity GABA receptors in the anterior pituitary (AP)(GRANDISON and GUIDOTTI, 1979, Endoc. 105, 754) suggest a regulatory role of GABA directly at the AP level. Thus, we have investigated the effect of GABA on the spontaneous and TRH-induced TSH release *in vitro*.

Quartered AP from adult male rats were superfused in oxygenated medium 199 (GIBCO) containing BSA (0.25 %) ; Ascorbic acid (2 mg %) and bacitracin (3 mg %), to prevent TRH degradation. TSH was measured by a specific RIA (from NIH). After 2 hours of superfusion for stabilization of the system, samples were taken every 3 min for 30 min in order to measure spontaneous release of TSH.

The effect of GABA (at concentrations ranging from 10^{-8}M to 10^{-4}M) was tested 30 min before and during a 6 min pulse of TRH (10^{-8}M) which stimulates TSH release by 220 %. GABA did not modify the spontaneous release of TSH at any dose tested but exhibited a dual effect on the stimulated TSH response according to the dose : at 10^{-8}M, GABA increased the TRH-induced response by 200 % ($p < 0.001$),then by only 30 % at 3.10^{-8}M and 6.10^{-8}M ; in contrast, from the concentration of 10^{-7}M to 10^{-4}M GABA suppressed the stimulatory effect of TRH. The inhibitory effect of GABA (10^{-7}M) was reversed by the antagonists bicuculline (10^{-5}M), picrotoxine (10^{-5}M), and by a specific GABA-A antagonist SR-95103 (CHAMBON et al., 1985, Proc. Nat. Acad. Sci. USA 82, 1832). In addition, Diazepam (7.10^{-9}M) that we have previously shown to inhibit the TSH response to TRH, potentiated (by 100 %) the GABA-stimulated TSH response to TRH (for a GABA concentration of 6.10^{-8}M).

Our results suggest a dual GABAergic control of TRH-induced TSH release, likely mediated by GABA-A receptors type, at the AP level.

OPIATE-THYROID HORMONE INTERACTIONS IN THE REGULATION OF TSH SECRETION IN THE RAT. 63

L.A. Berglund, W.J. Millard, S.M. Gabriel and J.W. Simpkins, Department of Pharmacodynamics, College of Pharmacy, University of Florida, Gainesville, FL 32610.

Studies were undertaken to determine the role of thyroid hormone in the suppression of TSH by opiates. Serum samples were collected by decapitation 1, 3, 6, 12, 14 or 48 hours after ovariectomized female rats were implanted with one sustained release 75 mg morphine (MORP) or placebo (PLAC) pellet. Serum TSH, T_3 and T_4 levels were measured by RIA. MORP decreased TSH by 44% at 1 hour, 83% by 3 hours and TSH remained depressed by 38% through 48 hours. T_4 levels were significantly (p.0.05) reduced from 12 to 24 hours after MORP and T_3 levels were not affected.

In a second experiment thyroidectomized (THX) or control male rats were implanted with MORP or PLAC 24 hours before serum collection. MORP significantly decreased TSH in controls but had no effect on TSH in THX rats. T_3 and T_4 levels were significantly decreased in THX rats. MORP significantly decreased T_3 and T_4 levels in control rats but had no effect in THX rats. Thus it appears that the suppression by morphine of TSH release requires circulating thyroid hormone.

In a third experiment, THX rats were chronically treated with MORP or PLAC, then injected (s.c.) with saline or 1, 10, or 100 fg T_4/Kg BW 24 hours prior to serum collection. MORP treatment alone did not affect serum TSH in THX rats, as observed in the second experiment. T_4 replacement causes a dose-dependent decrease in TSH in both MORP and PLAC rats. However, the 10fg T_4/Kg BW dose decreased TSH significantly more in MORP than in PLAC rats. Also, TSH was significantly lower (73.61%) in MORP than in PLAC treated rats after the 100fg/Kg dose of T_4. Thus, while chronic MORP treatment is ineffective in suppressing TSH in THX rats, MORP interacts with thyroid hormone to reduce TSH release. These data suggest that morphine exerts its inhibitory effect on TSH secretion by increasing hypothalamic sensitivity to thyroid hormone negative feedback. (Supported in Part by AG 02021 and HD14075).

THE SECRETION OF TSH IN ACROMEGALY MEASURED BY A SENSITIVE TSH ASSAY 63a

P.C. Eskildsen, A. Kruse, C.B. Kirkegaard
Medical Dept.C, Neurosurg.Dept.H, Glostrup Hospital and Medical Dept.E, Frederiksberg Hospital, Copenhagen, Denmark

Unresponsiveness of serum TSH to iv TRH has been seen in about 25% of acromegalic patients, and so far explained either by the occurrence of a nodular goiter, or by a possible selective pituitary TSH insufficiency. The problems of measuring TSH values < 3µU/ml with the traditional TSH assay supervened, but they are now solved by the commercial super sensitive, double antibody TSH assay (Sucrosep, Boots-Celltech, detect.limit 0.05µU/ml)

By this assay we measured basal and peak values of serum TSH after 200µg TRH iv in 13 active acromegalics (8♂ + 5♀, aged 37-80 years) and in 4 nonsubstituted pituitary insufficient patients (1♂ + 3♀, aged 40-63 years) using 40 normal controls as reference material.

While the pituitary insufficient patients had undetectable basal TSH (<0.05µU/ml) and no response to TRH, the acromegalics showed a 5-20 (median 6.7) fold increase of serum TSH from basal levels of 0.07-1.9µU/ml. Four of these acromegalics were "non-responders" with the traditional TSH assay, but showed a marked response to TRH, measured with the sensitive assay, but from low basal levels (0.07-0.31µU/ml) compared to normal controls (0.41-2.4µU/ml). The thyroid hormone levels of these 4 acromegalics were not different from the levels of the remaining 9 (T 4: 69-95 vs 63-106 nmol/l T 3:1.31 - 2.12 vs 0.91-2.24 nmol/l).

By this sensitive TSH assay it has been possible to demonstrate that euthyroid patients with active acromegaly do respond to TRH, but sometimes from a low basal level of serum TSH.

CHOLINERGIC SUPPRESSION OF TSH SECRETION: THERAPEUTIC APPLICATIONS 64

H.G. Fein, A.J. Ahmann, J.E. Hennessey, N.E. Butkus, D.M. Kornhauser, B.G. Petty, R.C. Smallridge
Depts. of Medicine, Walter Reed Army Institute of Research, Washington, D.C. 20307 and Johns Hopkins Medical Institutions, Baltimore, MD 21205

We previously showed that acetylcholine, through muscarinic receptors, suppressed basal and TRH--stimulated TSH secreted by cells cultured from two human thyrotropic pituitary adenomas. A 39 yr old man recently presented with hyperthyroidism due to a TSH-secreting macroadenoma (Free Thyroxine Index FTI : 7.04, nl:2.13-5.66; TSH:3.4 µU/ml). TRH did not increase TSH. Since it has been suggested that drugs which block calcium influx or H2 receptors may suppress TSH, we performed separate 3-hr iv infusions of verapamil (15 mg) and ranitidine (75 mg). Neither affected basal or TRH-stimulated TSH.

Tissue obtained at surgery was enzymatically dispersed into 11 microwells at 370,000 cells/well. The cells rapidly monolayered and secreted TSH for more than 35 days (initially: 38.7 ± 6.7 µU/well/day). As in vivo, TSH release was not responsive to either 100 nM TRH (90.8% of secretory rate in control wells, NS), 100 µM verapamil (79.6%, NS), or 100 µM ranitidine (96.7%, NS). However, 10 µM acetylcholine with 10 µM physostigmine suppressed TSH to 50.2% of controls ($p<0.005$); this was blocked by addition of 1.0 µM atropine (100.1% of controls). TSH-induced hyperthyroidism persisted after partial adenomectomy despite subsequent megavoltage radiotherapy. Attempts were made then to lower TSH using drugs that increase cholinergic tone. Single oral doses of pyridostigmine were administered every 1-2 days and blood collected hourly. Twenty and 40 mg blocked the afternoon rise in TSH seen on a control day; 60 mg lowered TSH from 3.1 to 2.4 µU/ml at 6 h. Oral bethanechol (100 mg qid for 12 days) lowered thyroid hormones (FTI: 5.66) and TSH (1.8). No major side effects were noted.

Muscarinic agonists thus appear to suppress TSH secretion. The use of cholinergic agents may provide a new means of treatment for patients with TSH-secreting pituitary macroadenomas that cannot be controlled by more conventional modes of therapy.

SERUM TSH REDUCTION IN RESPONSE TO hpGRF ADMINISTRATION IN PATIENTS WITH PITUITARY DWARFISM 65

T.Hashimoto, T.Sato, K.Kawai, N.Ohba, F.Matsubara. Central Clinical Laboratory and Department of Pediatrics, Kanazawa University Hospital, Ishikawa, 920, Japan.

Although hpGRF-44 is believed to stimulate GH secretion selectively, a recent report by Smals et al. showed a transient PRL rise in young adults after hpGRF injection. Highly sensitive immunoradiometric assay (IRMA), which is now available, allows us to examine the specific effect of hpGRF on other pituitary hormones. We concentrated on TSH secretion. We examined the effects of intraveneous injection (1µg/kg) of synthetic hpGRF-44 on serum levels of anterior pituitary hormones in 13 patients with pituitary dwarfism (11 males and 2 females; aged 11-22 yrs.). Blood samples were collected before and 15, 30, 60, 90 and 120 min after GRF injection. Serum TSH was measured using a highly sensitive IRMA kit. Serum GH, PRL, LH, FSH, FT_3 and FT_4 were measured by conventional RIA kits. Serum GH levels increased in 11 out 13 patients. In contrast, serum TSH levels significantly decreased after GRF injection in all the patients tested. The mean reduction was 19.8 % at 30 min ($p<0.02$), 16.5 % at 60 min ($p<0.05$), 24.8 % at 90 min ($p<0.05$). Serum PRL levels showed a transient increase. FT_3 levels were significantly lowered at 90 min. ($p<0.05$). FT_4 levels did not change during the observation period. This study clearly demonstrates evidence of TSH reduction after administration of synthetic hpGRF-44. It is unlikely that this suppression is mediated through a decrease in TRH secretion in the hypothalamus. It is possible that the responses of TSH and PRL to hpGRF reflect an increase of dopamine in the hypothalamus. Further investigations are required to clarify the mechanism.

NEURO-HORMONAL REGULATION OF HUMAN TSH-SECRETING ADENOMA IN CELL CULTURE. 66

P. Jaquet, G. Gunz, I. Pellegrini, J. Hassoun
INSERM U 297, UER de Médecine Nord 13326 Marseille Cedex 15 FRANCE.

The present study describes the hormone release and its regulation by TRH, T3, dopamine, somatostatin and GRF from 9 different TSH-secreting pituitary adenomas cells cultured upon extracellular matrix in serum free conditions. The 24-hour hormone release into the medium by 10^6 cells varied according to cases (5-679ng for TSH, 14-1600ng for the alpha-subunit). The alpha-subunit/TSH ratio was 10±2.5 (M ± SE). Furthermore 5 tumors also released PRL (n=3) or GH (n=2). In these mixed tumors, the morphological studies with protein A gold immunotechnique demonstrated the colocalization in the same granules of GH or PRL and the alpha-subunit. The pharmacological studies yielded the following results : 1) T3, after 4-6 days of culture, produced a dose-dependent inhibition of TSH, TSH-alpha (half maximal concentration : $2\text{-}8 \times 10^{-11}$M) 2) TRH ($10^{-8}$M) elicited a 150-220% increase of TSH, TSH-alpha release in 3/9 cases. In 3 non responsive adenomas, the prolonged exposure of the cells (12 days) to TRH restaured its stimulatory effect upon TSH and TSH-alpha release. 3) Somatostatin and bromocriptine produced a dose-dependent inhibition of TSH, TSH-alpha release. Maximal inhibition varied from 20-50% with 10^{-8}M bromocriptine and 36-70% with 10^{-9}M somatostatin. 4) Finally in 3 different tumor cell cultures (2 TSH+GH, 1 TSH only secreting tumors) GRF produced a dose-dependent increase of TSH and TSH-alpha. Maximal stimulation of 260-458% was obtained at 10^{-10}M GRF. It was reversed by coincubation with somatostatin. From these datas it is concluded that : 1) the TSH secreting adenoma cells recover in vitro a near to normal responsiveness to thyroid hormone and TRH regulation. These data argue against the hypothesis of a primary resistance of the tumor cells to the thyroid hormone action. 2) The colocalization of GH (or PRL) and TSH-alpha in the same tumor cell associated with an unusual regulation of TSH release by somatostatin and GRF allows to hypothetize that in such patients the elevated plasma TSH levels can be, at least partly, related to GRF stimulation despite high plasma values of thyroid hormones.

THYROID-HYPOPHYSO-HYPOTHALAMIC AXIS OF THE GENETICALLY HYPOPROLACTINEMIC RATS (IPL NUDE RATS) 67

D. Jordan (1), I. Sabbagh (2), P. Guillaumot (3), M. Veisseire (1), J. Bertrand (3), H. Cohen (3)
(1) INSERM U 197, Faculté de Médecine Alexis-Carrel, 69372 Lyon ; (2) Institut Pasteur, Lyon ; (3) INSERM U 34, Hôpital Debrousse, 69322 Lyon, France.

The IPL nude rat, a mutant from Sprague-Dawley, is characterized by delayed puberty and an absence of lactation. We have previously reported that male and female rats are hypoprolactinemic. Among the postulated prolactin (PRL) releasing factors described, TRH seems to be the major one. As far as both TRH and thyroid axis hormones are involved in the regulation of PRL secretion, the present study estimates the thyrotropin function of the IPL nude versus normal rats, either at hypothalamic, pituitary or peripheric levels. Radioimmunoassayable hormones (TRH, TSH, T3, T4) were measured at different times over the 24 hour period (09, 11, 17, 20, 23, 02 h) in sacrificed male rats.

The following results were obtained : 1) Hypothalamic TRH content in the IPL nude rat showed comparable variations during the day whereas a slight increase was observed during the night characterized by a significant difference at 20 h. 2) Pituitary weight and TSH content were doubled in IPL nude rats. However, when expressed as µg TSH/µg protein or DNA, a significant increase was found only at 17 h and 20 h. 3) Serum TSH, T3 and T4 depicted similar variations except for minute but significant modifications, i.e. an increase of TSH at 17 h and 23 h and a decrease of T4 at 11 h in IPL nude rats.

In conclusion, the slight increase in hypothalamic TRH and pituitary TSH contents and the absence of main associated variations of serum TSH, T3 and T4 do not send support to the initial hypothesis. On the contrary, observed thyrotropin axis variations appeared rather as the consequence of hypoprolactinemia in the IPL nude rats.

ANTERIOR PITUITARY HORMONE RESPONSES DURING EUGLYCEMIC INSULIN CLAMP. 68

T.Hashimoto, I.Miyamoto, Y.Noto, F.Matsubara
Central Clinical Laboratory and the 1st Department of Internal Medicine, Kanazawa University Hospital, Ishikawa, 920, Japan.

In order to study the effect of insulin on anterior pituitary hormone release, we raised and maintained serum insulin at a high physiological level using the euglycemic insulin clamp, and kept serum glucose unchanged for four and a half hours with combined infusions of glucose and insulin. This technique eliminates the complication of hypoglycemic stress.

Four normal subjects and 8 patients with chemical diabetes mellitus were studied. Actrapid insulin was infused at 0.5mu/kg/min for 90min, 3.0mu/kg/min for 90 min and 10mu/kg/min for 90 min using a Biostator. The serum insulin concentration was acutely raised and maintained at approximately 50µu/ml by 0.5mu/kg/min infusion (0-90min) then raised to about 400µu/ml by 3.0mu/kg/min infusion (90-180min) and then raised again to about 800µu/ml by 10mu/kg/min infusion (180-270min). The serum glucose level was held constant at basal level during euglycemic clamp. Blood samples were taken before and 30 mins. after application of the insulin clamp, and at 30 min. intervals thereafter up to 270 mins. Serum TSH levels determined by highly sensitive immunoradiometric assay (Hoechst Co. West Germany) demonstrated a significant decrease ($p<0.001$) over the period from 30 min to 270 min. Serum GH, PRL, LH, FSH and cortisol levels did not change. The observations in this study clearly demonstrate that insulin suppresses pituitary TSH secretion. The absence of any reduction of PRL levels suggests that this suppression is not mediated through a decrease in TRH secretion in the hypothalamus. In conclusion, it is likely that TSH secretion is not regulated just by the thyroid feedback mechanism alone, but is under the inhibitory influence of endogenous insulin.

HYPOTHALAMIC CONTROL OF 5'-DEIODINASE ACTIVITY IN RAT ANTERIOR PITUITARY 69

M. Murakami, K. Tanaka, M.A. Greer Section of Endocrinology, Oregon Health Sciences University, Portland, Oregon 97201

The conversion of thyroxine (T_4) to triiodothyronine (T_3) by Type-II iodothyronine 5'-deiodinase (5'-D) in the adenohypophysis appears to be of physiological importance in the control of TSH secretion. Type-II 5'-D is believed to be the primary regulator of the T_3 concentration in the thyrotroph responsible for negative feedback inhibition of TSH secretion. Although Type-II 5'-D activity is markedly increased in hypothyroidism, the role of hypothalamic factors in the regulation of this enzyme is not established. Reduction with hypothalamic lesions of the amount of TRH reaching the adenohypophysis from the PVN decreases plasma TSH, T_4 and T_3 concentration 50% and increases the inhibitory effect of a given dose of T_4 on TSH secretion. These effects might be due to an increase in pituitary Type-II 5'-D which would increase intracellular generation of T_3 from T_4. We have evaluated this hypothesis.

Complete (CHD) or anterior (AHD) hypothalamic deafferentation, or ablation of the paraventricular nuclei (PVN) were made in male hypothyroid rats using standard or C-shaped Halasz knives in 2 separate experiments with 5-10 rats per group. Seven days postoperatively adenohypophysial Type-II 5'-D was measured. Compared to sham-operated control rats, CHD and PVN reduced plasma TSH by 50% ($P<0.01$), AHD reduced it only slightly ($P>0.05$); CHD decreased Type-II 5'-D activity by 45% ($P<0.01$). However, enzyme activity was not significantly altered by PVN or AHD. No increase in adenophypophysial Type-II 5'-D occurred in any of the groups with various hypothalamic lesions.

Conclusions: 1) There is no increase in adenohypophysial Type-II 5'-D in hypothyroid rats with a marked reduction in hypothalamic TRH stimulation of TSH secretion. 2) It thus seems unlikely that this enzyme mediates the alteration of negative feedback sensitivity of TSH secretion to T_4 which is induced by TRH.

DOPAMINE SYNTHESIS IN THE HYPOTHALAMUS AS WELL AS DOPAMINE AND PROLACTIN CONCENTRATIONS IN THE ADENOHYPOPHYSIS ARE INFLUENCED BY THYROID STATUS IN THE RAT 70

M.J. Reymond, Th. Lemarchand-Béraud
Division of Endocrinology, Department Internal Medicine, C H U V, 1011 Lausanne, Switzerland

There have been conflicting reports on the influence of thyroid function on PRL secretion in the rat with scarce mention of effects on hypothalamic dopamine (DA).

In the present investigation DA synthesis in TIDA neurons - estimated by DOPA accumulation in the median eminence after inhibition of DOPA decarboxylase - as well as DA and PRL concentrations in the adenohypophysis were studied in male rats thyroidectomized (TX) or sham TX for 2 weeks, in TX rats treated for 7 days with T4 (20 µg/Kg BW daily) or vehicle as well as in intact rats treated similarly with T4 or vehicle.

In TX rats compared to sham TX rats an increase of DA synthesis in TIDA neurons ($p<0.001$) was observed in association with an accumulation of DA ($p<0.001$) and a reduction of PRL concentration ($p<0.001$) in the adenohypophysis.

Treatment of TX rats with T4 for 7 days reversed these effects, DA synthesis in TIDA neurons of TX rats treated with T4 being even less than in neurons of sham TX rats ($p<0.02$). DA and PRL concentrations in the pituitary gland of TX rats treated with T4 were similar to those found in sham TX rats.

Treatment of intact animals with T4 did not affect DA synthesis in TIDA neurons nor DA or PRL concentrations in the adenohypophysis.

The steady-state concentrations of DA in the median eminence were not altered by the various treatments.

The present results are supportive of a modulatory influence of thyroid status on the secretory activity of the hypothalamic TIDA neurons and consequently on PRL secretion in the rat.

ARGININE-VASOPRESSIN MODULATES β-ENDORPHIN RELEASE FROM RAT BRAIN STRUCTURES 71

I. Barna, V.M. Wiegant, H.D. Veldhuis, D. De Wied, Rudolf Magnus Institute for Pharmacology, University of Utrecht, Utrecht, The Netherlands

Much literature is available on the regulation of β-endorphin (βE) releasing cells in the anterior and intermediate lobes of the pituitary, substantiating a role as secretagogues for corticotropin releasing factor (CRF), arginine vasopressin (AVP) and β-adrenergic agonists in these tissues. The mechanisms regulating central β-endorphinergic cells, however, are still largely unknown. The aim of the present study was to investigate the effects of intracerebroventricular (icv) administration of pituitary βE secretagogues on βE-like immunoreactivity (βELIR) in the cerebrospinal fluid (CSF) as a reflection of the releasing activity of central nervous structures.

Male Wistar rats were implanted under Hypnorm® anesthesia with two permanent cannulae, one into the lateral ventricle allowing for icv injections (3 μl), the other into the cisterna magna for withdrawal of CSF samples (50 - 100 μl) from the animals without anesthesia. One day following surgery, the βELIR concentration in CSF was increased, but it returned to basal on the third day. Thus, all further experiments were performed three days after the operation.

Icv injection of isoprenaline (ISO; 3 - 300 pg) or CRF (1 - 3000 pg) did not influence βELIR levels in CSF. In the highest dose tested, CRF induced a slight increase in plasma βELIR 20 - 35 min after the injection. AVP dose dependently (1 - 1000 pg) elevated βELIR concentrations in CSF. The effect was maximal 20 min after the injection of the peptide. At 60 min, βELIR had returned to basal. No effect of AVP was found on plasma βELIR. The βELIR concentration in CSF and plasma was not affected by icv administration of AVP-(4-8) and oxytocin (100 pg).

Our data indicate that AVP is a potent releaser of βE from certain structures in the central nervous system. While CRH is the main factor which regulates the release of peptides derived from proopiomelanocortin (POMC) from the pituitary, vasopressin may be the main factor for the release of POMC-peptides from the brain.

OXYTOCIN RESPONSES TO STRESS IN LACTATING AND HYPERPROLACTINAEMIC RATS 72

D.A.Carter & S.L.Lightman. Medical Unit, Charing Cross & Westminster Medical School, Page St.,London, SW1P 2AP

It was recently shown that the posterior pituitary response to stress is characterized by a preferential release of oxytocin (OT) compared to arginine-vasopressin (AVP) (Lang et al, 1983). We have shown that the OT response is sexually dimorphic, being determined by organizational rather than activational effects of gonadal steroids (Carter & Lightman, 1985; Williams et al, 1985). In order to further investigate the hormonal and behavioural factors which modulate the stress related release of OT we have now made a comparative study of OT responses to immobilization in lactating rats and hyperprolactinaemic virgin rats.

Six days after the birth of litters lactating Sprague-Dawley rats were either immobilized for 1 min and then decapitated, or decapitated immediately following separation from the pups. Trunk blood was collected, and plasma levels of OT were determined by RIA. The previously observed OT response to immobilization was absent in lactating rats (plasma OT: control, 9.4 ± 2.2 pmol/l; immobilized, 9.0 ± 1.1pmol/l).

Hyperprolactinaemia was induced by treatment with the dopamine antagonist domperidone (DOM, 4mg/kg s.c. twice daily for 5 days and 2h before stress on day 6) and confirmed by subsequent RIA. Plasma levels of OT in immobilized, DOM-treated rats (16.5 ± 3.6pmol/l) were significantly lower ($p<0.05$) than in vehicle treated immobilized animals (25.2 ± 3.0pmol/l). In two further experiments hyperprolactinaemia was induced by similar treatment with either the neuroleptic haloperidol (0.4mg/kg) or ovine prolactin (2mg/kg). In both cases the level of OT in immobilized rats (HAL, 15.3 ± 3.5pmol/l; O-PRL, 14.6 ± 2.6pmol/l) was significantly lower ($p<0.02$ both) than in vehicle treated rats (29.0 ± 5.6pmol/l).

We suggest that hyperprolactinaemia may be partly responsible for the inhibition of OT stress responses in lactating rats; the neuroendocrine factors which mediate this effect are now under investigation.

Carter, D.A. & Lightman, S.L. (1985) J.Physiol. 369, 119P
Lang, R.E., Heil, J.W.E., Ganten, D.et al (1983) Neuroendocr.37, 314-316
Williams T.D.M. et al, (1985) Endo.116, 738-740

A CORRELATIVE NEUROPHYSIN IMMUNOHISTOCHEMICAL AND FINE STRUCTURAL STUDY OF NEUROSECRETORY AXON REGENERATION INTO INTRAHYPOTHALAMIC NEURAL LOBE ALLOGRAFTS. 73

H.-D. Dellmann, L.-F. Lue, S.I. Bellin
Department of Veterinary Anatomy, Iowa State University, Ames, Iowa, 50011.

To test the capability of neural lobe tissue to induce and sustain regeneration of severed neurosecretory axons in an area where such regeneration usually fails to occur, allografts of halved neural lobes were made stereotactically into the hypothalamo-neurohypophysial tract in the region between the paraventricular and supraoptic nuclei. Animals were sacrificed between 5 and 71 days post operationem; alternate 50 μm vibratome-cut sections were processed for neurophysin immunohistochemistry and for conventional electron microscopy, respectively. There was a temporal increase in the number and density of neurophysin + axons in the neural lobe grafts. At the fine structural level, phagocytosis of endogenous neurosecretory axons in the grafts by pituicytes or macrophages was completed by 5 days provided that grafts were vascularized. At this time, single host neurosecretory axons and especially numerous axonal growth cones were observed in association with pituicyte processes and/or scalloped basal lamina scaffolds. Axon terminals containing both neurosecretory granulated vesicles and microvesicles were present occasionally at 5 days and became more numerous subsequently; these terminals, partially wrapped by pituicyte processes, contacted basal lamina-delineated, wide perivascular spaces containing numerous collagen fibrils that tended to decrease after 30 days. Neurosecretory axons were also invaginated deeply into pituicytes. Macrophages and phagolysosomes within pituicytes were still present at 20 days but absent at 30 days. At 71 days, the fine structural characteristics of the grafted neural lobes were virtually indistinguishable from those of intact controls, except for the presence of many non-fenestrated capillaries, and occasional astrocyte processes. The neural lobe provides an ideal microenvironment for intrahypothalamic regeneration of neurosecretory axons. Supported by NSF grant BNS 84-04183 and Basic Research Grant No. 1-900 from the March of Dimes Birth Defects Foundation.

ARGININE VASOPRESSIN (AVP) AND CORTICOTROPIN RELEASING FACTOR (CRF) IN THE ANTERIOR PITUITARY: NO CORRELATION WITH PRESUMED SECRETION RATE. 74

J.Dohanics[1], E.A.Linton[2], T.Janaky[3], F.A.László[3] and G. B. Makara[1]
[1]Institute of Experimental Medicine, Hungarian Academy of Sciences, Budapest, Hungary
[2]Pituitary Hormone Laboratory, St.Bartholomews Centre for Clinical Research, London, U.K.
[3]Endocrine Unit, 1st Department of Medicine, University Medical School, Szeged, Hungary

Arginine vasopressin (AVP) and corticotropin releasing factor (CRF) content in the anterior pituitary (AP), stalk-median eminence (SME) and neurointermediate lobe (NIL) and plasma ACTH concentration were measured with RIA and IRMA methods. AVP measurements in the AP showed scatter and none of the subsequent interventions caused a change in AVP content of the anterior pituitary. An anterolateral cut (ALC) that disrupts all fibers running from the supraoptic and paraventricular nuclei (PVN) to the SME and NIL caused almost total disappearance of AVP from both of these regions, while plasma ACTH was low. Selective destruction of the PVN resulted in a small, but statistically significant decrease in AVP content in both the SME and NIL. 2 weeks after adrenalectomy (ADX) a slight increase in the AVP content of the SME was observed and plasma ACTH was high. Similarly, CRF measurements of the AP showed no differences between the various groups, although ALC sharply reduced CRF content of the SME as well as that of the NIL, whilst the decrease in CRF content due to PVN lesion was less, but still significant. Adrenalectomy 14 days prior to sacrifice was without effect on SME or NIL content of CRF. Dexamethasone, given to ADX animals 6 h prior to decapitation, failed to alter CRF content in these regions although completely suppressing the previously-elevated plasma ACTH concentration. The results show that AVP and CRF are present in the anterior pituitary in detectable quantities; however, the AVP and CRF content of the anterior lobe failed to correlate with either that of the SME or NIL or with ACTH release rate.

CALCIUM IONS AND OXYTOCIN-INDUCED CONTRACTIONS OF THE MALE MOUSE ANOCOCCYGEUS 75

A. Gibson and M. Ginsburg

Dept. of Pharmacology, Kings College London, Chelsea Campus, London SW3 6LX, UK.

Anococcygeus muscles, isolated from male mice, contract in response to low concentrations of oxytocin (OT). Using selective agonists and antagonists the receptor involved has been shown to be similar, but perhaps not identical, to the OT receptor of the uterus. We are now investigating the mechanisms which link OT receptor activation to contraction, and report here some initial studies on the role of calcium ions (Ca).

In normal Krebs, repeated additions of 10 nM OT gave reproducible increases in tension of the mouse anococcygeus (between 90 - 95% of maximum). In Ca-free Krebs, there was a progressive decrease in these responses, such that by the sixth addition 10 nM OT failed to cause contraction. When Ca was added to the quiescent organ 2 min after the application of 10 nM OT in Ca-free Krebs contractions were evoked. The effective range of Ca concentration was 0.125 - 2.5 mM ; the highest concentration produced increases in tension equal to those caused by 10 nM OT in normal Krebs. Ca had no contractile effect in the absence of OT.

The organic Ca-channel antagonists verapamil (0.1 - 10 μM) and nitrendipine (0.001 - 1 μM) had little or no effect on Ca-induced contractions in the presence of OT. However, the inorganic Ca-channel antagonist Mn (0.01 - 0.5 mM) produced a marked inhibition of the responses.

We conclude that OT-induced contractions of the mouse anococcygeus require extracellular Ca, which is made available to the intracellular contractile elements through channels which are blocked by Mn. However, these channels can be distinguished from the voltage-operated Ca-channels found in smooth muscle by their insensitivity to block by verapamil or nitrendipine.

CONVERGING EXCITATORY INPUTS TO PARVOCELLULAR PARAVENTRICULAR NEUROSECRETORY CELLS AFTER NOXIOUS AND HYPOVOLEMIC STIMULI 76

M. Hamamura, T. Onaka, K. Yagi

Dept. of Physiol., Jichi Med. Sch., Tochigi, Japan

Noxious and hypovolemic stimuli potentiate corticotropin (ACTH) secretion in a synergistic fashion. Neurosecretory cells immunoreactive to corticotropin-releasing factor exist in the parvocellular region of the hypothalamic paraventricular nucleus (PVN). It is thus possible that parvocellular neurosecretory (PC) cells in the PVN receive converging excitatory inputs after noxious and hypovolemic stimuli. The present study aimed to test this hypothesis in anesthetized rats.

Those PVN units, which showed an antidromic spike after median eminence stimulation but not after posterior pituitary stimulation with the intensity up to 0.45 mA and were proved to be located within the parvocellular region of the PVN, were identified as PC cells. Saphenous nerve (SP) stimulation at 4 Hz elevated plasma ACTH level and produced an excitation in 13 of the 52 PC cells tested. Post-stimulus time histograms of spike discharges of these cells were constructed during 1-Hz SP stimulation and disclosed the existence of an excitatory synaptic inputs after the stimuli. Hemorrhage through a catheter attached to the femoral vein (4 ml/kg b.w.) was tested in 10 of the 13 excited cells and found to produce an excitation in 7 cells. Histological examination showed that these 7 PC cells were located within the medial parvocellular and periventricular part of the PVN.

These data show that PC cells in the PVN receive converging excitatory synaptic inputs after noxious and hypovolemic stimuli and suggest that these converging inputs may be involved, at least in part, in the synergistic potentiation of ACTH secretion as has been shown to occur after these stimuli.

VASOPRESSIN-STIMULATED TURNOVER OF PHOSPHATIDYLINOSITOL IN SENSORY GANGLIA OF THE RAT 77

A.M.Horn and S.L.Lightman. Medical Unit, Charing Cross & Westminster Medical School, Westminster Hospital, 17 Page Street, London, SW1P 2AP, UK.

Arginine vasopressin (AVP) causes a rapid hydrolysis of phosphatidylinositol (PI) in the superior cervical ganglion (SCG) of the rat via activation of V1 receptor sites (Hanley et al, 1984). We have detected AVP immunoreactivity in the trigeminal ganglion (TG) of the rat and have now investigated whether AVP can effect PI turnover both in the TG and in dorsal root ganglia (DRG).

Tissue was pre-labelled with ^{3}H-inositol in vitro and then incubated with AVP, in the presence of 10mM Li^+. Total ^{3}H-inositol-phosphates were extracted with $HClO_4$, and then separated from free ^{3}H-inositol by Dowex anion-exchange chromatography. Total ^{3}H-inositol content of tissue was measured after a chloroform extraction of ^{3}H-labelled lipid. To allow for differences in incorporation of ^{3}H-inositol, IP dpm are expressed as a standard incorporation of IP dpm/1000 lipid dpm. Results are given as a ratio of test/control.

AVP caused a dose-dependent accumulation of IP in both TG and DRG; maximum stimulation of 1.7 fold of control ($p<0.01$), at a concentration of 3×10^{-7}M in TG, and a maximum stimulation of 2.5 fold of control at a concentration of 3×10^{-8}M in DRG ($p<0.01$). The response to AVP in both tissues was maintained in Ca^{2+}-free buffer. The V2 agonist, DDAVP, at concentrations up to 3×10^{-6}M, had no effect on the accumulation of IP in either tissue. The V1-antagonist, $(CH_2)_5$MeTyrAVP, at a concentration of 2×10^{-5}M, inhibited the response to doses of AVP which had given a maximal stimulation in each tissue.

We conclude that the rat TG and DRG, have functional AVP receptors, and that these receptors are of the V1 sub-type.

Ref: Hanley et al, 1984. Nature, 309, 258-261

HYPOTHALAMIC SARCOIDOSIS WITH PARTIAL HYPOPITUITARISM: A study of 3 cases. 78

M. Kamelman Levitin, I. Molocznik, H. A. Ruggiero, J. E. Argonz, E. Caputti, A. Sanchez, R. Driollet Laspiur, R. Artese.

Costa Buero Institute, Department of Neuroendocrinology, Medical School, U. B. A., Buenos Aires, Argentina.

Hypothalamic sarcoidosis with clinical and neuroendocrinological pituitary alterations had seldom been reported.

An attempt to establish possible (case I) and positive (cases II and III) hypothalamic-hypophyseal sarcoidosis is presented.

Case I: Male, aged: 39; Symptoms: diabetes insipidus (8 lts.), gravative asthenia, sexual impotence, hypogenitalism and peripheral neuropathy. Hormonal studies evidenced basal hyperprolactinaemia, secondary hypothyroidism and hypogonadotropic hypogonadism. Radiological and scintigraphical studies: pathological rib image. Biopsy: bone sarcoidosis.

Case II: Male, aged: 39; Symptoms: severe obesity, hyperphagia, diabetes insipidus (10 lts.), gynaecomastia, sexual impotence, hypogenitalism, visual hallucinations, headaches and desorientation. Hormonal studies showed basal hyperprolactinaemia, hypogonadotropic hypogonadism and partial secondary hypocortisolism. Necropsy: hypothalamic and systemic sarcoidosis.

Case III: Female, aged: 60; Symptoms: diabetes insipidus (7 lts.), obesity, arterial hypertension, thyroid enlargement and visual disturbances (bitemporal quadrantopsia). Hormonal studies showed basal hyperprolactinaemia, hypogonadotropic hypogonadism and secondary hypothyroidism. Chest C.A.T.: pulmonary nodes. Biopsy: lung sarcoidosis. Brain C.A.T.: intra and suprasellar tumour. Biopsy: pituitary stalk sarcoidosis.

Hypothalamic sarcoidosis associated with partial hypopituitarism confirmed by provocative neuroendocrinological tests are rarely referred in medical literature.

INHIBITORY INFLUENCE OF EXOGENOUS OXYTOCIN (OT) ON CORTISOL AND ACTH IN MAN: EVIDENCE FOR REBOUND EFFECT AND REPRODUCIBILITY

79

J.J. Legros, P. Chiodera, V. Geenen
Psychoneuroendocrine Unit, University of Liege, Sart Tilman, B23, B-4000 Liège, Belgium

In previous works we demonstrated that OT induces a decrease of basal as well as stimulated ACTH and cortisol in normal humans (JCEM, 55, 1035 (1982); JCEM, 58, 105 (1984)). In the present work, we have tested the influence of low dose of OT perfusion (32 mIU/min) on ACTH and cortisol plasma levels in 8 normal male volunteers (age 18-26). The one hour OT perfusion periods were preceded and followed by two one hour saline control periods. During the first control period, there was a slight ACTH concentration decrease in 4 individuals. OT perfusion induced a clear cut plasma ACTH decrease in 7 out of 8 volunteers and a slight decrease in the remaining one. During the second saline infusion, there was a marked ACTH increase in 7 out of 8 volunteers and a weak increase in one ($F\ 2,14 = 28.86$, $p < 0.00001$). A similar pattern was observed for plasma cortisol levels ($F\ 2,14 = 72.88$, $p < 0.00001$). Further the reproducibility of this inhibitory influence was retested in 4 volunteers: the tests were repeted under the same conditions 7 days later. There were no global differences between the two sets of tests both for ACTH (1,3 = 0,57 p NS) and cortisol (1,3 = 0,03 NS).

The present results confirm the inhibitory influence of low dose OT perfusion on ACTH and cortisol levels in normal males. Moreover the demonstration of a rebound effect during the second control saline infusion and the reproducibility of the inhibitory effect at a one week interval in 4 volunteers bring new arguments for the specificity of OT action on ACTH release in normal human.

THE ANTIBODY RAISED AGAINST NEUROPEPTIDE: IS IT A NEW MEAN TO ACT IN VIVO ON PEPTIDERGIC NEURONS ?

80

Burlet A. Leon-Henri B. Arahmani A. Robert F. Burlet C.
Laboratoire de Biologie cellulaire, Faculté de Médecine, BP184.- F-54505-Vandoeuvre-les-Nancy.

The specific antibodies prepared against cerebral antigens might have biological effects when they were injected into the brain. In some experiments, it has been demonstrated that these effects were due to the uptake of antibodies into the neurons, inducing specific immunolesions. We attempted to evaluate the possibility of using antibodies directed against neuropeptides to act, in vivo, on peptidergic neurons. The study was performed from the neurons synthezising vasopressin (VP): monoclonal anti-VP antibodies (VP-MAbs, ascites fluid) were injected in vivo into the paraventricular nucleus (PVN) of the rat brain and detected by immunocytochemistry.

Depending on the post-survival time, the VP-MAbs were stained in various groups of the VP neurons: the most anterior neurons after the shortest time (10min) and the most posterior one after the longest survival time (90min). The neuronal capture of VP-MAbs was specific: it appeared neither into the oxytocinergic neurons nor into the neurons of the Brattleboro rat brain where the VP processsing is genetically impossible. The prior incubation of VP-MAbs with VP (2.3pM/ml) abolished the neuronal capture. In addition, the VP neurons never caught monoclonal antibodies prepared against the bovine thyroglobulin. Several data proved that the VP-MAbs were enclosed by living neurons. The VP-MAbs were carried to different levels of the VP neurons according to the post survival time : from the cytoplasm (10 min to 3h after injection) to the eminential fibres and the granular layer of the Gyrus Dentatus (1 to 24h post-injection). The neuronal capture and the carrying of VP-MAbs were abolished when the rats were injected with colchicine 24h before experiment. The moderate heating (56°C for 30min) of the ascites fluid containing the VP-MAbs did not alter the antibodies; however, their neuronal uptake was totally inhibited. Finally, when the rats received intracisternally 40 µCi of ^{35}S-cysteine 30min before the VP-MAbs injection, the rate of radioactive tracer incorporated into the neurons labelled by VP-MAbs was significantly modified.

These results suggest that the antibodies prepared against VP may be a specific mean to act on VP neurons in vivo.

VASOPRESSIN AND OXYTOCIN INCREASE ACTH BUT REDUCE PROLACTIN SECRETION. STUDY OF THE RECEPTOR(S) INVOLVED

81

P. Mormède[1], J.D. Vincent[2], B. Kerdelhue[3], R. Dantzer[1], M. Le Moal[1]
[1]INSERM-INRA U-259, [2]INSERM U-176, Domaine de Carreire rue Camille Saint-Saëns, 33077 Bordeaux, [3]CNRS Laboratoire des Hormones Polypeptides, 91190 Gif-sur-Yvette, France

Subcutaneous administration of arginine vasopressin (AVP) to conscious rats induces ACTH/β-endorphin release but reduces PRL secretion in both basal and stress conditions.

Dose-response studies of ACTH release by analogs with various activities in the different neurohypophysial hormone receptors showed that two mechanisms can be operative in this action. Non-pressor agonists, such as dDAVP or oxytocin, release ACTH in vivo with a characteristic, low-slope dose-response curve and this effect is not related to their activity on the vasopressor (V1), antidiuretic (V2), or oxytocic receptor. Furthermore dDAVP (V2 agonist)-induced ACTH release could be blocked neither by V1-nor by V2-receptor antagonists. This is suggestive of a direct action on the pituitary gland, as its AVP receptor was described in vitro as being different from other known neurohypophysial hormone receptors. Vasopressor (V1) agonists, on the other hand, release ACTH with a different, high-slope dose-response curve. We suggest that this latter effect is mainly indirect, and results from the aversive properties of the hypertensive crisis. No antagonist tested so far was able to reduce ACTH release induced by novel environment stress.

In the same experimental design, AVP reduced plasma prolactin (PRL) levels, in both basal and stress conditions and this effect was also obtained with oxytocin but not with specific V1 or V2 agonists. None of the antagonists tested so far was able to modify PRL levels. The mechanism of this action and the receptor type(s) involved remain to be discovered.

These results suggest that it should be possible to design AVP/oxytocin analogs with a specific action on ACTH and/or PRL secretion.

OPOSITE EFFECTS OF ARGININE VASOTOCIN AND LYSINE VASOPRESSIN INJECTED INTO THE CEREBRAL VENTRICULES ON VISUAL EVOKED POTENTIALS IN CAT.

82

V. Neştianu, M[x]. Coculescu, M. Iancău, St. Mihăilescu
Dpt. of Physiology, Craiova University School of Medicine and Dpt.[x] of Endocrinology, Bucharest Faculty of Medicine, Romania.

As shown by our previous work, arginine vasotocin (AVT) and lysine vasopresin (LVP) intravenously (iv) injected can modulate transmission through the visual pathways, the effect of AVT being similar to that of the pineal gland extract injected in the same animal (1). Since the transport of synthetic nonapeptides through the blood-brain-barrier is controversial (2) we are studying their effects on visual evoked potentials (VEP) after administration into the lateral cerebral ventricules (iLCV). In 9 cats operated on under ether anaesthesia, which were further curarized and locally anaesthesied by procain, the VEPs of the visual cortex were recorded, as shown elsewhere (1). Synthetic AVT (Ferring) or LVP (Sandoz) in doses of 0.2-4 ng/kg b.w. and a volume of 0.1 ml were injected into LCV or infused iv in doses up to 20 ng/kg b.w., within 1 min. AVT, either iLCV or iv produced an increase in the amplitude of positive waves and a decrease of the negative ones, while LVP showed opposite effects. Small amounts of AVT, of 0.2 ng/kg b.w. showed no effects when iv infused, while the same doses injected iLCV produced a decrease of the ratio of the amplitude-sum of negative versus that of positive waves from 1.33 ± 0.4 to 0.140 ± 0.06 ($x \pm SEM$). The same amounts of LVP iLCV increased the ratios from 1.7 ± 0.4 to 85.7 ± 2.3 (p 0.001).

The much stronger effects of nonapeptide when injected within the brain as compared to their systemic infusion suggests a physiological role of the locally produced AVT and vasopressin on the visual system, the first one inhibiting and the facilitating the visual transmission.

1. Neştianu V., Coculescu M., et al., Proc. Int. Cong. "Endocrinology '85", ICS No 685, Elsevier, 1985.

2. Coculescu M., Oprescu M., Acta Endocrinol. (Kbh), suppl. 256, 103, 243, 1983.

HISTAMINE AS A NEUROMODULATOR OF THE VASOPRESSINERGIC SYSTEM 83

H. Niigawa, R. Cacabelos, A. Yamatodani*, H. Wada*, K. Tada, S. Hariguchi, T. Nishimura.
Departments of Neuropsychiatry and Pharmacology II*, Osaka University Medical School, Osaka 553, Japan.

It is believed that histamine (HA) is a potent re-leaser of vasopressin (VP), but little is known about its mechanism of action. To gain more information, we have studied the effects on VP in the hypothalamo-hypophyseal system and plasma of L-histidine, HA, mepyramine (Mep), famotidine (Fam) and alpha-fluoromethylhistidine (FMH), a specific K_{cat} inhibitor of histidine decarboxylase.

The chronic administration of L-his (200 mg/day;i.p.) increased the concentration of VP both in the posterior hypothalamic region (PHR), where the HA-secreting neurons are located, an in adenohypophysis (Ah). At the same time, VP decreased in the anterior hypothalamic region (AHR) and median eminence (ME) with no apparent changes in the neurohypophysis (Nh) and plasma.

HA (0.6 mmol/Kg; i.p.) produced an elevation of VP in the PHR, ME, Ah and plasma, along with a clear decrease in Nh-VP. The administration of HA + Mep (0.3 mmol/Kg; i.p.) enhanced the HA-induced VP release in the ME and clearly reduced VP in the PHR and Ah. The same drug combination increased VP two-fold in the Nh. Inverse results were obtained in the ME and Ah after administration of HA + Fam (0.4 mmol/Kg; i.p.). In the PHR, Mep as well as Fam abolished the HA-induced VP response.

After the chronic administration of FMH (100 mg/Kg/day; i.p.), a clear impairment of the synthesis and release of VP in HhS was observed.

These results lead us to conclude that neuronal HA is indispensable to the normal functioning of the vasopressinergic system. Its effects on VP seem to be mediated through the H_1-receptors in the Ah, the H_2-receptors in the Nh and ME, and both the H_1- and H_2-receptors at the hypothalamic level.

Effects of Leu-Enkephalin and Met-Enkephalin on vasopressin release from perifused rat hypothalamo-neurohypophyseal complex 84

Y. Oki, I. Tanaka, S. Ohgo, Y. Ikeda, M. Sakamoto, M. Nanno, T. Yoshimi
Hamamatsu University School of Medicine, Hamamatsu, Japan

The effects of leucine enkephalin (L-Enk) or methionine enkephalin (M-Enk) on the release of vasopressin from the perifused rat hypothalamo-neurohypophyseal complex (HNC) were examined in vitro.

The HNC was obtained from a male Wistar rat weighing about 200g by the method of Sladeck et al. The HNC was placed in a incubation chamber in a water bath at 37°C and the perifusion was performed. The flow rate of the medium consisting of Krebs Ringer bicarbonate buffer containing 10mM glucose, 0.1% ascorbic acid and 0.1% bovine serum albumin saturated with 95%O_2-5%CO_2 was 0.2ml/min and every 5 min fraction was collected. During the perifusion, L-Enk or M-Enk were added to the perifusion medium at a concentration of 10^{-8}M. The collected samples were lyophylized and reconstituted with the assay buffer and subjected to radioimmunoassay (RIA) for arginine vasopressin (AVP). The minimum detection limit of the RIA for AVP was 0.1pg/tube. The antiserum against AVP did not cross-react to oxytocin, L-Enk and M-Enk.

About 120 min after the start of the perifusion, a stable release of AVP from the perifused rat HNC was observed and the rate of the AVP release was 4 - 10 pg/min/block. An increase in NaCl in the medium by 20mM caused a significant increase in the release of AVP from HNC. Both L-Enk and M-Enk caused a marked decrease in the basal release of AVP and inhibited the AVP release stimulated by the increase in NaCl in the medium. These effects of L-Enk or M-Enk were completely antagonized by naloxone.

These findings suggest that L-Enk and/or M-Enk have an important role in the control of the release of AVP probably as an inhibiting factor.

VASOPRESSIN RESPONSES TO CORTICOTROPIN-RELEASING FACTOR IN CONSCIOUS DOGS: GLUCOCORTICOID SUPPRESSION 85

H. Raff, D. Merrill, M. Skelton, A.W. Cowley, Jr.
Medical College of Wisconsin, Milwaukee, WI 53226 and St. Luke's Hospital, Milwaukee, WI 53215.

We demonstrated previously that infusion of ovine corticotropin releasing factor (oCRF) resulted in a significant increase in plasma vasopressin (AVP) in conscious dogs (AJP:R281, 1985). Since glucocorticoids can suppress AVP responses to other stimuli (Endocrinology 114:1245, 1984), the present study investigated the effects of maximal glucocorticoid negative feedback on AVP responses to oCRF in conscious dogs.

6 dogs with indwelling catheters received no pretreatment (NO-DEX) or 1.5 mg DEX im at 1600 h of day 1. At 0700 of day 2 (15 hr later) and after a control sample, oCRF was infused at 20 ng/kg/min for 45 min. Plasma samples were analyzed for osmolality (OSM), sodium (Na^+), and hormones (AVP and ACTH by RIA). oCRF did not alter blood pressure or heart rate. Data (mean±SE) at 0 and 45 min of oCRF infusion are as follows:

PRE-TREATMENT	TIME min	OSM mosm/kg	Na^+ meq/l	ACTH pg/ml	AVP pg/ml
NO DEX	0	291	145.5	46‡	1.9
		±2	±0.5	±8	±0.5
	45	291	146.0	224*‡	4.8*‡
		±2	±0.4	±32	±1.2
DEX	0	298‡	146.6‡	18	1.8
		±2	±0.4	±3	±0.2
	45	297‡	148.2*‡	19	2.7
		±2	±0.3	±3	±0.5

*45 diff from 0 min, ‡DEX diff from NO-DEX; $p<0.05$

DEX significantly increased control OSM and Na^+ and decreased control ACTH but not AVP. oCRF induced a small increase in Na^+ with DEX pretreatment only. oCRF significantly increased ACTH and AVP; these responses were blocked with DEX pretreament.

We conclude that oCRF stimulation of AVP is sensitive to glucocorticoid negative feedback.

NEURAL GRAFTING IN THE THIRD CEREBRAL VENTRICULAR LUMEN OF THE BRATTLEBORO RAT WITH CHRONIC AUTOSOMOL DIABETES INSIPIDUS (DI). 86

D.E. Scott and R. Wolkowitz, Eastern Virginia Medical School, Norfolk, Virginia and University of Missouri-Columbia School of Medicine, Columbia, Missouri.

Microangiographic, ultrastructural (SEM-TEM) and immunocytochemical investigations have confirmed that when fragments of normal fetal hypothalamic tissue (17 days post coitus) are stereotaxically introduced into the third cerebral ventricle of male DI rats, that growth is vigorous and survival rates of indwelling neurografts are high. During recovery experimental and controls are kept in metabolic cages and assessed for urine osmolarity and daily water consumption. Fetal neurografts in rats killed 3 and 9 days post-surgery demonstrate a rapid invasion by surrounding host vessels. Grafts derive vascular input from a variety of periventricular regions including the median eminence, the paraventricular nuclear complex and the entire periventricular stratum. Upon entry into fetal graft parenchyma, hypophyseal portal vessels from the median eminence lose their fenestrated appearance and assume that of normal cerebral capillaries. The neuronal density within grafts vary. The largest population of neurons in animals killed 10 and 20 days following surgery appear to be dopaminergic as observed with immunocytochemistry employing antisera against tyrosine hydroxylase. ICC with antisera against arginine vasopressin (AVP) revealed relatively few neuronal perikayria despite impressive numbers of AVP positive varicosities and afferent fields. Large numbers of supraependymal neurons (CSF contacting) are observed to emerge upon the lumen of the cerebral ventricular system of host rats in close anatomical juxtaposition to the fetal neurografts. This emergence of CSF contacting neurons following neural grafting argues for the existence of a mechanism of dynamic plasticity and reorganization which may be a compensatory response to changes in the neuroendocrine milieu of the host cerebral ventricular system. Supported by NIH grant NS19197-03.

VASOPRESSIN ACTIVATION OF PHOSPHATIDYLINOSITOL METABOLISM IN RAT ANTERIOR PITUITARY IS MODIFIED BY CHANGES IN THE HYPOTHALAMO-PITUITARY ADRENAL AXIS

87

K. Todd and S.L. Lightman. Medical Unit, Charing Cross & Westminster Medical School, Westminster Hospital, 17 Page Street, London, SW1P 2AP, UK

Arginine vasopressin (AVP) activates phosphatidylinositol (PI) turnover in rat anterior pituitary tissue *in vitro* (Ref.1). Since AVP has activity as a corticotrophin releasing factor, we have now investigated whether changes in activity of the hypothalamo-pituitary adrenal axis modify this PI response to vasopressin.

Quartered anterior pituitaries from sham adrenalectomized rats were pre-incubated with 15μCi [H^3] inositol for 2.5 hr. Subsequently, in the presence of 10mM Li^+, incubation with vasopressin (3×10^{-7}M) resulted in a 1.77 fold stimulation of inositol phosphate accumulation measured by Dowex ion-exchange chromatography. Pituitary quarters from rats which had been adrenalectomized four days earlier showed no stimulation of inositol phosphate accumulation in response to vasopressin (Sham operated rats AVP 21.81 ± 1.84, Control 12.34 ± 0.58, dpm in phosphates/10^2 total dpm; Adrenalectomized rats AVP 15.25 ± 0.53, Control 14.77 ± 0.16, dpm in phosphates/10^2 total dpm). Daily administration of dexamethasone (40μg/day) did not alter the response to AVP of pituitary quarters from sham operated controls; it did however reverse the effect of adrenalectomy, vasopressin resulting in a 1.85 fold stimulation of inositol phosphate accumulation. This action of dexamethasone was not seen when dexamethasone (40μg/ml) was added to the incubation medium of adrenalectomized rat pituitary quarters - AVP still failed to stimulate inositol phosphate production.

We have demonstrated that the absence of circulating adrenal corticosteroids results in a desensitisation of the pituitary PI response to vasopressin. We suggest that this may be secondary to changes in portal blood vasopressin concentrations following adrenalectomy.

Ref.1: Lightman & Todd. J. Physiol, 371, 277P, 1985

β-ENDORPHIN AND DYNORPHIN SUPPRESS VASOPRESSIN RELEASE IN RATS UNDER VARIOUS CONDITIONS

88

Tj.B. Van Wimersma Greidanus, J.A. Ten Haaf
Rudolf Magnus Institute for Pharmacology, University of Utrecht, Vondellaan 6, 3521 GD Utrecht, The Netherlands

Opioid peptides have been shown to influence the release of several hormones from the pituitary in animals and men. With respect to the posterior pituitary it appears that β-endorphin (βE) and dynorphin-(1-13) exert a strong inhibitory effects on the secretion of vasopressin. Intracerebroventricular (icv), but not subcutaneous (sc), administration of these opioid peptides results in a decrease of plasma vasopressin levels. Time-effect relationship studies reveal that the suppressive effect is most pronounced at 30 min after icv administration of the peptides. Dose-effect relationship studies show that 1 μg of either peptide is approximately the lowest dose to induce a significant decrease of basal vasopressin levels. However, in water deprived rats icv administration of much lower doses (30-50 ng) of the opioid peptides induce a significant suppression of vasopressin levels in plasma. Sc, but not icv injection of the opiate antagonist naloxone results in a counteraction of the suppressive effects of βE and of Dyn-(1-13) on basal vasopressin levels as well as on vasopressin levels elevated after water deprivation. A similar dose of this opiate antagonist by itself does not affect the vasopressin levels.

In addition it appears that icv administration of βE markedly reduced the acute stimulation of vasopressin secretion by icv administration of histamine. Again naloxone, by itself not effecting thus stimulated vasopressin levels, counteracts this effect of βE.

From these data it is suggested that the opioid peptides used exert a suppressive effect on basal as well as on chronically or acutely stimulated vasopressin levels, probably by an action on the brain. The observation that systemic rather than central administration of naloxone counteracts this suppressive effect of βE and of Dyn-(1-13) points to an interaction of the opiate antagonist at the level of the pituitary.

MODULATION OF HORMONE SECRETION BY FOLLICULO-STELLATE CELLS IN RAT ANTERIOR PITUITARY CELL AGGREGATES

89

W. Allaerts and C. Denef
Laboratory of Cell Pharmacology, School of Medicine, University of Leuven, Belgium .

Previous work has demonstrated that functional communication between hormone secreting cells of the anterior pituitary can be studied in pituitary cell aggregates.In the present investigation we wanted to know whether or not the activity of hormone secreting cells could be modulated by interaction with folliculo-stellate cells (FS-cells),a cell type not secreting hormones but for which no apparent function has been clearly demonstrated yet .

We succeeded in isolating a highly-enriched population of FS-cells by using the technique of unit gravity sedimentation.FS-cells were identified by immunohistochemical staining of the nervous tissue-specific S100 protein.A population of 65.6%±4.2 was recovered from thetop fraction of the gradient,when dispersed cells from adult female rats were used.In other fractions only very small numbers were found.The influence of FS-cells on PRL and LH release was studied by coaggregating the FS-cell fraction with enriched populations of lactotropes and gonadotropes.In coaggregates containing 40% FS-cells the following effects induced by FS-cells were seen:1)a 50-70% inhibition of the PRL response to 0.1nM Angiotensin II(AII);2)a slight reduction(30%)of the PRL response to 0.1nM TRH; 3)a 60% reduction of the PRL response to 100 nM AII and TRH;4)a 66% inhibition of the LH respons to LHRH.In coaggregates with a smaller proportion of FS-cells(20%)there was a slight decreaseof the PRL response to 0.1nM AII.However,at 100nM AII,PRL secretion was considerably higher in the coaggregates than in the aggregates not mixed with FS-cells.These results suggest that FS-cells exert a complex regulatory control on hormone secretion in addition to other proposed functions such as supporting function,trophic functions and phagocytosis.

ARTERIES ARE PRESENT IN HUMAN PROLACTINOMAS

90

J.E. SCHECHTER, R.I. WEINER
University of Southern California, School of Medicine, Los Angeles, California and University of California San Francisco, School of Medicine, San Francisco, California.

Considerable evidence suggests that human prolactinomas have escaped dopamine inhibition *in vivo*, however, the tumors are responsive to the action of dopamine *in vitro*. An additional mechanism by which focal regions of the anterior pituitary could escape dopamine inhibition would be by a direct arterial blood supply to the region. We now report the presence of arteries in prolactinomas. Pituitaries from 6 patients with pituitary prolactinomas have been compared with 3 non-tumorous pituitaries. Prolactinomas included 2 males, ages 28 and 53, and 4 females, ages 25-30. Non-tumorous pituitaries were obtained by: 1) autopsy, male, age 14, 2) hypophysectomy, male, age 68 with prostatic cancer, and 3) hypophysectomy, female, age 45 with breast cancer. Well formed arteries were identified by electron microscopy within the anterior pituitary tissues of 4 of the 6 prolactinomas (1 of 2 males, 3 of 4 females). The arteries were comprised of a thin, continuous endothelium enveloped by a few to multiple layers of well differentiated smooth muscle cells. Transitional vessels between arterioles and capillaries were also seen, i.e., a single layer of smooth muscle surrounding a fenestrated capillary endothelial cell. Non-tumorous pituitaries contained only thin walled fenestrated capillaries characteristic of the anterior pituitary and no arteries. Arteries within the anterior pituitary, present either congenitally or newly developed, may bypass the normal hypothalamic dopamine inhibition of pituitary mammotrophs, and thus stimulate mammotroph hypertrophy, hyperplasia and tumorigenesis.

(Supported by NIH #35904 JES and NIH-HD #08935 RIW).

DOPAMINE (DA) D_2 RECEPTORS IN DA-RESISTANT PROLACTIN-SECRETING RAT PITUITARY TUMORS 7315a AND MtTW15: STRUCTURAL STUDIES 91

C. Bouvier, J. Lafond, G. Beauregard, M. Potier, R. Collu
Research Unit on Reproductive and Developmental Biology, and Section of Medical Genetics, Hôpital Sainte-Justine and University of Montreal, Montreal, Canada, H3T 1C5

Previous studies performed with an estrone-induced, prolactin (PRL)-secreting rat pituitary adenoma have allowed us to conclude that D_2-type DA receptors present in normal lactotrophs have a molecular weight of 143,000 ± 3,000 when attached to membranes and of 106,000 ± 4,000 when solubilized. In addition, they have indicated the presence of a GTP-binding protein (Gi or Go) in membrane-bound but not in solubilized receptorial preparations. More recently, we have investigated the structure of D_2 receptors present in 7315a and MtTW15 tumors which are resistant to the inhibitory control by DA. D_2 receptors were found to have high affinity binding sites for $[^3H]$spiperone when membrane-bound or solubilized by CHAPS. Molecular weights determined by radiation inactivation were: 7315a, membrane 101,000 ± 6,000, solubilized 103,000 ± 7,000; MtTW15, membrane 204,000 ± 13,000, solubilized 184,000 ± 7,000. Guanine nucleotides had no effect on the displacing potency of the agonist N-propylnorapomorphine evaluated with membrane-bound or solubilized receptors obtained from either tumor, which suggests the absence or inactivation of a guanine-nucleotide binding protein in the receptorial complex. These data indicate the existence of a structural anomaly in the D_2 receptors of two PRL-secreting pituitary tumors and are the first to show a possible mechanism for resistance to DA inhibitory activity. They suggest, furthermore, that the receptorial defect is different in the two tumors.

THE PROLACTIN RELEASING ACTION OF TRH BUT NOT VIP IS POTENTIATED FOLLOWING THE BRIEF INTERRUPTION OF DA INHIBITION. 92

G. Martinez-Escalera, J. Guthrie, R. Weiner.
Reprod. Endo. Center, UCSF, San Francisco, CA 94143.

The amplitude of PRL release stimulated by TRH from cultured anterior pituitary (AP) cells was dramatically increased following the brief interruption of dopamine (DA) inhibition. We have extended these observations to determine: if the response to VIP is also modified; and if the potentiated stimulation is mediated via a Ca^{++}/C-kinase pathway or adenylate cyclase. Enzymatically dispersed AP cells from ovariectomized, E_2-treated (1 cm silastic capsules for 14 days) were plated on extracellular matrix coated coverslips and cultured in DME H-21, 500 nM DA, 100 μM ascorbic acid (DME + DA) and 10% calf serum. After 20 hrs. the coverslips were placed in Sykes-Moore chambers and superfused with DME + DA at a rate of 0.3 ml/min. for 1 hr. prior to the collection of 2.5 min. samples. The cells were challenged for 10 min. with VIP, A-23187 (a Ca^{++} ionophore), TPA (a C-kinase activator), forskolin (an adenylate cyclase activator) or 8-Br-cAMP either during continual (+DA) or 20 min. after a 10 min. interruption of DA (±DA). PRL was measured by RIA. The stimulation of PRL release by TRH or activation of the Ca^{++}/C-kinase pathway was potentiated following the brief removal of DA.

AGENT	DOSE (M)	n	MAX. ↑ (%) +DA	±DA	TIME MAX. ↑ (MIN.)
TRH	10^{-7}	3	313±125	1400±450	3-5
VIP	5×10^{-7}	4	117±1	104±30	20-30
A-23187	2×10^{-5}	2	383±14	636±111	3-5
TPA	5×10^{-8}	3	341±111	837±144	15-20
8-Br-cAMP	2.5×10^{-3}	4	430±110	372±88	30-40
Forskolin	10^{-5}	3	145±29	103±45	30-40

However stimulation of PRL release by VIP or activation of adenylate cyclase showed no potentiation. These findings are consistent with the known mechanisms of action of TRH and VIP and suggest a lack of convergence of C-kinase and adenylate cyclase mediated pathways on potentiated PRL release. The work was supported by NIH grant HD08924 and the Mellon Foundation.

LIVER FACTOR(S) STIMULATES CASEIN RELEASE IN VITRO IN THE ABSENCE OF ADDED PROLACTIN 93

J.P. Hoeffler and L.S. Frawley, Zoology Dept Iowa State University, Ames, IA 50011

Recent evidence by Nicoll et al. (Endo 116:1449, 1985) suggests that liver tissue from rats with elevated serum prolactin (PRL) secretes a factor(s) that synergizes with PRL to enhance mammary mitogenic activity. In the present study, we attempted to resolve whether this factor also possessed lactogenic activity. This was accomplished by employing a reverse hemolytic plaque assay to measure casein release from individual rat mammary cells in culture (Frawley et al., Abstract, Endocrine Society, 1986). Briefly, assay chambers containing monolayers of mammary cells (from day-10 lactators) and indicator RBCs were preincubated for 17h and then subjected to a casein plaque assay. Addition of 25 or 100 pg/ml rat PRL at the beginning of the preincubation increased the percentages of all mammary cells that released casein from a control value of 19.4±0.3% to 24.5±0.5% and 32.9±0.7%, respectively ($\bar{X}$±SE, triplicate determinations in a single experiment representative of 3 separate experiments), whereas addition of medium that bathed liver slices (3h) from day-12 lactators had no effect. In contrast, treatment with rPRL or liver incubation medium (1:32) increased the average size of the plaques that formed (an index of the relative amount of casein released per cell). Plaque sizes ($\mu^2 \times 10^{-3}$) from the same experiment described above are summarized in the following table.

MEDIUM	0 pg/ml rPRL	25 pg/ml rPRL	100 pg/ml rPRL
Control	18.8±1.3	32.7±3.1	40.8±1.4
Liver	60.8±1.6	76.7±5.0	90.4±5.8

Surprisingly, medium bathing liver slices from lactators was much more potent than rPRL in stimulating casein release and the combined effects of these treatments were additive rather than synergistic. Incubations of kidney tissue from lactating rats, liver tissue from male or virgin female rats, and IGF-1 had no activity in this assay system. Taken together, our results demonstrate that liver tissue from lactating rats produces a substance(s) which partially mimics the actions of PRL; it increases the amount of casein released per mammary cell but not the number of cells committed to casein release.

SIMULTANEOUS BILATERAL COLLECTION OF BLOOD FROM INFERIOR PETROSAL SINUSES OF PATIENTS WITH PROLACTIN-SECRETING ADENOMAS. 94

L.Annunziato, B.Merola, P.Miletto, A.M.Colao, M.Taglialatela, C.Nappi, G.De Chiara and G.Lombardi. Institute of Endocrinology, Pharmacology and Gynecology, 2nd School of Medicine, University of Naples, Via S.Pansini 5, 80131 Naples, Italy

Anterior pituitary hormones leave the pituitary gland by small hypophyseal veins that drain into the inferior petrosal sinuses (IPS) via the intercavernous plexus. The recent increased use of intercavernous phlebography for the diagnosis of pituitary adenomas has enabled the collection of selective venous sampling of IPS, where prolactin (PRL) levels can be measured before the hormone becomes excessively diluted in the systemic circulation.
In the present study, plasma PRL levels were studied in the right and/or left IPS and simultaneously in the peripheral circulation of 3 groups of patients: 1. Normoprolactinemic patients affected with different pituitary function diseases (17), 2. Hyperprolactinemic patients with negative radiological (RT) and CT signs of adenoma (11), 3. Adenomatous hyperprolactinemic patients (11).
1. In the normoprolactinemic patients plasma PRL concentration in the IPS were 3.5 times higher than peripheral circulation.
2. In the 2nd group of patients, there was a central to peripheral gradient for PRL of 2.5. No significant difference was detected between PRL concentrations in the left or right IPS.
3. Adenomatous hyperprolactinemic patients exhibited a central to peripheral gradient for PRL of 3.8 on the side of the tumor; furthermore plasma PRL concentrations in the IPS ipsilateral to the adenoma was significantly higher than controlateral.
The results of the present study show, for the first time, that a clearcut gradient of concentration does exist between plasma PRL levels in the IPS and the peripheral circulation of normoprolactinemic and hyperprolactinemic patients with negative RT and CT signs of adenoma. This gradient is also observed in adenomatous patients if blood is withdrawn from the IPS ipsilateral to the tumor. This indicates that the persence and the side of prolactinoma may be preoperatively identified by venous sampling of IPS.

(Partially supported by CNR Grant 840062644 to L.A.)

CONCORDANCE BETWEEN LH AND PRL PULSES IN OVARIECTOMIZED RATS IN THE PRESENCE AND ABSENCE OF DOPAMINE INHIBITION 95

C.R. Pohl, R.I. Weiner, M.S. Smith. University of Pittsburgh, Pittsburgh, PA 15261 and University of California at San Francisco, San Francisco, CA 94143.

Recent evidence suggests that hypothalamic substances controlling LH release (GnRH, GAP) may also affect PRL secretion. To investigate a possible relation between the regulation of these two hormones, serial blood samples were collected at 6-min intervals from OVX rats bearing chronic jugular catheters and analyzed for plasma concentrations of LH and PRL. Release patterns were assessed using the PULSAR computer program. Some animals were pre-treated (30 min before blood sampling) with the dopamine antagonist domperidone (DOM), and others were further pre-treated (4 hours before blood sampling) with a potent GnRH antagonist (GnRH-A). The following results (means ± S.E.M.) were obtained:

Treatment	LH Pulses Per 4HR	LH IPI (min)	LH Pulse Amp (ng/ml)	Mean LH (ng/ml)
Vehicle	9±0.6	32±3	443±46	352±46
DOM	10±0.6	26±2	448±50	549±68
DOM+GnRH-A	1±0.6	-	15±10	14±3

Treatment	PRL Pulses Per 4HR	PRL IPI (min)	PRL Pulse Amp (ng/ml)	Mean PRL (ng/ml)
Vehicle	3±0.6	125±25	57±11	24±3
DOM	7±0.7	37±3	241±39	220±59
DOM+GnRH-A	8±0.5	31±3	132±45	159±46

Treatment with DOM had no effect on LH pulses in the OVX animals. However, DOM significantly increased the number of PRL pulses observed, in addition to raising mean PRL concentrations. The PRL IPI was somewhat longer than the LH IPI (37 vs 26 min). In both DOM-treated and control rats, 73% of the PRL pulses were synchronous with LH pulses. Assuming that GnRH and GAP are released simultaneously, these data do not support a physiological role for GAP as a PIF in this animal model. Furthermore, treatment with GnRH-A had no effect on the number of PRL pulses even though LH pulses were virtually abolished. However, PRL concentrations were reduced in the presence of low basal LH levels. Whereas these data support a relation between LH and PRL release, it appears that neither GnRH nor GAP can account for the PRL release patterns observed. (Supported by AA 05913 and HD 14643.)

EFFECT OF PLACENTAL LACTOGEN ON CIRCULATING PROLACTIN AND HYPOPHYSIAL STALK PLASMA DOPAMINE LEVELS. 96

J.L. Voogt, W.J. deGreef, J.T.M. Vreeburg. Univ. of Kansas Med. Ctr., Kansas City, KS 66103 and Erasmus Univ., Rotterdam, Netherlands.

The first half of pregnancy in the rat is characterized by twice daily surges in prolactin (PRL). The disappearance of these surges at midpregnancy is thought to be due to increasing concentration of placental lactogen (PL). However, no one has been able to demonstrate that injection of PL will terminate these surges. To mimick the continuous presence of PL rather than the acute change which occurs with an injection, we infused fluids containing PL via a jugular cannula from midnight until 0700h into pregnant rats hysterectomized (HS) 1 day earlier. Infusion of spent media (day 12 trophoblasts) or spent media in which PL was concentrated using ultrafiltration, resulted in significant inhibition of the nocturnal PRL surge. To ascertain whether both PL and PRL might act similarly to inhibit PRL via an increase in dopamine (DA) release into the stalk blood, the following experiments were done. Male rats with pituitary tumors secreting large amounts of PRL were used so that plasma PRL levels were comparable to PL levels seen at midpregnancy. The DA concentration (ng/ml) in the stalk plasma of these tumor bearing rats was a mean of 15.1±2.7, compared to 6.0±1.5 for the controls (P<.02). To see if endogenous secretion of PL also increased DA in the portal blood, day 12 intact pregnant rats were compared to mated rats HS on day 6 and injected with 3 mg/Kg CB-154 (to inhibit PRL) or vehicle 24 hours before stalk blood collection on Day 12. To our surprise, DA concentrations did not differ in the 3 groups (intact, 11.1; HS plus vehicle, 11.4; HS plus CB-154, 10.4). These results support the hypothesis that long term elevation of peripheral PRL levels inhibit PRL release by increasing DA secretion into the pituitary stalk vessels, but do not support this as a mechanism to explain the PL-induced inhibition of PRL surges at midpregnancy. However, it is important to note that DA levels in the stalk blood of all groups of pregnant intact or HS rats were much higher than control male rats.

CENTRAL NERVOUS SYSTEM SITES OF ACTION OF ATRIAL NATRIURETIC FACTOR. 97

W.K. SAMSON, J. ANTUNES-RODRIGUES, C.A. DUDLEY AND R.L. MOSS. Southwestern Medical School, Dallas, Texas 75235

A family of peptides, atrial natriuretic factors (ANFs), isolated from mammalian atria, possesses potent renal, adrenal, and vascular activities and has been hypothesized to play an important role in the physiologic control of fluid volume and electrolyte homeostasis. The recent demonstrations of ANF-like immunoreactivity in neuronal elements within the CNS, together with quantitation of ANF content of discrete brain regions, suggest that in addition to their effects in the periphery these peptides exert hypothalamic actions as well. We have observed the ability of synthetic ANF (atriopeptin III) to alter membrane excitability of single neurons in the septum, bed nucleus and preoptic areas when applied by either microiontophoresis or pressure-ejection. The majority (89%) of these neurons exhibited dose-related decrements in spontaneous firing rates during application of ANF, an effect which often outlasted the period of application.

Profound neuroendocrine and behavioral effects were observed following third intracerebroventricular (3V) administration of ANF in conscious rats. Basal vasopressin (AVP) secretion was inhibited significantly by 3V infusion of 1.0 (p<0.05) and 2.0 (p<0.01) nmoles ANF. In vitro studies failed to demonstrate a significant action of ANF on AVP release from neural lobe explants; however, a significant inhibitory action was seen in cultured hypothalamo-neurohypophysial complex explants. Similar doses of ANF significantly inhibited dehydration and angiotensin II-induced water intake, as well as salt-preference in the euvolemic, hyponatremic rat. These hypothalamic actions seem well coordinated with the actions of ANF in the periphery and comprise, perhaps, the CNS component of a coordinated mechanism by which ANF controls fluid volume and electrolyte homeostasis.

NON-Ca^{++}-DEPENDENT REGULATION OF *IN VITRO* ATRIAL NATRIURETIC FACTOR RELEASE BY EXTRACELLULAR OSMOLALITY 98

D.M. Gibbs
Dept. of Reproductive Medicine, UCSD School of Medicine, La Jolla, CA 92093

Recent reports have described modulation of atrial natriuretic factor (ANF) secretion by atrial stretch, increased Na^+ concentration, and a variety of hormones and neurotransmitters. One problem in the study of ANF secretion has been the isolation of stimulatory effects from interference due to rhythmic myocardial contraction. To avoid this problem, rat atria were dispersed with collagenase and DNAse, the myocytes were suspended in a polyacrylamide gel matrix, and the resulting cell column was perifused with a physiologic buffer. The secretion of ANF immunoactivity was markedly stimulated by increases in extracellular osmolality, regardless of the solute (NaCl, KCl, or glucose). This effect did not require extracellular Ca^{++}, nor could it be mimicked by depolarizing concentrations of K^+ in an isotonic medium. Functional viability of this model was demonstrated by significant, dose-related increases in ANF release in response to as little as 1 nM epinephrine. The dissociation of ANF secretion from depolarization-induced changes in Ca^{++} flux is unusual and may represent an adaptation to the dual roles of the atrial myocyte, contraction and secretion.

Supported by Office of Naval Research contract N00014-85-0306 and NIH grant AM-32517.

PRESENCE OF AN ENKEPHALIN-CONVERTING ENZYME (ENDO-OLIGOPEPTIDASE A) IN ENDOCRINE TISSUES 99

E.B.Oliveira*, M.S.Medeiros*, A.C.M. Camargo*, K.M. Metters+, J. Rossier+
* Instituto Ciências Biomédicas-USP, São Paulo, Brasil
+ Laboratorie de Physiologie Nerveuse, C.N.R.S. 91190 Gif-sur-Yvette, France

Biologically active peptides are initially synthesised as part of large inactive precursors molecules and subsequently generated by protrolytic cleavages. The observation that many biologically active sequences are bracketed by pairs of basic aminoacids has lead to the proposal that these peptides are liberated by the action of a trypsin-like endopeptidase followed by a carboxypeptidase B-like exopeptidase. However, in this study, we provide evidence that this combination of trypsin-like and carboxypeptidase B-like enzymes may not be the only mechanism for liberating enkephalin from low molecular weight enkephalin-containing peptides (ecp^s). Our data demonstrate that brain endo-oligopeptidase A can produce, by a single cleavage, Leucine^5-enkephalin (LE) and Methionine^5-enkephalin (ME) from small ecp^s. Thys cysteinyl-endopeptidase, highly purified from the soluble fraction of bovine, rat and human brain homogenates by immunoaffinity chromatography also hydrolyse the Phe^5-Ser^6 bond of bradykinin, the Arg^8-Arg^5 bond of neurotensin and produce ME and LE from several ecp^s as previously reported. When the same procedure of immunoaffinity chromatography was applied to the soluble fraction of human pituitary, pineal, hypothalamus, ovarium, testicle, thyroid and adrenal gland homogenates, a variable amount of a similar enzyme was determined.

EVIDENCE FOR PROGNRH IN RAT PERIPHERAL TISSUES: IMMUNOSTAINING WITH ANTIBODIES AGAINST GNRH AND THE GNRH-ASSOCIATED PEPTIDE 100

C.A. Padula, K. Nikolics, P.H. Seeburg, P.C. Goldsmith
Reproductive Endocrinology Center, Dept. of Ob/Gyn and Repro. Sci., University of Calif., San Francisco, CA 94143

Enzymatic cleavage of the prohormone for GnRH (proGnRH) produces a single copy of the GnRH decapeptide and a 56 amino acid GnRH-associated peptide (GAP) with some unexpected neuroendocrine properties. Antisera raised against portions of human GAP 27-40 (39A) and rat hypothalamic GAP 1-11 (24A) can immunostain GnRH neurons and axon terminals in the rat (Philips et al., Nature 316:542, 1985) and rhesus macaque (Goldsmith et al.; Song et al., this meeting). In view of earlier reports of GnRH or proGnRH-like peptides in rat placenta, hypothalamus, brain cortex, ovary, and mammary gland, we used antisera 24A and LR1 (anti-GnRH, R. Benoit) and the PAP technique to investigate the presence of GAP and proGnRH in paraffin sections of these and other paraformaldehyde perfused tissues. Solid and solid + liquid phase absorption with GAP confirmed the specificity of immunostaining.

GAP immunopositive (GAP+) staining was present in rat **placenta:** syncytiotrophoblast > cytotrophoblast, **ovary:** interstitial cells and large corpus luteal cells, **testis:** Leydig cells > bases of Sertoli cells, **kidney:** ascending thick limbs of the loops of Henle and distal convoluted tubules, **adrenal:** zona glomerulosa > z. fasciculata (not z. reticularis), **lactating mammary gland:** apical surface of glandular cells, and **brain:** cerebral cortex. GAP+ staining was questionable in **uterus:** basal part of most endometrial cells, **liver:** cells at center of lobules, **thymus:** center of lobules and reticular cells, and **spleen:** white pulp. It was negative in **anterior pituitary** and **heart.** GnRH+ staining with LR1 was evident in steroid producing cells, but was light or absent from other locations.

Consistent results with 24A and LR1 support the presence of proGnRH better than either antiserum alone. Further studies are necessary to confirm proGnRH synthesis by these tissues, and to examine differential proGnRH processing. It is strikingly coincidental that GnRH binding sites have also been identified in corpus luteum, adrenal cortex, and human breast carcinoma. The association between proGnRH+ cells and others in these organs may reveal new sites of GAP action, paracrine interaction, or suggest additional properties of proGnRH.

Supported by HD 11979 and HD 10907 (PCG).

IMMUNOHISTOLOGICAL STUDIES ON NEUROPEPTIDES IN THE RAT OVARY 101

T.J. Gorcs[1], A. Arimura[1], D.H. Coy[2]
U.S.-Japan Biomedical Research Laboratories, LMNED, Tulane University Hebert Center, Belle Chasse, LA 70037[1] and Department of Medicine, Tulane University School of Medicine, New Orleans, LA 70112[1,2]

Paraformaldehyde(4%) fixed rat ovaries were cut at 15 um thickness with a cryostat and processed for the immunohistochemical detection of the following peptides using the indirect immunofluorescent technique. The following antisera were used in this study: oxytocin, Arg-vasopressin, beta endorphin, $ACTH_{1-24}$, Met-enkephalin, Leu-enkephalin, sulfated CCK_{26-33}, GnRH decapeptide, synthetic peptide corresponding to GnRH-associated peptide $(GAP)_{14-25}$(Nikolics et al. Nature 316: 511-517, 1985), substance P, neurotensin, TRH, VIP, PHI, somatostatin 14, somatostatin 28_{1-14}(leader peptide), and rat atrial natriuretic $peptide_{5-27}$(rANP II).

The following peptide-like immunoreactivities were demonstrated in the luteal cells: oxytocin, Arg-vasopressin Leu-enkephalin, $ACTH_{1-24}$, GAP_{14-25}, and rANP II. Weak oxytocin, rANP II, and GAP_{14-25}like immunostaining were also found in the granulosa cells. All the immunoreactivities were absorbed by the addition of the respective peptides in the concentration of 50 ug/ml 1:500 dilution of the primary antisera, suggesting that these immunoreactivities were specific.

No immunoreactivity was detected with different region specific antisera against GnRH decapeptide. This raises the possibility that there is an ovarian peptide which shares a structure similar or same as GAP_{14-25}, but does not contain the GnRH decapeptide region.

(This research was supported in part by NIH grant HD 014761)

HYPOTHALAMIC CYCLIC AMP AND cGMP RESPONSE TO INTRAVENTRICULAR SUBSTANCE P AND/OR NEUROTENSIN IN THE RAT. 102

E.VIJAYAN, ANAHITA MISTRY
School of Life Sciences, University of Hyderabad, Hyderabad - 500134, India.

A variety of neuropeptides/neurotransmitters exert their action through cyclic nucleotides. Substance P (SP) and neurotensin (NT) have been localized in most parts of the central nervous system including the hypothalamus. Hypothalamic cAMP and cGMP levels in ovariectomized (OVX) and OVX-estrogen primed rats were evaluated, by radioimmunoassay, at 5,15,30 and 60 min after intracerebroventricular (ivt) injection of SP or NT in conscious rats.In one experiment intraventricular SP administration was followed by an equal dose of NT, ivt, and the hypothalamic nucleotide levels were assayed 15 min after the peptide injection.

Intraventricular SP significantly elevated hypothalamic cAMP and decreased cGMP levels. In contrast ivt administration of NT significantly stimulated cGMP and decreased cAMP levels. However, ivt injection of SP immediately followed by an equal dose of NT had no effect on the hypothalamic cAMP or cGMP levels. These results demonstrate an interesting observation that SP and NT, two closely related neuropeptides present abundantly in the hypothalamus, possibly exert their action through two different mechanism(s), viz.,SP stimulates cAMP while NT enhances cGMP production in the hypothalamic tissue.

(Supported by Grants from the Dept. of Science and Technology, Govt. of India).

HYPOTHALAMO-HYPOPHYSIAL SYSTEM: HIDDEN MICROVASCULAR BLOOD FLOW PATTERNS REVEALED IN VIVO BY FLUORESCENT MICROSPHERES 103

A.J. Baertschi
University of Virginia, Charlottesville VA 22908

Anatomical studies have demonstrated intricate vascular relationships between the arcuate hypothalamic area, median eminence and pituitary gland (Am. J. Anat. 148: 345, 1977; Science 204: 18, 1979), but the direction of blood flow between these structures is not fully understood. The hypothalamo-hypophysial complex of 15 anaesthetized rats was exposed by a retropharyngeal approach, and fluorescein-labelled microspheres (0.84-1.00 µm Ø) were injected intra-arterially or i.v.. The motion of the microspheres in the microvasculature was observed to a depth of 200 µm through a Nikon fluorescence microscope (x11 objective), image-intensified (SIT-66), video-displayed (x500) and magnetically recorded (10-20msec resolution). In the hypophysial stalk, the direction of blood flow was without exception from median eminence to pituitary gland. The same result was obtained with urethane anaesthesia, where blood pressures are low, and chloralose anaesthesia, where blood pressures are high. Large hemorrhage slowed the velocity of the microspheres, but did not change the direction of blood flow. Injection of 3-100mU vasopressin caused a large increase in blood pressure, biphasic changes in the velocity of microspheres, but no change in the direction of blood flow. Retrograde blood flow was only observed in dying animals, or when a pituitary vessel had been damaged during dissection. In conclusion, pituitary-brain transport of pituitary hormones is unlikely to take place by a vascular route, although transport via cerebrospinal fluid is not excluded. In-depth focusing of the median eminence area revealed significant outflow towards the arcuate and retrochiasmatic area, supporting the hypothesis that hypothalamic factors may modulate the activity of hypothalamic endocrine neurones. This method offers a new approach to study the hypothalamo-hypophysial microcirculation and the role of vasoactive peptides (vasopressin, CRF, atrial natriuretic factor) in pituitary control. (Supported by NIH HL31133).

SELECTED NEUROPEPTIDES IN AMYOTROPHIC LATERAL SCLEROSIS PATIENTS 104

J.Szulc-Kuberska, H.Stepien, A.Klimek, D.Cieslak
Dept.Neurology and Inst.Endocrinology, Medical Academy in Lodz, Poland

The etiopathogenesis of amyotrophic lateral sclerosis /ALS/ remains unclear and recently attention was payed to the role of neuropeptides in the disease. Corticotropin releasing factor /CRF/ widely distributed in the brain and spinal cord neurons and besides hormonal have also neuromodulatory function. Epidermal growth factor /EGF/ a mitogenic peptide is also widely distributed in the brain and play also neuromodulatory function.

5 patients in average age 59.6 with undoubt diagnosis of ALS were studied. The control group consisted of 7 patients in average age 56.6 with discopathy on the level L4-L5 or L5-S1 confirmed by myelography. In all patients the lumbar puncture was performed before tretment. The concentration of CRF in the cerebro-spinal fluid /CSF/ was measured by radioimmunoassay technique using kits produced by Peninsula Lab. The concentration of EGF was measured by using EGF radioreceptor assay kits purchased by Biomedical Technologies Inc.

The CRF level in ALS patients was 22.9 +7.61 pg/ml and this value was significantly lower than in control group, 51.3+6.97 pg/ml. The EGF level in Csf in ALS patients was 662.4 + 207 pg/ml as compared to controls 1013 +182.8 pg/ml, and was also significantly lower.

The low Crf and EGF level in CSF in our patients could imply neurosecretory damage in ALS and suggest some role of the neuropeptides in the pathogenesis of the disease.

SIMULTANEOUS DISTRIBUTION OF OVARIAN LHRH AND β-ADRENERGIC RECEPTORS DURING SEXUAL MATURATION IN THE RAT: ROLE OF OVARIAN INNERVATION 105

B. Marchetti, M. Cioni, U. Scapagnini, *G. Pelletier
Dpt. Pharmacology, Catania University, 95125 Italy and *Molecular Endocrinol. Laval University, Quebec, Canada

The hypothalamic peptide LHRH has direct antigonadal actions in the rat ovary and specific receptors (R) for the neurohormone have been localized in the ovaries of immature and adult rats. Recently, the importance of ovarian adrenergic innervation has been substantiated by the characterization of specific β-adrenergic R of the β_2-type, responsible for adrenergic stimulation of ovarian steroid secretion. In the present study we have used in vitro autoradiography and quantitative binding studies to localize simultaneously ovarian LHRH and β-adrenergic R during sexual maturation. Between 12 and 20 days of age, the distribution of LHRH and β-adrenoceptors shows a marked concentration of silver grains at the interstitial gland. Around puberty LHRH R are primarily localized around the follicles, while β-adrenoceptors are present mostly on corpora lutea. Quantitative studies show a marked drop of LHRH-R activity at puberty, accompanied by a significant increase in the number of β-adrenergic binding sites. Complete removal of adrenergic innervation performed by cutting the superior ovarian and plexus nerves markedly decreases both LHRH and β-adrenergic R levels measured by autoradiography and quantitative binding assay, within the operated ovary with no effect taking place in the intact contralateral gland. These data indicate that changes of receptor levels and distribution within the different ovarian compartments take place during sexual maturation. Furthermore, results obtained following unilateral nervotomy suggest a direct participation of ovarian innervation in receptor regulation, possibly as a direct result of changes of central adrenergic activity.

ANGIOTENSIN II : A GROWTH HORMONE RELEASING FACTOR IN THE DEVELOPING RAT ? 106

Wim Robberecht and Carl Denef
Laboratory of Cell Pharmacology, School of Medicine, University of Leuven, Belgium

In vivo Angiotensin II (AII) has an inhibitory effect on growth hormone (GH) release in rats (Steele et al. Endocrinology 109, 893 (1982)), while in vitro it is reported to have only a slight (ibidem) or no effect at all (Aguilera et al. Endocrinology 111, 1025 (1982)) ; these studies were performed with adult rats. We investigated the effect of AII in the regulation of GH release in anterior pituitary cellaggregates from 9-day-old, 14-day-old and adult male and female rats. Aggregates were cultured in serum free medium supplemented with glucocorticoids and thyroid hormone. In 9-day- and 14-day-old males and females AII was found to release GH in a dose dependent way (10^{-11}M-10^{-9}M). Increases above baseline values (in %) were : 9-day-old males : 10^{-10}M : 195 % ; 10^{-9}M : 576 % ; 14-day-old males : 10^{-10}M : 204 % ; 10^{-9}M : 407 % ; 14-day-old females : 10^{-10}M : 212 % ; 10^{-9}M 413 %. In adult animals, AII had no effect on GH release at all, even when concentrations of 10^{-7}M were used. Adult spontaneously hypertensive females however did respond to AII 10^{-8}M. In additional studies GRF was used as a comparison : 10^{-12} M GRF caused a mean increase of 226 % and 10^{-11} M stimulated the release of GH to 1132 % above baseline values. No major differences in GRF-responsiveness were found between the 3 age groups.

These results suggest the possibility of a role of AII in the regulation of GH release during a restricted period of development. It is known that the regulation of GH release significantly varies during the rat's lifespan : pituitary cell responsiveness to GRF in vitro decreases with age (Szabo and Cuttler, Endocrinology 118, 69 (1986)) while the role of somatostatin only seems to be established after 10 days of age (Wehrenberg, Endocrinology 118, 489 (1986)). AII immunereactivity is known to be present in the pituitary gland, particularly in gonadotrophes (Deschepper et al. Neuroendocrinology 40, 471 (1985), Healy and Prinz, Hypertension 6 S I, I 130 (1984)). Since gonadotrophes seem to exert paracrine actions (Denef and Andries, Endocrinology 112, 813 (1983)), it is tempting to speculate that AII is a paracrine GH releasing factor in the growing animal.

DEVELOPMENTAL CHANGE IN THE SENSITIVITY TO SOMATOSTATIN IN THE OVINE FETUS AND LAMB. 107

J.Daaboul, F.de Zegher, S.L.Kaplan, M.M.Grumbach, Dept. of Pediatrics, University of California San Francisco, San Francisco, CA 94143

In the ovine fetus circulating GH levels are high in midgestation, fall at term, and are low in the neonatal lamb. Moreover, the ovine fetus exhibits a GH hyper-response to GRF compared to the neonate. The mechanisms underlying these changes are unknown. We examined the hypothesis that one factor in these ontogenetic changes is an alteration in pituitary sensitivity to somatostatin (SRIF) between midgestation and neonatal life.

Four chronically catheterized fetuses (gestational ages 115-130 days; term 147d) and five lambs (ages 4-16d) were studied singly or sequentially. After 30 min of baseline sampling SRIF was given as a 30 μg/kg IV bolus, followed by SRIF 125-150 μg/kg as an IV infusion over 75 min. Thirty minutes after the start of the SRIF infusion, GRF 1 μg /kg was given as an IV pulse. In the control studies a saline infusion and GRF were used.

In fetuses 115-122d a significant difference was not detected between controls (n=3, 5 studies) and SRIF infused animals (n=3, 5 studies), either in the mean maximal increment in GH (ΔGH) after GRF (555±212 vs 526±227 ng/ml) or the integrated incremental GH area over the 45 min following GRF (9693±1002 vs 10544±4437 ng/ml.min). In the control lambs (n=5, 7 studies) the Δ GH evoked by GRF was 118±89 ng/ml; SRIF significantly suppressed the ΔGH to 0±3 ng/ml (mean±SD; p <0.01). The integrated incremental GH area after GRF in control lambs, was 2037±1611 ng/ml.min, whereas in SRIF infused lambs this area was -42±128 ng/ml.min, which is strikingly lower (mean±SD; p <0.005). In fetuses 126-130d (n=3, 3 studies) the ΔGH and integrated incremental GH area in the presence of SRIF were intermediate (172±118 ng/ml and 2942±2483 ng/ml.min).

These data support the hypothesis that pituitary sensitivity to SRIF increases between midgestation and the neonatal period, and suggests that the hyper-response to GRF in the fetus is mediated in part by decreased sensitivity to SRIF.

DIFFERENTIAL EFFECTS OF THE PERINATAL STEROID ENVIRONMENT ON SEXUALLY DIMORPHIC PARAMETERS IN THE RAT BRAIN 108

A. Siddiqui, D.P. Gilmore, J.S. Clark
Institute of Physiology, University of Glasgow, Glasgow, G12 8QQ.

Evidence is now accumulating to indicate that sex steroids play a significant role in modulating postnatal neuronal maturation and neuronal circuit formation.

In this study the developmental influence of perinatal androgens on catecholaminergic and serotoninergic neuronal systems has been examined in the rat. Male rats (n=8 in each group) were either castrated, or sham-operated, on Day 1 postnatally. One group (n=8) of female rats was administered 100 μg of testosterone in corn oil daily for the first 5 neonatal days, a second group (n=8) received vehicle only. The animals were decapitated at 60, 75, 90, 120 and 180 days of age. The brain was dissected out and the hypothalamus, amygdala and corpora quadrigemina surgically isolated. These discrete regions were homogenised in 0.1M HCl and centrifuged. 20μl of the supernatant was injected onto a reversed-phase high performance liquid chromatography column coupled to an electrochemical detector. Noradrenaline (NA), dopamine (DA), serotonin (5-HT) and 5-hydroxylindoleacetic acid (5-HIAA) levels were measured in samples from each region. Differences observed in treated animals when compared to controls are outlined below:

Deprivation of testosterone in the neonatal male resulted in a significant depletion (P<0.001) of NA, DA, 5-HT and 5-HIAA levels at 60 and 75 days in all 3 regions. By 90 days the differences between experimental and control animals were no longer significant. At both 120 and 180 days the situation had become reversed with the concentrations of all 4 neurotransmitters being significantly higher (P<0.001) in the brain regions of the experimental animals.

In the female rats the levels of all the neurotransmitters measured at 60 and 75 days were either higher or unchanged in those treated with androgens. However, this situation was reversed at 90, 120 and 180 days.

These experiments demonstrate the manner in which all 3 neurotransmitter systems respond to perinatal androgens.

AROMATASE ACTIVITY IN BRAIN REGIONS OF STANLEY-GUMBRECK PSEUDOHERMAPHRODITE MALE RATS AND NORMAL LITTERMATES 109

C.E. Roselli, R. L. Salisbury, J.A. Resko
Oregon Health Sci. Univ., Portland, Oregon and the Univ. of Akron, Akron, Ohio

We used gonadally intact Stanley-Gumbreck pseudohermaphrodite (PSH) and normal littermate (NL) male rats to study the regulation of brain aromatase activity (AA). AA was measured in homogenates of brain tissue by using a radiometric assay that quantifies the production of ^3H_2O from [1β-^{3}H] androstenedione as an index of estrogen formation.

Initially, we assessed the capability of block-dissected tissues to aromatize androgens. We found that AA was 2 to 4 times higher (p < .001) in the amygdala, preoptic area, and basal hypothalamus of NL versus PSH rats. To pinpoint specific sites where AA is affected in PSH rats, we measured AA in ten hypothalamic and limbic nuclei that were dissected from 300 μm frozen brain sections. AA was highest in the bed nucleus of the stria terminalis (NL = 340 ± 11 (SEM) vs PSH = 117 ± 10 fmol/h•mg protein; p < .001); medial amygdala (NL = 353 ± 66 vs PSH = 289 ± 40 fmol/h•mg protein; p > .1), and periventricular preoptic area (NL = 161 ± 16 vs PSH 38 ± 6 fmol/h•mg protein; p < .001). Although testosterone levels were 6-fold higher in PSH rats tnan NL siblings (PSH = 17.8 ± 2 vs NL = 4.4 ± 1 ng/ml; p < .001), NL rats had higher levels of AA in all microdissected brain regions except for the medial and cortical amygdala (p < .01).

This study demonstrates that brain AA is deficient in PSH male rats and may explain why these animals are insensitive to the effects of testosterone on masculine sexual behavior. Since it has been demonstrated previously that brain androgen receptor concentrations are severely reduced (85-95%) in PSH rats, we interpret our data as providing further evidence to support the hypothesis that brain aromatase is an androgen-receptor regulated gene product. Supported by HD 18196

APPRAISING THE INSTANTANEOUS SECRETORY RATES OF LUTEINIZING HORMONE AND TESTOSTERONE IN RESPONSE TO SELECTIVE MU OPIATE RECEPTOR IN LATE PUBERTAL BOYS. 110

N. Mauras, A.D. Rogol, J.D. Veldhuis
The University of Virginia Medical Center
Charlottesville, Virginia 22908

We have examined the pulsatile properties of gonadotropin and testosterone release before and after chronic mu opiate receptor blockade with naltrexone, 50 mg every other day, in 4 normal boys in late puberty (ages 14 8/12 - 15 1/12 years). The nature of spontaneous secretory events was appraised for immunoactive LH, and testosterone in blood withdrawn every 20 min for 24 hr, using a novel discrete deconvolution algorithm to estimate apparent instantaneous secretory rates. The application of this methodology revealed that the frequency of discrete LH secretory episodes increased after mu opiate-receptor blockade (p=0.011). More strikingly, all parameters of testosterone secretory events responded significantly to mu opiate-receptor blockade; viz, there were increases in mean estimated secretory rate, testosterone pulse frequency and amplitude; and, correspondingly, decreases in testosterone interpulse secretory intervals, and secretory pulse duration and interpulse valley duration.

The marked increase in LH and testosterone secretory activity after opiate-receptor blockade suggests an integral interaction between the endogenous opiate system and the gonadal axis in the later stages of puberty in males.

REMOVAL OF A CENTRAL INHIBITORY COMPONENT AND HYPOTHALAMIC MATURATION AT THE ONSET OF PUBERTY 111

N.J. Schultz, E. Terasawa
Wis. Reg. Primate Res. Ctr., Univ. WI, Madison, WI 53715

Previously, we have hypothesized that in nonhuman primates there is a developmental period during which a central inhibition predominates over the activity of the LHRH neurosecretory apparatus, and the release from this central inhibition as the result of hypothalamic maturation appears to precede the onset of puberty. Our recent studies have provided further evidence for this hypothesis: 1) In female rhesus monkeys ovariectomized neonatally, LH levels were suppressed during the prepubertal period until 25 mo. of age, when LH levels started to increase. The increase in basal LH continued and a 100% elevation from prepubertal levels was attained at 26 mo., and a 200% elevation at 30 mo. of age. An appearance of diurnal variation in LH (nocturnal LH increase) preceded the initial LH increase by 4-5 mo. 2) Lesions of the posterior hypothalamus at 17-18 mo. of age, which we previously reported to be effective in advancing the time of menarche and first ovulation by several months in ovarian intact monkeys, induced an increase in basal LH levels and the diurnal LH variation within 1 mo. postoperatively in ovariectomized monkeys. Basal LH levels in these ovariectomized monkeys further increased reaching a 100% elevation of the prelesion levels by 20 mo. and a 200% elevation by 23 mo. of age. All these LH changes with posterior hypothalamic lesions occurred significantly earlier than those in control animals. 3) Lesions of the posterior hypothalamus at 13-14 mo. of age in ovariectomized monkeys also resulted in an increase in LH and the diurnal LH variation within 1.5 mo. postoperatively and both these changes occurred significantly earlier than those of animals receiving lesions at 17-18 mo. of age. However, 100% and 200% LH elevations did not occur until 20 mo. and 23 mo. of age, respectively, ages similar to those of animals receiving lesions at 17-18 mo. of age. These results indicate that 1) lesions of the posterior hypothalamus seem to remove an inhibition to activity of the LHRH neurosecretory system that is essential to the onset of puberty, 2) hypothalamic maturation in addition to removal of a central inhibition is a prerequisite for the pubertal process to proceed.

β-ENDORPHIN AND DYNORPHIN-17 LEVELS IN RAT PITUITARY AND HYPOTHALAMUS: AGE STUDIES 112

Elizabeth M. Dax*, Coral Reichman, Meryl Fullerton and John W. Funder
National Institutes of Aging, Francis Scott Key Medical Center, Baltimore 21224, and Medical Research Centre, Prince Henry's Hospital, Melbourne 3004, Australia.

Previous studies (1) have documented progressive changes in pituitary and hypothalamic content of immunoreactive β-endorphin (ir-βEP) and immunoreactive dynorphin (ir-DYN) over the first 3 months of life. Other studies (2) have compared mature versus old animals. In the present study we have extended these observations to examine animals from 3 to 24 months in a cross-sectional study. Male outbred Wistar rats (9-14 per group) were housed under standard conditions at the NIA, and killed by decapitation at 3, 6, 12, 18 and 24 months of age. Hypothalami and pituitary glands were removed, the anterior pituitary (AP) separated from the neurointermediate lobe (N-IL), and tissues rapidly frozen on dry ice and maintained at -70°C until assay. Tissues were extracted in 0.1 M HCl and assayed for ir-βEP and ir-DYN1-17. In both AP and N-IL no significant or consistent change in level of ir-βEP was seen with age; in the hypothalamus, however, levels of ir-βEP fell progressively from 3-18 months, but were restored at 24 months to levels indistinguishable from those at 3 months. For ir-DYN, levels in AP similarly progressively declined to half, with plateau levels at 18-24 months. In the hypothalamus a significant, but less marked, fall was seen to plateau levels at 12 months; in contrast, in the N-IL no consistent changes in ir-DYN were seen. We interpret these studies as evidence (i) that there are tissue-specific, age-related changes in synthesis and/or release of endogenous opioid peptides in the hypothalamo-pituitary axis and (ii) that such changes may be reflected by age-related changes in putative neuromodulator opioid actions in the hypothalamus, or in putative paracrine actions of dynorphin in anterior pituitary.

1. Seizinger et al: Endocrinology 115, 926, 1984.
2. Rogers et al: Neurobiology of Aging 6, 1, 1985.

STRUCTURE AND ACTIVITY OF THE GnRH PRECURSOR 113

P.H. Seeburg, J. Ramachandran and K. Nikolics
Genentech, Inc., So. San Francisco, CA 94080

The gene for GnRH and its precursor was cloned and analyzed from human, rat and mouse. The deduced protein sequences of the respective precursor molecules specify a common tripartite structure consisting of: signal sequence, GnRH with proteolytic and amidating processing site and the sequence of a 56 residue long peptide which we termed GAP for GnRH-associated peptide. The presence of GAP in rat hypothalamic perikarya and nerve terminals was shown by immunocytochemistry [Phillips et. al., Nature 316, 542-545 (1985)] and pulsatile GAP released from neurosecretory cells was detected in portal blood (Clarke et.al, in preparation). Bacterially synthesized human GAP was purified to homogeneity and used to assess its hypophysiotropic actions in primary rat pituitary cells. GAP was found to stimulate LH and FSH release and to be a potent inhibitor of prolactin release from lactotrophs. Rabbits immunized against GAP sequences showed highly elevated circulating prolactin levels and GAP showed *in vivo* activity in the hypogonadal mouse and lactating rats (in collaboration with A.V. Schally). These data support the notion that GAP is a physiological regulator of prolactin secretion. The release of GnRH and GAP from the same neurosecretory cells suggests a coupled inverse regulation of circulating gonadotropin and prolactin levels.

TRANSCRIPTIONAL REGULATION OF PROOPIOMELANOCORTIN GENE EXPRESSION IN NEUROENDOCRINE CELLS 114

James L. Roberts
Columbia Univ. College of Physicians & Surgeons, NY, NY

Proopiomelanocortin (POMC) is an important neuroendocrine peptide precursor. Depending upon its site of expression in the brain and pituitary it is cleaved into different biologically active peptides. In addition, its expression varies in the different tissues. For example, the POMC gene is negatively responsive to glucocorticoids in the anterior pituitary while it is nonresponsive to them in the intermediate pituitary. In contrast, the POMC gene is not responsive to estrogen in either lobe of the pituitary, whereas it is negatively regulated by it in the hypothalamus. In addition to being regulated by steroids, POMC gene expression is regulated by a variety of different peptide hormones such as corticotropin releasing hormone and catecholamines. A series of transcriptional studies have shown that all factors which physiologically regulate POMC secretion have parallel effects on POMC transcription. We have isolated the gene encoding the rat POMC molecule and have completely characterized its 5' flanking sequences. Nucleotide sequence analysis reveals a region of strong homology to a cyclic AMP regulatory element at approximately -275 and a glucocorticoid regulatory element at approximately -580 region of the promoter area. A series of deletion mutants in the 5' region of the gene have been constructed and are currently being tested for altered gene expression by transient transfection analysis. For analysis of POMC gene transcription in the complex hypothalamic system, it is of value to be able to make measurements in individual cells. Thus, we have used intervening sequence-specific DNA probes in an *in situ* hybridization assay. We can quantitate levels of transcription in individual neurons in response to various hormonal and environmental changes. These studies have shown that transcriptional regulation of specific neuropeptide genes is an important element in the function and response of the organism to changing behavioral, environmental, and hormonal influences.

STRUCTURES AND REGULATIONS OF THE PREPROTACHYKININ GENES 115

S. Nakanishi
Institute for Immunology, Kyoto University Faculty of Medicine, Kyoto, 606 Japan

The peptides of the tachykinin family exhibit similar biological activities and include one of the best characterized peptidergic neurotransmitters, substance P (SP). The primary structures of three types of the SP precursors (preprotachykinins A or PPTs-A) were elucidated by determining their cloned cDNAs. α-PPT-A contains a single SP sequence, while β- and γ-PPTs-A include an additional novel tachykinin sequence named substance K (SK). SK was chemically synthesized and different pharmacological profiles between SK and SP were demonstrated, indicating that SK represents a second mammalian tachykinin. The single PPT-A gene encodes the above three PPT-A mRNAs and SK is specified by a discrete internal exon sequence within the gene. Furthermore, the generation of α- and β-/γ-PPT-A mRNAs is regulated in a tissue-specific manner by alternative RNA splicing through the inclusion or exclusion of the SK-coding exon sequence.

cDNA and genomic DNAs for the precursor containing the third tachykinin neuropeptide termed neuromedin K (preprotachykinin B or PPT-B) were also isolated and characterized. The structural organization of the PPT-B gene closely resembles that of the PPT-A gene, suggesting that the two PPT genes have evolved from a common ancestor gene. Furthermore, the PPT-A and PPT-B mRNAs differ in their major expression sites. Thus, it can be concluded that the mammalian tachykinin system has acquired its diversity through various cellular mechanisms including gene duplication, differential expression of duplicated genes and alternative RNA splicing for the generation of multiple mRNAs from a single gene.

HOW GENE TRANSFER METHODS HELP US TO UNDERSTAND REGULATION OF EXPRESSION OF OPIOID PEPTIDES 116

E. Herbert, M. Comb, G. Thomas, D. Liston, J. Douglass, B. Thorne, M. Martin
Institute for Advanced Biomedical Research, The Oregon Health Sciences University, 3181 SW Sam Jackson Park Road, Portland, Oregon 97201

The 15 or more peptides that comprise the family of opioid peptides are synthesized from three different precursor proteins: proopiomelanocortin (POMC) which contains the sequences of ACTH, melanocyte stimulating hormones and β-endorphin, proenkephalin (proenk A) which contains 7 copies of the enkephalins, and prodynorphin (proenk B) which contains dynorphins. Each precursor is expressed in a number of tissues where it may undergo differential processing and tissue specific regulation. For example, the production of POMC peptides in the anterior pituitary is stimulated by corticotropin releasing factor (CRF), whereas in the intermediate lobe of the pituitary, POMC production is controlled by catecholamines and not by CRF.

We have cloned and sequenced the genes and the cDNA encoding the 3 opioid precursors and the cDNA encoding 2 enzymes that may be involved in proteolytic processing of these precursors. The genes and cDNA encoding the precursors are being introduced into various types of secretory and nonsecretory cells to determine how they function in different cellular environments. One example is the introduction of the gene encoding human proenk into mouse pituitary cells (AtT-20) that normally express POMC but not mouse proenk. Stably transformed AtT-20 clones have been isolated which express the human proenk mRNA and protein at very high levels and process the protein accurately and completely to Met-enk which is secreted in parallel with ACTH under the control of CRF. Transcription of the transfected proenk gene can be stimulated by CRF and cAMP and suppressed by methylation of sequences in the DNA. Further experiments with fusion gene constructs have enabled us to pinpoint the location of the regulatory elements in the proenk gene that are responsible for suppression of transcription by methylation and for cAMP and phorbol ester stimulation of transcription.

ENDOGENOUS OPIATES AND GONADOTROPIN SECRETION IN THE NON-HUMAN PRIMATE 117

M. Ferin
College of Physicians & Surgeons, Columbia University, New York, NY 10032

Opiates are known to modify the secretion of several hypophyseal hormones. In this seminar, we will review the evidence which supports a physiological role for endogenous opioid peptides, and for B-endorphin in particular, on gonadotropin secretion in the female rhesus monkey. An interaction between endogenous opiates and LH release is indicated by the observations that intraventricular administration of B-endorphin results in a decrease in LH secretion and that antagonism of endogenous opiate activity following naloxone increases LH release. This regulatory mechanism, however, is a complex one which involves gonadal steroid hormones: for instance, a rapid LH response to naloxone is seen only during the luteal phase of the menstrual cycle when progesterone concentrations are elevated. The effectiveness of naloxone in releasing LH is related to the secretory activity of the hypothalamic opiate system, which fluctuates significantly throughout the menstrual cycle: maximal release of B-endorphin by the hypothalamus occurs during the luteal phase in the presence of estrogen and progesterone, while relative ovarian steroid deficiency such as at menstruation, is characterized by absent or diminished brain B-endorphin release. Further data indicate that endogenous opioid peptides regulate pulse frequency of the GnRH (gonadotropin-releasing hormone) pulse generator, as demonstrated during the luteal phase of the menstrual cycle. Experimental evidence in the rhesus monkey suggests that changes in GnRH-LH pulse frequency that occur during the luteal phase may be an important determinant of cyclicity: prevention of these frequency changes exerts subtle effects on anterior pituitary secretion which may lead to abnormalities in subsequent menstrual cycles including luteal phase defects and anovulation. Supported by NIH HD 10873 and HD 05077.

NEUROPEPTIDES IN THE MEDIAN EMINENCE 119

M. Palkovits
First Department of Anatomy, Semmelweis University Medical School, Budapest, Hungary

The median eminence (ME) plays a key role in the neuroendocrine regulatory mechanisms constituting a link between the central nervous system and the pituitary gland. More than 20 neuropeptides have been localized in the ME by radioimmuno- or immunohistochemical techniques. The major group of the peptidergic fibers terminate around the pericapillary space from where neuropeptides can reach the portal blood and exert their neurohormonal effects on anterior pituitary cells. An other group of peptidergic fibers (vasopressin, oxytocin, leu-enkephalin, dynorphin, neo-endorphin, cholecystokinin, galanin, angiotensin II containing axons) pass through the ME on way to the neuronal and intermediate lobes.

Peptidergic fibers enter the ME from two major directions: (1) Fibers from anterolateral direction through the lateral retrochiasmatic area: LH-RH containing fibers arise from the medial preoptic nucleus, TRH-, CRF-, NPY-, VIP-, ANF-, PHI-27- and CCK-containing fibers from the paraventricular nucleus, somatostatin fibers from the periventricular nucleus, dynorphin, neo-endorphin, enkephalin, galanin, angiotensin II, vasopressin and oxytocin containing fibers arise from both supraoptic and paraventricular nuclei. (2) Short tuberoinfundibular fibers arise mainly from the arcuate nucleus. They contain GRF, ACTH, α-MSH, β-endorphin, NPY, substance P and neurotensin.

Presynaptic regulation of neurohormone release has been described in the ME.

INTRINSIC AND SYNAPTIC REGULATION OF VASOPRESSINERGIC NEURONS 120

L.P. Renaud
Neurosciences Unit, Montreal General Hospital and McGill University, Montreal, Quebec, Canada.

An understanding of the neuroregulatory role of peptides may be surmised through analysis of their biochemical, behavioral and electrical actions consequent to exogenous application. An alternate complementary strategy is to examine the intrinsic and synaptic factors that regulate the excitability of peptide-secreting neurons themselves. Electrophysiologists seldom utilize this approach as it necessitates the confident identification of the peptidergic cell. In the mammalian nervous system, this rare possibility is offered by the hypothalamic vasopressin (VP)-secreting magnocellularneurosecretory neuron.

During in-vivo extracellular recordings in the rat, VP neurons in the supraoptic and paraventricular nuclei demonstrate activation by (a) local osmotic stimuli; (b) circulating angiotensin II, through a pathway that requires the subfornical organ; (c) stimulation of carotid chemoreceptors, hepatic portal osmoreceptors and renal nerve nociceptive fibers, probably mediated through ventrolateral medulla noradrenergic afferents. Depressant influences include a GABA-mediated input activated through peripheral baroreceptor stimulation, and afferent pathways arising in amygdala and lateral septum.

Intracellular observations in-vitro reveal the intrinsic nature of their phasic activity, a variety of membrane conductances and their modulation by osmotic stimuli, synaptic influences and applied neurotransmitters. The influence of these factors can be expressed by changes in VP released in the neurohypophysis. As such the VP neuron may be viewed as a model for the study of other peptide-secreting neurons.

THE RENIN ANGIOTENSIN SYSTEM (RAS) IN THE BRAIN 121

D. Ganten
German Institute for High Blood Pressure Research and Dept. of Pharmacology, University of Heidelberg, Heidelberg, FRG

The biosynthetic pathway and the functions of the hormonal plasma renin angiotensin system are well recognized. Since the components of the RAS were first described within the brain (Ganten et al., Science 1973: 64, 1971), evidence has accumulated supporting the existence of a complete RAS endogenous to the brain and playing a role in cardiovascular and volume homeostasis. Other functions e.g. on memory or reproductive behaviour are presently being studied.

The high molecular weight peptide precursor angiotensinogen has been cloned and the complete sequence of angiotensinogen is determined. Using molecular biological techniques it has been demonstrated that the same angiotensinogen molecule is synthesized in the brain and in the liver. The regulation of transcription of the gene, however, appears to be tissue specific. Angiotensin I and the active octapeptide angiotensin II (ANG II) have been characterized in brain. The distribution of ANG II in the central nervous system has been investigated by chemical as well as by immunohistochemical techniques. The main locations of ANG II are the hypothalamus, the limbic system, the medulla oblongata and the spinal cord; there is good agreement with the localization of ANG II receptors. The key enzymes of the peptide system, i.e. renin, converting enzyme and angiotensinases, have equally been shown to be present in the brain and pharmacological inhibition of the synthesizing enzymes leads to reduced angiotensin synthesis and inhibition of function, e.g. blood pressure reduction (Ganten et al., Science 221: 869, 1983). Since the genes for the RAS proteins are now known, studies at the cellular and molecular level have become possible. The availability of pharmacological interferences at the sites of peptide generation and peptide action to an extent not equalled for other enzyme peptide systems makes the RAS one of the well studied peptide systems in the brain.

MODULATION OF PITUITARY HORMONE SECRETION BY INTERCELLULAR COMMUNICATION. 122

C. Denef, M. Baes and P. Carmeliet
Laboratory of Cell Pharmacology, University of Leuven, Medical School, Belgium.

Homeostasis in the anterior pituitary appears to be preserved not only by hypothalamic hypophysiotropic hormones and peripheral hormones but also by intercellular messengers produced in the pituitary itself. We have shown, using rat pituitary reaggregate cell cultures, that certain cell types transmit regulatory signals to other cell types in a selective fashion. Gonadotrophs produce a factor(s) with prolactin (PRL) releasing activity. Gonadotrophs mediate the stimulation of PRL release by LHRH and modulate the PRL response to angiotensin II and B-adrenergic agents. Another cell type so far not fully identified, strongly potentiates growth hormone (GH) secretion stimulated by B-adrenergic agents and, to a smaller extent, by GRF and VIP. The glial-like folliculostellate cells interact with several cell types. Coaggregating folliculo-stellate cells with enriched populations of lactotrophs, somatotrophs or gonadotrophs results in a significant inhibition of the PRL response to angiotensin II, TRH and VIP,the GH response to GRF and B-adrenergic agents and the LH response to LHRH. Most recently we found evidence for the existence of an intrinsic cholinergic system in the pituitary aggregates. Blocking muscarinic receptors resulted in a significant rise of basal as well as B-adrenergic stimulated GH and PRL secretion. Most of these intercellular messenger systems are strongly dependent on steroid and thyroid hormones.

References: Denef,C. and Andries, M. Endocrinology 112, 813 (1983)
Denef, C., Baes, M. and Schramme, C. In: Frontiers in Neuroendocrinology, Vol 9, Ganong WF and Martini L, eds) Raven Press, New York, 1986.

STRESS, ADRENAL STEROIDS AND THE HIPPOCAMPUS 123

B.S. McEwen, R.M. Sapolsky, A. Harrelson and R.E. Brinton
Rockefeller University, New York, NY 10021

Communication between nerve cells involves far more than the direct excitation and inhibition of neuronal firing by released neurotransmitters. Other chemical messengers liberated by neurons or glial cells, and hormones reaching the brain via the blood, are responsible for modulating neuronal function. Modulation may involve phosphorylation of various proteins via second messengers and also the regulation of genomic activity and expression of gene products involved in neuronal activity. The consequence of modulation is to alter the functional capacity and response profile of the neuron in carrying out its normal activity.

The hippocampus is an excellent tissue for studying physiologically relevant neuromodulation, for this structure is an interface between cognition and affect, as well as waking and dreaming, and is involved in regulating pituitary-adrenal activity. Glucocorticoid receptors abound, and adrenal steroids influence various aspects of hippocampal function. We have divided these actions into 3 aspects: "activational", "adaptive" and"degenerative". Activational effects are involved in coordinating and optimizing the animal's daily activity in terms of synaptic efficacy for learning, exploratory activity and obtaining food. Superimposed on these actions are stress-induced adaptational effects in which the glucocorticoids alter the neurochemistry of the hippocampus and other brain regions in ways that allow the animals to cope. When stress persists, and also during aging, degenerative glucocorticoid effects may emerge which represent the inability of coping mechanisms to fully protect the organism. Hippocampal, and possibly other, neurons are destroyed and with this destruction a "feed-forward" cascade emerges which results in progressively higher levels of glucocorticoids and resultant peripheral metabolic and immune disturbances.

(Supported by PHS grant MH41256).

FUNCTIONAL SIGNIFICANCE OF PEPTIDERGIC THYROID NERVES. 124

G.A. Hedge, L.J. Huffman, and J.M. Connors
Department of Physiology, West Virginia University Medical Center, Morgantown, WV, USA

Thyroid nerves impinging upon both follicle cells and blood vessels are known to contain various neuropeptides (NPs), including vasoactive intestinal peptide (VIP), peptide histidine isoleucine (PHI), and neuropeptide Y (NPY). Therefore, we have investigated these NPs for simultaneous effects on thyroid hormone secretion and blood flow (BF) in anesthetized adult rats. Changes in plasma concentrations of T_3 and T_4 (by RIA) were used as an index of hormone secretion, while BF to the thyroid and other tissues was determined by the reference sample version of the radioactive microsphere technique (^{141}Ce). VIP (2-4 min infusion) caused an increase in thyroid BF in proportion to the log of the dose over a range of 0.006 - 0.6 µg/rat. Beyond this range, BF decreased in association with hypotension, but vascular conductance (VC) plateaued or continued to increase. Among the VIP homologs, the order of potency was VIP>PHI>secretin>> growth hormone releasing hormone. Some NPs of this family also increased VCs in pancreas (>5x) and salivary gland (>10x), but not in other tissues (e.g., adrenal, spleen, kidney, testis, small intestine, and brain). T_3 and T_4 levels were not changed by any of these NP treatments, but were significantly increased by bolus injections of TSH. Prolonged infusion of VIP (15µg/1.1ml/h for 2 h) increased plasma T_3, but not T_4, levels. NPY (not a VIP homolog) decreased VCs in thyroid and pancreas under time and dose conditions (0.06 - 6 µg/rat) in which systemic pressure was not different from control. VCs in other tissues (e.g., adrenal, testis, kidney, and salivary gland) were not changed by NPY. This NP was also without effect on plasma thyroid hormone levels. We conclude that various NPs, known to occur in thyroid nerves, can increase or decrease thyroid VC (and BF) in the absence of alterations in systemic blood pressure and at doses that do not alter thyroid hormone secretion (Supp NIH AM35037).

EFFECTS OF GONADAL STEROIDS AND BROMOCRYPTINE ON LACTATION AND SUCKLING-INDUCED PROLACTIN SECRETION. 125

S. El Arab, M.I. El-Ghamry, B. Abou Hozaifa, and J.W. Simpkins, Department of Pharmacodynamics, College of Pharmacy, Univ. of Florida, Gainesville, FL 32610

Lactating female rats were treated daily with estradiol benzoate (EB, 5µg/kg), progesterone (P_4, 1mg/kg), EB and P_4 or the corn oil vehicle for each hormone beginning on the 1st day of lactation. At 1, 7, 14 or 20 days of lactation, the pups were removed from the mother for 5-7 hours then returned to test for suckling-induced prolactin (PRL) release. Treatment with EB or with the combination of EB and P_4 decreased the rate of growth of pups from 7 to 20 days of lactation relative to either vehicle or P_4-treated rats. EB or P_4 treatment alone did not modify the suckling-induced PRL release, but the combination of EB plus P_4 suppressed suckling-induced PRL release from 1 to 14 days of treatment. Thus, the combined steroid treatment, but not EB alone, reduced lactation by suppressing suckling-induced PRL release.

To evaluate the effects of bromocryptine (BROM) on lactation, rats were treated daily with EB (5µg/kg), BROM (0.1 mg/kg), EB plus BROM or the vehicles for both drugs. EB decreased pup growth rate from 7 to 13 days of lactation. In contrast, BROM completely suppressed pup growth and pup died by 7 days of lactation. Interestingly, EB enhanced lactation in the BROM-treated rats as evidenced by an EB-induced increase in the growth rate of pups treated with BROM. BROM treatment reduced basal PRL levels to 3.5% of controls. In contrast, EB treatment of BROM-exposed rats returned basal serum PRL levels to 50% of control values. This elevation in basal PRL levels maintained some lactation and was responsible for improved growth rate of pups.

In summary: (1) EB reduces lactation, but does not block suckling-induced PRL release, (2) EB plus P_4 appears to suppress suckling-induced PRL release and (3) bromocryptine causes a profound suppression of PRL, blocks suckling-induced PRL release and appears to completely suppress lactation. (Supported by AMIDEAST, AG02021 and HD14075).

FEMALE PROLACTINOMAS: A study of 77 cases. 126

J. E. Argonz, R. Artese, I. Molocznik, H. Benencia, E. Raida, R. Driollet Laspiur
Costa Buero Institute, Department of Neuroendocrinology, Medical School, U. B. A., Buenos Aires, Argentina. (1121)

Seventy-seven female patients with prolactin (PRL) producing pituitary tumours were studied: 28 cases (microadenomas, Stage I), 24 (intrasellar macroadenomas, Stage II), 16 (expansive adenomas, Stage III) and 9 (invasive adenomas, Stage IV). Evolution time: Stage I and II: 2-5 years; III: 5-15 years; IV: 10-20 years. Mean age: Stage I: 25 years; II: 33, III: 40 and IV: 42. Mean basal PRL concentrations: Stage I: 100-200 ng/ml; Stage II: 200-300 ng/ml; Stage III: 300-1000 ng/ml and Stage IV: 500-1500 ng/ml.

Neuroradiological studies were abnormal in all cases except in 8: 5 cases (Stage I) and 3 (Stage II) Transphenoidal surgery was performed in all the cases from Stage I and II, 9 cases from Stage III and 3 from Stage IV. Frontal surgery was performed in all others. Radiotherapy: 9 of 28 cases (Stage I), 10 of 24 (Stage II), 15 of 16 (Stage III) and 8 of 9 (Stage IV). Anatomopathological studies confirmed diagnosis in all cases. Post-surgical follow-up: 62 cases. Follow-up time: 7.5 (0.1-12) years. Mean basal PRL levels were normalized spontaneously in 17 of 25 cases (Stage I), 9 of 21 (Stage II), 2 of 11 (Stage III) and 2 of 5 (Stage IV). Menstrual cycles were recovered in 20 of 24 cases (Stage I), 11 of 21 (Stage II), 4 of 9 (Stage III) and 1 of 9 (Stage IV). Expected pregnancies: 8 of 11 cases (Stage I) and 6 of 13 cases (Stage II) with normal deliveries.

We conclude from present results that the surgical procedure should be performed in earlier stages since the recovery of the PRL axis with restauration of cycles and expecting pregnancies are greater.

GALACTORRHEA AS ONLY SYMPTOM OF HYPOTHALAMIC–CHIASMATICAL GLIOMA 127

J. E. Argonz, A. Martino, I. Molocznik, S. Damilano, A. Mosto.

Optic chiasm tumours usually show neuro-opthalmological manifestations being those of endocrine origin rarely mentioned.

It is described an uncommon case of a hypothalamic-chiasmatical glioma associated with galactorrhea as its unique symptom. The case of a 19 year old female patient who consulted for moderated obesity is presented. Physical examination revealed centrifuge obesity, arterial hypertension (150/100 mmHg) and minimal provocative unilateral galactorrhea.

Hormonal studies showed: Increased plasmatic prolactin (PRL) levels (basal pulses every 10 minutes): 33-36-38-40-36-29 ng/ml; Conserved diurnal PRL rhythm: 44-19-48 ng/ml (8,14 and 20hs.); PRL stimulation with T.R.H. (200 ug, i.v.): basal: 50,30 min.: 120 ng/ml (normal response) and Metoclopramide (10 mg, i.v.): basal: 66,30 min.: 105 ng/ml (limited response). Gonadal, thyroid and suprarrenal axis explorations were normal. Neuro-opthalmological studies were normal. Hypocyclic sellar tomography evidenced a slight ballooned sella turcica.

Ventricular dilatation was observed in pneumocisterntomography and C.A.T. showed a small hyperdense image in the trird ventricle.

Initially the patient was exposed to a ventricule-peritoneal shunt to resolve hydrocephalous. Consecuently a small mass in close contact with posterior optic chiasm was partially removed. Pathological specimen study: gliomatous tumour.

Conclusions: 1) To emphasize about the exceptional condition of an hypothalamic-chiasmatic glioma with galactorrhea as its unique specific clinical manifestation. 2) To enhance the decisive role of the hypothalamic-hypophyseal-prolactin axis study (normal T.R.H. and limited Metoclopramide response) which allowed us to diagnose this severe pathology in a precocious stage.

MALE INVASIVE PROLACTINOMAS: A study of 15 cases.

128

J. E. Argonz, I. Molocznik, R. Artese, J. Razumny, S. Damilano, M. Kamelman Levitin, J. Oviedo.

Costa Buero Institute, Department of Neuroendocrinology, Medical School, U. B. A., Buenos Aires, Argentina.

Fifteen men with invasive prolactin (PRL) producing pituitary tumours (Stage IV) were selected from thirty-eight cases studied between 1977-1984.

Mean age: 33.6 (18-53) years. Evolution time: 2.5 (0.5-5) years. Clinical symptoms: Headaches and visual disturbances in 93% of the cases; Sexual impotence, hypotrichosis and hypogenitalism in 80% ; Astenia, adynamia and arterial hypotension in 40% ; Galactorrhea in 40% ; Gynaecomastia in 33% ; Ophthalmoplegia in 20% . Neuro-ophthalmological studies were abnormal in all the cases except one. Neuroradiological studies were abnormal in all the cases.

Mean basal PRL concentrations: 3727 (range 140-18000) ng/ml.

Treatment: Surgical in all the cases: transphenoidal (20%), transfrontal (80%) and followed by radiotherapy.

Before surgical procedure three cases were treated with bromocriptine with dramatic tumoral shrinkage.

Evolution: follow-up time: 2.7 (0.2-7) years. Sexual function was normalized in 60% of the cases. Neuroradiological studies showed tumoral persistence in 26% of the cases.

Residual hyperprolactinaemia was found in all the cases and therefore bromocriptine was administered (Mean dose: 7.5 (2.5-30) mg/day. We achieved serum PRL levels normalization in 20% of the cases and a significant disminution in 48% ($<$ 100 ng/ml).

We conclude that bromocriptine treatment for a limited period of time could be useful to improve posterior surgical results and also to lower residual higher PRL levels.

P-TYRAMINE INHIBITS PROLACTIN SECRETION "IN VITRO".

129

D. Becu-Villalobos, M.I. Vacas, C. Libertun

IBYME and CEFAPRIN; Obligado 2490, (1428) Buenos Aires, Argentina.

In a previous work we demonstrated that p-tyramine , a natural amine, inhibited prolactin secretion in a series of experimental models in which prolactin levels were elevated (Endocrinology, 116: 2044, 1985). As p-tyramine was effective in median eminence lesioned rats we decided to test the effect of the drug "in vitro". Incubations of hemipituitaries were carried out in Medium 199 (pargyline 10 μM, ascorbic acid 0.1%) which was maintained at ph 7.4 by the addition of 35 mg/100 ml of $NaHCO_3$ and constant gassing with 95% O_2,5% CO_2.

Each hemipituitary served as control of the corresponding half which was incubated in the same medium with the addition of either tyramine HCl (10^{-6}M or 10^{-4}M) or dopamine HCl (10^{-6}M). After a preincubation, and a 3.5 hr incubation, medium was separated from pituitary tissue and frozen for RIA determinations. Dopamine effectively inhibited prolactin secretion (78.85 vs. 179.66 ng/mg tissue (n= 17), $p < 0.01$), and so did tyramine at the two doses used (10^{-4}M : 85.57 vs. 273.98 ng/mg tissue (n= 17), $p < 0.01$; 10^{-6}M : 113.5 vs. 192.6 ng/mg tissue (n= 18), $p < 0.05$). Tyramine did not modify the secretion of LH or TSH.

It was also investigated whether tyramine could displace ^{3}(H) spiperone from its binding to D2 receptors at the pituitary. Incubations were carried out in Tris HCl 50 mM buffer (2 mM Cl_2Ca, 120 mM ClNa, 5 mM KCl, 1 mM Cl_2Mg, 1 mM EDTA, 0.1% ascorbic acid, 12 μM pargyline) in the presence of 1.5 nM ^{3}(H) spiperone and the displacing drugs (either spiperone, dopamine or tyramine) at doses ranging from 10^{-4}M to 10^{-10}M. Spiperone and dopamine displaced ^{3}(H) spiperone binding (IC50 5.25 10^{-8}M and 1.4 . 10^{-5}M respectively) while tyramine was ineffective even at the dose of 10^{-4}M.

It is concluded that tyramine can inhibit prolactin not only "in vivo" but also "in vitro", and the mechanism of action does not seem to be an agonist action at the dopamine D_2 receptor of the pituitary.

Supported by CONICET, SECyT and UBA. Argentina.

PITUITARY REGIONS DIFFER IN THE PROPORTIONS OF CELLS THAT RELEASE PROLACTIN (PRL) ALONE OR BOTH GROWTH HORMONE (GH) AND PRL.

130

F.R. Boockfor and L. Stephen Frawley, Zoology Dept., ISU, Ames, IA 50011

Recent evidence demonstrates that PRL cells located in the narrow peripheral rim (outer zone) of the lactating rat pituitary are more responsive to hypophysiotropic input than are those from the larger central area (inner zone)(Nikitovitch-Winer et al., Proc. IV Int. Cong. PRL, p17, 1985; Boockfor and Frawley, Abst, Endo. Soc., 1986). In the present study, we used fixed sequential plaque assays that enabled the identification of cells which released PRL only, GH alone or both PRL and GH (mammosomatotropes) to determine whether the proportion of single and dual-hormone secretors also differed between these pituitary regions. In this assay, GH and PRL antisera were applied either separately or sequentially to monolayers of dispersed pituitary cells and indicator erythrocytes. The proportions of single and dual-hormone secretors were then determined by comparing the sum of the percentages of plaque-forming cells detected when the antisera were used separately to that found when these antisera were employed sequentially. Results (% plaque formers, $\bar{X}$±SE) from 4 separate experiments are summarized as follows:

	Antisera used			
	GH	PRL	PRL and GH	Sum
Outer Zone	24.0±1.2	49.7±0.4	50.5±1.1	73.7
Inner Zone	26.6±1.2	36.8±1.4	53.7±0.4	63.4

Although the percentage of GH cells did not differ between these two areas, more PRL secretors were detected in the outer zone than in the inner zone. Moreover, as evidenced by the greater degree of functional overlap (Sum - PRL and GH), the outer zone contained a much larger proportion of dual-hormone secretors than the inner zone. These data demonstrate regional differences in the proportions of single and dual-hormone secretors in pituitary glands of lactating rats. When taken together with the responsiveness differences reported to exist between PRL cells derived from these same pituitary regions, our findings raise the possibility that the release of PRL from mammotropes and mammosomatotropes is regulated differently.

(Supported by NIH AM-33943)

DOPAMINERGIC CONTROL OF PRL SECRETION IN THE RAT VARIES DURING THE ESTROUS CYCLE IN RELATION TO ESTRADIOL AND PROGESTERONE LEVELS

131

A.M. Brandi, D. Bression, M. Michard, M. Le Dafniet, F. Peillon

INSERM U. 223, Faculté de Médecine Pitié-Salpétrière, 105 Boulevard de l'Hôpital, 75013 Paris, France.

Pharmacological doses of 17β estradiol (E_2) and progesterone (P) influence PRL inhibition by dopamine (DA). E_2 decreases the sensitivity of lactotrophs to DA while P antagonizes this effect. We present evidence that this steroid regulation may have a physiological significance during the estrous cycle.

When pituitaries are collected on rats at different stages of the estrous cycle and perifused in the presence of increasing doses of DA, we observed variations in PRL inhibition.

In proestrus, at 1100 h (n = 4), when E_2 levels are high (160 ± 55 pg/ml) and P levels low (5 ± 5 ng/ml ; E_2/P : 30) PRL inhibition appears at 10^{-8}M DA and is evident at 10^{-7}M (45 % inhibition). In estrus (n = 3) and diestrus I and II (n = 7), when the ratio E_2/P is lower than in proestrus (E_2/P <10) the lactotrophs are sensitive to doses of DA as low as 10^{-11}M. The inhibition observed at 10^{-9}M is around 40 % and equivalent to that observed in proestrus at 10^{-7}M.

When rats in estrus, diestrus I or II, have been injected the day before with E_2 (a single injection, sc, 50 μg/rat in 0.5 ml sesame oil), the sensitivity of the lactotrophs decreases to that observed in proestrus, at the moment of the E_2 surge.

These results demonstrate that there is a modified sensitivity of the lactotrophs throughout the estrous cycle. In proestrus, the lactotrophs are less sensitive to DA than in the other stages of the cycle. This decreased sensitivity agrees with the fewer number of DA receptor sites described in proestrus and seems to be related to variations in the E_2/P ratios.

EVIDENCE THAT OPIATE STIMULATION OF PROLACTIN SECRETION INVOLVES VASOACTIVE INTESTINAL POLYPEPTIDE (VIP) 132

G. Burns, B.L. Brown, P.R.M. Dobson
Department of Human Metabolism & Clinical Biochemistry, University of Sheffield Medical School, Beech Hill Road, Sheffield S10 2RX, UK.

It has been known for some time that both morphine and the endogenous opioid peptides (enkephalins and endorphins) raise plasma prolactin concentrations in vivo. We and others have provided evidence to suggest that these agents act, at least in part, at the level of the hypothalamus. Changes in the release of dopamine into the hypophysial portal system have been implicated in the effect of opiates on prolactin secretion although Arita & Porter (Neuroendocrinol. 38, 62-67, 1984) suggested that such changes were insufficient to account for all the effects. We have investigated whether the neuropeptides, VIP and TRH, both putative prolactin releasing factors, might be involved. Rat hypothalamic fragments were perifused in Krebs Ringer bicarbonate medium (pH 7.4, 37°C) at 0.2 ml/min and the output of both VIP and TRH were measured by radioimmunoassay. The TRH antiserum was a gift from Dr. H. Frazer and initial supplies of a VIP antiserum were a gift from Prof. S. Bloom. Subsequently, an antiserum to VIP, which was usable in the range of 4-1000 fmoles/ml, was raised in a rabbit. Met-enkephalin (10^{-7} - 10^{-6}M) caused a dose-dependent rise in the rate of VIP release; an 85.2% (± 28.6 SD n=4) increase over basal being observed during a 15 min. pulse with 10^{-6}M met-enkephalin. Similarly, B-endorphin (10^{-8} -10^{-6}M) stimulated VIP release, but leu-enkephalin was without effect. Neither met-enkephalin, leu-enkephalin, nor B-endorphin affected TRH release from the hypothalamic fragments. Depolarizing concentrations of K^+ stimulated TRH release but did not affect VIP. The possibility that the lack of effect of K^+ on VIP release was due to the release of an inhibitor was investigated. However, none of the cholinergic, dopaminergic, or adrenergic antagonists tested restored a response to K^+. These results suggest that opiate stimulated prolactin secretion may, at least in part, be due to increased release of VIP.

EVIDENCE FOR AN INTRINSIC CHOLINERGIC SYSTEM IN THE ANTERIOR PITUITARY. 133

Peter Carmeliet and Carl Denef
School of Medicine,University of Leuven, Belgium

It is known thath Acetylcholine (Ach) has a direct effect on GH and PRL release in Anterior Pituitary (AP) in vitro but its physiological significance remains unknown. Recently, Fink showed evidence for endogenous Ach production in the AP in situ. The present work was intended to find evidence for a paracrine role of Ach, using AP cell aggregates,which were cultured in serum free medium,supplemented with T3 and/or dexemethasone (dex). Hormone secretion was studied in superfusion experiments.

Application of atropine (At) increased the basal release of both GH and PRL in a concentration dependent fashion (1-1000 nM). With 100 nM At the increase of GH was 32% ($p<0.01$) and of PRL 16% ($p<0.025$) in 4 nM dex/ 0.05 nM T3. This increase was higher in aggregates cultured in 80 nM dex/0.05 T3 ; GH: 84% ($p<0.01$) and PRL 39% ($p<0.01$). The At analogue dexetimide gave similar results, while its inactive enantiomer levetimide was completely inactive.

Further evidence was given by the finding that At potentiated the stimulation of GH and PRL release by isoproterenol (Iso) in aggregates cultured in 0.05 T3/80 nM dex. Iso-stimulated GH release increased from 4986% without At to 8037% with At ($p<0.05$), whereas Iso-stimulated PRL release increased from 82% without At to 133% with At ($p<0.001$).

In contrast to previously reported uniform effects of the muscarinic agonist Carbachol (CAR)(stimulation of GH inhibition of PRL),we observed both stimulatory and inhibitory actions, depending on the hormones added to the culture medium. In 80 nM dex there was an inhibition of GH release (-65%) followed by a rebound, while a stimulation (270%) was seen in 1 nM T3. The stimulation by CAR of PRL was highest in medium without dex/T3 (240%). In medium with 1 nM T3 there was a 180% stimulation,while 80 nM dex diminished this increase to 20%.

These results suggest a paracrine action of Ach in AP cell aggregates, modulating the stimulation of GH and PRL release. The reciprocal effects of CAR, dependent on hormone conditions also suggest a complex intercellular communication.

MONOCLONAL ANTIBODY RECOGNIZING BOTH MAMMOTROPHS AND SOMATOTROPHS OF THE RAT 134

H.T. Chen and C.S. Pittman
Univ. of Alabama at Birmingham, Birmingham, AL 35294

Cell type-specific antibodies to anterior pituitary cells have been found in sera from patients with autoimmune diseases. Furthermore, the autoimmune nature of destructive lymphocytic hypophysitis has long been suspected. To facilitate studies on the possible role of pituitary cell-specific antibodies in autoimmune hypophysitis, we have applied hybridoma technology of Kohler and Milstein to generate monoclonal antibodies against rat anterior pituitary cells. In this abstract, we report the generation and partial characterization of a monoclonal antibody (WHC-2) which defines a cell surface antigen common to both mammotrophs and somatotrophs.

BALB/c mice were immunized with enzymatically dispersed anterior pituitary cells from adult female Sprague-Dawley rats. Spleen cells of immunized mice were fused with murine myeloma Ag8.653. Hybridomas were initially screened for antibodies to cell surface antigens by ELISA using rat anterior pituitary cells and aortic smooth muscle cells as positive and negative controls, respectively. Positive clones were further analyzed by immunofluorescence (IF) and immunocytochemical (ICC) stainings using NIADDK anti-rPRL-IC-1 and NIADDK anti-hGH-IC-3 to identify mammotrophs and somatotrophs, respectively.

Antibody WHC-2 is an IgM with K light chains and is cytotoxic in the presence of complement. Based on double IF staining, this antibody stained ~ 56% of the anterior pituitary cells. Among them, 50% were mammotrophs and the other half were somatotrophs. Antibody WHC-2 did not stain gonadotrophs, corticotrophs, or thyrotrophs. Only 65% of mammotrophs and 87% of somatotrophs were antibody WHC-2 positive. In general, results from IF were in good agreement with those from ICC. In addition to anterior pituitary cells, antibody WHC-2 also reacted with acinar cells in the pancreas and cells in the stomach.

These results provided immunological evidence for the heterogeneity among mammotrophs and somatotrophs. Monoclonal antibody WHC-2 should be useful in the development of an animal model for autoimmune hypophysitis.

(Supported by NIH Grant HD-18355)

CEREBROSPINAL FLUID PROLACTIME AND GONADOTROPINS IN HUMAN FOETUSES 134a

M. Coculescu[x)], C. Poiană[x)], D. Alessandrescu[xx)]
Dpt.[x)] Endocrinology and Dpt.[xx)] Obstretics-Ginecology, Faculty of Medicine, Bucharest, Romania.

There is some evidence about the similarity between the foetal pituitary cells and those of adult pituitary tumors. The blood-cerebrospinal fluid (CSF) barrier is explored.

Prolactine (PRL) and gonadotropins (LH and FSH) of simultaneously sampled CSF and serum were measured by RIA in basal conditions in the following groups: (F), 11 human foetuses aged 18-24 weeks of gestation, extracted by Caesarian section together with their intact amniotic membranes; group T, 12 patients with invasive pituitary tumors and group N, 7 adults with nonendocrine disorders. The same hormones were measured after stimulation with LRH 0.2 mg iv plus TRH 0.4 mg iv in two foetuses and in the adult groups.

The mean CSF concentrations (x ± SEM) of PRL (17.7 ± 2.5 ng/ml) and LH (59.0 ± 24.6 mIU/ml) in group F were significantly higher ($p < 0.05$) than those of both group T and group N. The serum/CSF ratios of PRL (2.7 ± 1.7), LH (3.7 ± 0.8) and FSH (2.1 ± 0.3) in human foetuses were not significantly different from those of group T, with invasive adenomas, but in both groups F and T the serum/CSF ratios of all hormones were significantly lower ($p < 0.05$) than those of group N. After releasing hormones (RH) iv, the CSF levels of PRL, LH, FSH increased in 4 out of 7 patients with invasive tumors, but was unchanged in normal foetuses and adults.

Our data suggest an increased permeability of the blood-CSF barrier for adenohypophysial hormones in human foetuses in comparison with normal adults. Although a similar increase in permeability was produced by invasive pituitary adenomas, the mechanisms are different as shown by the response to RH. An immaturity of the development of the blood-CSF barrier in foetuses, is probably involved.

EVIDENCE FOR A DIRECT ACTION OF CORTICOLIBERIN ON PROLACTIN RELEASE 135

A. Enjalbert, L. Proulx*, G. Pelletier*, P.M. Dubois**, G. Morel**
INSERM U. 159, 2ter rue d'Alésia, 75014 PARIS, France ; *MRC Endocrinology Moléculaire, CHUL, Québec, Canada ; **CNRS UA 559, Fac. Méd., 69600 Oullins, France.

Corticoliberin (CRF) has been isolated and characterized from ovine hypothalamus and synthesized. This peptide stimulates the secretion of adrenocorticotropin (ACTH) in vivo and in vitro. Injected in intact male rat (10 ug/rat) via indwelling jugular cannulae r-CRF modified ACTH and prolactin (PRL) release. Five minutes after injection ACTH and PRL release were increased 10 and 3 times respectively. Ninety minutes after injection PRL release was similar to the control (saline injected). In order to study the possible direct action of the r-CRF in the pituitary gland an in vitro study and an immunocytological method were performed. In vitro r-CRF did not modified PRL release from anterior pituitary cells of female rats. However, after 5 days of pretreatment with estradiol (10^{-9} M) PRL release was significantly increased by r-CRF. The immunocytological method studied the endogenous r-CRF in the pituitary gland fixed by glutaraldehyde and osmium tetroxide. Ultrathin sections were obtained by cryoultramicrotomy. Endogenous r-CRF-like immunoreactivity was observed in both corticotrophs and lactotrophs. These observations suggest a cellular specificity. The serum anti-r-CRF was used at the maximal dilution of 2.10^{-5} in lactotrophs and up to 2.10^{-8} in corticotrophs. Immunoreactivity was abolished if anti-r-CRF was incubated with homologous antigen but not with heterogenous antigen. In corticotrophs and lactotrophs, r-CRF was localized in both the cytoplasm and the nuculeus. In the cytoplasm, it was present in the cytoplasmic matrix and in the secretory granules. In the nucleus, it was primarily localized in the euchromatin. The immunocytological reaction was also observed at the plasma membrane level, but very scarcely.

These data 1) suggest that CRF has an effect on prolactin release, 2) bring evidence for endogenous CRF within corticotrophs and lactotrophs, 3) support the hypothesis that CRF acts directly in lactotrophs.

PROLACTIN IN THE CNS OF HYPOPHYSECTOMIZED RATS: COMPARISON WITH PITUITARY PROLACTIN 136

N.V. Emanuele, L. Metcalfe, L. Wallock, J. Tentler, T.C. Hagen, C. Beer, D. Martinson, P. Gout, L. Kirsteins, A.M. Lawrence
Hines Veterans Administration Hospital, Hines, Illinois 60141, Loyola University of Chicago Stritch School of Medicine, Maywood Illinois, 60152, Zablocki Veterans Administration Medical Center, Milwaukee, Wisconsin 53202, and Cancer Control Agency of British Columbia, Vancouver, B.C.

Pituitary hormone-like proteins, including growth hormone, thyrotropin-stimulating hormone, luteinizing hormone, and adrenocorticotropic hormone have been measured in the rat brain and have been shown not to be of pituitary origin. We have measured concentrations of an immunoactive and bioactive prolactin-like material (PLI) widely distributed in hypophysectomized rat brain and spinal cord, confirming and extending immunocytochemical reports of others. Measurable PLI is found in thalamus, caudate, cerebellum, and brainstem as well as hypothalamus. Unlike other brain-based pituitary-like proteins, which appear identical to their pituitary counterparts, chromatographic studies of brain and spinal cord PLI are quite different. For example, most of the immunoreactive PLI from brain and spinal cord extracts elutes from a Sephadex G-75 column before anterior pituitary prolactin. Furthermore, brain and spinal cord prolactin is less biologically active in the Nb_2 lymphoma bioassay for lactogenic hormones. Conclusion: Immunologic, chromatographic and biologic studies of prolactin extracted from the brain and spinal cord show certain similarities to prolactin of anterior pituitary origin. However, clear discrepancies between the two prolactin-like proteins support the hypothesis that CNS prolactin probably represents a synthesized protein pool which is distinct from pituitary prolactin. As this material from the brain and spinal cord appears to be of a larger molecular size, and shows less biologic activity than pituitary prolactin, it is possible that prolactin extracted from the CNS represents an alternative processing of the post-translational product of messenger RNA for prolactin which has previously been identified in the rat brain, by other workers.

FOLLICULAR CELLS OF THE BOVINE ANTERIOR PITUITARY HAVE BETA ADRENOCEPTORS THAT STIMULATE ADENYLATE CYCLASE 137

P.R. Findell, M. Jacobs and R.I. Weiner

Follicular cells are a highly organized non-secretory component of the anterior pituitary (AP). We have developed a culture technique which yields polarized monolayers of bovine follicular cells (Methods in Enz. 124:255, 1986). β-adrenergic agonists increase the transepithelial potential across these monolayers. We asked if there are both β_1 and β_2 adrenergic receptors in follicular cells and if they are positively coupled to adenylate cyclase. First or second passage cultures of bovine follicular cells were harvested and homogenates were prepared in 50 mM Tris buffer with 5 mM $MgCl_2$ and the protease inhibitors bacitracin (50 μg/ml) and PMSF (0.1 nM). β-adrenergic binding was examined in homogenates with the β-ligand (^{125}I) iodocyanopindolol (ICYP). Specific binding was defined by 100 μM propranolol. Saturation analysis described high affinity (Kd=0.1 nM) and low capacity (βmax=24 fmol/mg protein) binding sites. Competition experiments with ICYP and the β_1-selective antagonists metroprolol and nordefrin and the β_2-selective antagonist ICI 118.551 were resolved with computer modeling into two-site interactions with high (nM) and low (μM) affinities. Additionally the β_1-selective agonist prenalterol and the β_2-selective agonist zinterol both competed for ICYP in a biphasic manner in the presence of 100 μM Gpp-(NH)p, a non-hydrolyzable GTP analog. These data demonstrated the presence of both β_1 and β_2 subtypes with a majority of β_2 sites. Adding β-agonists (isoproterenol, epinephrine and norepinephrine) to homogenates containing ^{32}P-ATP stimulated in a dose dependent fashion the formation of ^{32}P-cAMP measured by sequential Dowex-alumina chromatography. Isoproterenol and epinephrine were ten-fold more potent than norepinephrine in stimulating cAMP consistent with interactions at a predominence of β_2 sites. High affinity β adrenergic receptors positively coupled to cAMP on follicular cells is consistent with data suggesting a role for follicle cells in ion transport or paracrine regulation of PRL. This work was supported by NIH grant HD08924.

Specific Effect of CV 205-502, a Potent Dopamine Agonist, on Prolactin Secretion 138
Combined Pituitary Function Test With TRH, CRH, GRH and LHRH.

R.C. Gaillard[1], J. Brownell[2] and K. Abeywickrama[2]
University Hospital Medical Clinic, Geneva[1] and Clinical Research Department[2], SANDOZ LTD., Basle, Switzerland

CV 205-502, an octahydrobenzo[g]quinoline, is a unique dopamine agonist compound, which, despite a potent and sustained suppression of prolactin (PRL) secretion, is well tolerated, producing few adverse reactions. In order to investigate the site of action of CV 205-502 and to assess the effect of the hypothalamic releasing hormones on the pituitary-thyroid, -adrenal and -gonadal axes while under steady-state influence of the drug, pituitary challenge tests were given. Three groups of 5 men ($\bar{x}$ 25 years) were treated once-daily with CV 205-502 (0.04, 0.06 or 0.08 mg per day--doses which suppress PRL by 60 - 80 % for 24 h); on day 6 a combined anterior pituitary function test using i.v. administration of four hypothalamic releasing hormones (TRH, 200 μg, GRH 100 μg, CRH, 100 μg and LHRH, 100 μg) was performed. One month later the challenge tests were repeated to obtain control values. The following hormones were measured by RIA in plasma: TSH, ACTH, cortisol, PRL, GH, LH, FSH and testosterone. All subjects responded normally with marked increases in all hormones, both following CV 205-502 treatment and after the 1-month washout, with the exception of PRL. PRL concentrations increased markedly on the control day, while this response was largely attenuated during treatment with all 3 doses of CV 205-502 (percent inhibition was 76, 93 and 94 %, respectively).

The results confirm the strong dopamine agonist properties of CV 205-502, and implicate the pituitary as a major site of endocrine action. These data suggest also that the lactotropic cells are the only adenohypophyseal cells whose secretory activity is altered by a direct action of dopaminergic drugs. CV 205-502 did not change either the basal values or responses of the other cells to their respective hypothalamic releasing hormones.

INTERACTION OF CHLORDIAZEPOXIDE WITH TRH BINDING AND BIOLOGICAL EFFECTS IN GH3/B6 RAT PITUITARY CELL STRAIN. 139

D. GOURDJI, J.M. SEQUIER, N. BUISSON and A. TIXIER-VIDAL.
Groupe de Neuroendocrinologie Cellulaire et Moléculaire UA CNRS 1115, Collège de France, PARIS , FRANCE

The specificity of the TRH receptor is well known to be extremely stringent, and no competitive antagonist has been described so far to the exception of chlordiazepoxide (CDZ), a benzodiazepine (BZ) shown to compete with ^{3}H-TRH binding in brain and anterior pituitary homogenates as well as to antagonize some TRH-induced biochemical events in tumor-derived rat pituitary GH3 cells (Drummond et al. 1985).Here we have investigated the ability of CDZ to interfere with TRH binding and actions in GH3/B6 PRL and GH secreting cells, a model system in which ^{3}H-TRH elicits a rapid release of stored hormones , a delayed and long-term augmentation of PRL synthesis and a down regulation of its own receptors.

We observed that CDZ interact with ^{3}H-TRH binding sites, being able to both inhibit ^{3}H-TRH binding in a dose-dependent manner (IC_{50} : 10 uM) and chase prebound ^{3}H-TRH from intact GH_3B_6 cells. At 37°C the maximum inhibition never exceed 85-90% whereas total inhibition of the binding can be achieved when cells are challenged at 4°C. Co-incubation of increasing doses of ^{3}H-TRH with 5.10^{-5}M CDZ led to a 2-fold decrease on both binding capacity and affinity ($k_d$app 19 nM versus 9 nM).

In terms of biological actions , we observed that inhibition by CDZ of TRH-induced release occurs only when using pharmacological dose (100 uM) in combination with low dose of TRH (2 nM). Besides, the level of inhibition of the secretory response does not parallel that of the binding. Finally long-term concomitant exposure of cultures to CDZ plus TRH (24-48h) partially prevents the down-regulation of ^{3}H-TRH binding elicited by TRH alone.

Pharmacological studies using series of BZ and selective antagonists such as Ro 15-1788 and Ro 5-4864 suggests that neither the involvement of a classical BZ binding site (of central or peripheral type) nor a simple competitive interaction of CDZ with high affinity TRH binding sites could satisfactorily account for the above described TRH-CDZ interaction in GH3/B6 cells.

NEUROCHEMICAL AND ENDOCRINE INDICES OF TUBEROINFUNDIBULAR DOPAMINERGIC NEURONAL ACTIVITY FOLLOWING STIMULATION OF THE ARCUATE NUCLEUS. 140

J.W. Gunnet, K.J. Lookingland and K.E. Moore, Dept. Pharmacology/Toxicology, Michigan State Univ., East Lansing, MI 48824

Tuberoinfundibular dopaminergic (TIDA) neurons have cell bodies in the arcuate nucleus (ARN) and axons which project into the median eminence (ME). Dopamine (DA) released from TIDA terminals is carried by the blood to the anterior pituitary and there inhibits prolactin secretion. The activity of TIDA neurons has been estimated by measuring the rates of DA synthesis (DOPA accumulation following decarboxylase inhibition with NSD 1015) and turnover (α-methyltyrosine (α-MT)-induced decline in tissue DA concentrations). Such neurochemical measurements have been proven to reflect the activity of nigrostriatal DA neurons and have been assumed valid for determining TIDA neuronal activity. The purpose of the present study was to verify this assumption by measuring DA synthesis and turnover rates in the ME following direct electrical stimulation of TIDA neurons. Prolactin secretion was also monitored, a decrease in plasma prolactin levels is indicative of an increase in DA release.

Bilateral electrical stimulation (biphasic 1 msec pulses, 10 Hz, 200 µA peak-to-peak) was applied to the ARN of adult Long Evans rats. NSD 1015 (100 mg/kg, i.p.) was given at the onset of the 30 min stimulation. ARN stimulation increased DOPA accumulation in the ARN, ME and posterior pituitary. The stimulation produced comparable results in both male and female rats. DA turnover was determined by measuring the decline in DA concentrations 20 and 80 min after α-MT injection (250 mg free base/kg,i.p.). ARN stimulation was begun 20 min after α-MT injection and continued for 60 min. The stimulation induced a significant increase in DA turnover within the ARN, ME and posterior pituitary. Plasma prolactin levels were found to be significantly decreased within 15 min of ARN stimulation and remained low for 30 min. These results show that measurements of DA synthesis and turnover within the ME reflect TIDA neuronal activity. (Supported by USPHS Grant NS09174.)

CYTOSKELETAL ORGANIZATION IN LACTOTROPHS 141

J. Guthrie, G. Martinez-Escalera, R. Weiner
Reprod. Endo. Center, UCSF, San Francisco, CA 94143

To analyze the morphological basis of cytoskeletal involvement in PRL secretion, we have devised a technique for stabilizing, fixing, and immunostaining the microfilaments and microtubules in cultured lactotrophs. Anterior pituitary cells from ovex rats implanted with 1 cm E_2 silastic capsules for two weeks were enzymatically dispersed, plated at 200,000 cells/ml/well on 12 mm glass coverslips coated with extracellular matrix and cultured in DME-H21, 10% calf serum, $5X10^{-7}$M dopamine and 10^{-4}M ascorbic acid. The medium was changed after 16 and 19 hours. At 22 hours, the cells were incubated for 3 min. at 37° in extraction/stabilization buffer (0.1MK^+-PIPES, 1 mM MgC1, 5 mM EGTA, 0.1% TRITON-X-100, 30% glycerol, pH 6.8) then fixed with 100% methanol at -20°C for 2 min. Double immunolabelling for PRL and a cytoskeletal protein was done by incubation in rabbit-anti-rat-prolactin antiserum combined with a mouse monoclonal against the cytoskeletal element. This was followed by incubation in goat-anti-rabbit-IgG-fluorescein and goat-anti-mouse IgG-rhodamine. Coverslips were viewed under epifluorescence. α- and/or β-tubulin staining in lactotrophs (65% of rounded cells) appeared in three different conformations: 20% as an aster array radiating from the microtubule-organizing-center near the nucleus; 60% as a tangled mass of bundled microtubules that snaked through the whole cytoplasm and lay over the nucleus as well; and an intermediate conformation. An antibody to MAP_1 stained the nuclei, while antibodies to MAP_2 and tau did not stain lactotrophs. The staining of filamentous actin in lactotrophs, in contrast to fibroblasts, contained no stress fibers and was visualized in 3 planes of focus, consistent with a cortical web. The actin associated proteins, α-actinin and vinculin only appeared in adhesion plaques, while filamin stained in a diffuse haze over the entire cell. An antibody against the intermediate filament protein vimentin showed a staining pattern like microtubules. These studies demonstrate that lactotrophs have well-developed and highly organized microtubule, microfilament and intermediate filament systems. Work was supported by NIH grant HD08924 and ARCS Foundation.

EFFECTS OF DEXAMETHASONE AND MORPHINE ON PLASMA PROLACTIN LEVELS: A RAT MODEL FOR ENDOCRINE TESTS IN DEPRESSION RESEARCH 142

J.L. Haracz and E.G. Zimmermann
Brain Research Institute, UCLA, Los Angeles, CA 90024

Depression is associated with a blunted suppression of plasma cortisol levels by dexamethasone (DEX). This blunted feedback inhibition of cortisol secretion may reflect a glucocorticoid receptor deficiency. Since DEX also blocks stress-induced elevation of prolactin levels (PRL), a deficiency of glucocorticoid receptors might also lead to a diminished DEX suppression of the PRL response to opiates. To explore this DEX-opiate interaction, the present studies were performed to develop a rat model of endocrine tests for potential application in depression research.

Adult male rats were given 40 mg/kg s.c. morphine (MOR) 1 hr before jugular venipuncture. Plasma PRL levels were measured by RIA. Naloxone, 0.4 mg/kg, completely blocked the MOR-induced rise in PRL levels. Pretreatment with various DEX doses at 2 hr before MOR revealed that 100 µ/kg, but not 5 or 20 µ/kg, inhibited the PRL rise at 1 hr post-MOR. When injected 15 minutes after MOR, both the 100 and 400 µ/kg doses of DEX suppressed the PRL elevation at 1 hr post-MOR. DEX (100 µ/kg) given at a pretreatment interval of 21 hr was significantly less effective in suppressing the MOR-induced PRL rise then when given at at pretreatment intervals of 1, 2, 6, or 12 hr.

These findings indicate that DEX inhibition of MOR-induced release of PRL is dose- and time-dependent. The results are consistent with predictions of a receptor mediated interaction. Thus the rat may be used to explore the glucocorticoid receptor deficiency hypothesis of depression. (supported by USPHS Grants DA-826 and RR5756.

AN INCREASE IN THE RATIO OF SEROTONINERGIC TO DOPAMINERGIC ACTIVITY IN THE MEDIAN EMINENCE PRECEDES PREOVULATORY PROLACTIN AND LUTEINIZING HORMONE SURGES IN CYCLING FEMALE RATS. 142a

B. Kerdelhué [a], Ph. Lesieur[b], A. El Abed [a,c], F. Bojda[a], C. Pasqualini [a], V. Lenoir[a], P. Douillet[b], C.C. Chiueh[b] and M. Palkovits [b,d].

[a]Unité Neurobiol.Reprod.,INRA-CNRS, 78350 Jouy-en-Josas; [b]Lab. Clin. Sci. and Cell Biol., Natl. Inst. Mental Health, Bethesda, Md.20014, USA ; [c] Ecole Ntle d'Ingénieurs, 3038 Sfax, Tunisie ; [d]First Dpt Anatomy,Semelweiss Univ., Medical School, H-1450 Budapest, Hungary.

In the present work, we deal, using a high performance liquid chromatography (HPLC) system coupled with electrochemical detection, with a concurrent analysis of norepinephrine (NE), dopamine (DA) and 5-hydroxytryptamine (5-HT) and the major specific metabolites of DA and 5-HT, 3, 4-dihydroxyphenylacetic acid (DOPAC) and 5-hydroxyindole-3-acetic acid (5-HIAA),respectively, in the median eminence (ME) and the arcuate (AN) and medial preoptic (MPN) nuclei throughout the rat estrous cycle.

There was no significant change between afternoon (17h) and morning (10h) values for any biogenic amine, metabolite or ratio in AN or the MPN at any stage of the estrous cycle. On the contrary, significant changes were specifically recorded in the ME on proestrus day (PRO). NE, DA and 5-HT levels elevated and DOPAC decreased significantly.

The major fact was that there was a progressive decrease in the ratio DOPAC to DA with minimal values (50 % decrease, $p < 0.05$) at 16h. However, the ratio 5-HIAA to 5-HT changes with a composite pattern : it decreased until 12h but subsequently increased until 14h. Last but not least, the ratio of serotoninergic to dopaminergic metabolism elevated between 10h and 16h and then a decline was observed until 1900h. The rise of this ratio precedes preovulatory PRL and LH surges by 2h.

These studies emphasize the need to study discrete brain nuclei and to measure several parameters concurrently, and at very short intervals of time, in order to obtain a better understanding of the temporal events involved in PRL and LH preovulatory surges.

HISTAMINERGIC MEDIATION OF THE STRESS-INDUCED RELEASE OF PROLACTIN 143

Ulrich Knigge, Steen Matzen, Jørgen Warberg

Inst. of Medical Physiology C, The Panum Inst., University of Copenhagen, Copenhagen, Denmark.

Histamine (HA) has recently been identified as a neurotransmitter in the hypothalamus, and several studies suggest that HA participates in the regulation of pituitary hormone secretion.

We investigated the role of HA in the stress induced release of prolactin (PRL) in conscious male rats.

Restraint-stress applied for 5 min decreased the hypothalamic content of HA by 70% and of methylHA by 50%, suggesting an increased release and turnover of hypothalamic HA.

Restraint-stress (R) and ether-stress (E) increased PRL in plasma from 5 ± 1 to 84 ± 6 and 46 ± 5 ng/ml, respectively.

Icv infusion of the H2-antagonist cimetidine (CIM, 100ug) abolished the response to R and E, while icv infusion of the H1-antagonist mepyramine (MEP, 100ug) decreased the response to R by 80% but had no effect on the response to E.

Icv infusion of HA (30ug) stimulated PRL secretion to 53 ± 10 ng/ml. Prior icv infusion of CIM completely inhibited the response, while MEP had no effect. Similar findings were obtained in urethane anesthetized rats.

Hypophysial portal blood was collected in urethane anesthetized rats. HA (30ug) infused icv decreased the dopamine level from 870 ± 170 to 520 ± 60 pg/ml.

HA had no effect on PRL release from incubated adenohypophyses, and HA infused iv had no effect on PRL secretion in rats with transsection of the pituitary stalk.

We suggest that R and E cause a release of HA from hypothalamic neurons. The released HA, activating H2-receptors, stimulates PRL secretion, at least partially, via an inhibition of the secretion of dopamine to the portal blood.

Mechanisms involved in the regulation of prolactin gene transcription by thyroliberin. 143a

Laverrière JN, Tixier-Vidal A, Buisson N and Gourdji D. UA CNRS 1115, Collège De France, Paris, France.

Thyroliberin (TRH) induces two main effects when it interacts with prolactin (PRL) pituitary cells. First TRH increases in a rapid and transient manner the release of stored PRL. A large body of data indicates that this effect is mediated through an increase of cytosolic calcium concentration and activation of C-kinase dependent pathway. Secondly, TRH rapidly enhances the rate of PRL gene transcription (Laverrière et al. 1983) which results in a delayed and sustained increase of PRL production.

Here we attempted to determine whether the intracellular messengers involved in the TRH-induced stimulation of PRL release may be responsible of the TRH-induced stimulation of PRL gene transcription. We have tested at both levels the calcium ionophore A23187 and the tumor promoting agent (TPA) which increases the intracellular calcium concentration and activates C-kinase respectively. We have compared their effects with those of TRH. This was investigated by measuring acute release (30 min incubation) by RIA and gene transcription (4 h treatment) by run-on assay using GH3/B6 cells as a model system.

For PRL release the order of efficiency of the agents tested was found as follows : TPA > TRH > A23187 , corresponding to 4.0 folds, 2.6 folds and 1.6 folds stimulations respectively.

At the gene level the range of efficiency was found different : TRH > A23187 > TPA, corresponding to stimulations by 3.1 folds, 2.3 folds and 2.0 folds respectively. Besides, combined treatments (TRH+A23187, TRH+TPA, A23187+TPA) lead to conclude that increase in intracellular calcium concentration and C-kinase activation may participate to the regulation of the PRL gene transcription but cannot account for the complete response to TRH. Moreover experiments involving withdrawal of TRH after increasing time of treatment indicate that occupancy of TRH receptors is required for the full stimulation of transcription.

EFFECTS OF PROLACTIN AND STRESS ON DOPAC CONCENTRATIONS IN THE MEDIAN EMINENCE: EVIDENCE THAT DOPAMINE METABOLISM REFLECTS THE ACTIVITY OF TUBEROINFUNDIBULAR NEURONS 144

K.J. Lookingland, H.D. Jarry and K.E. Moore

Dept. of Pharmacology and Toxicology, Michigan State Univ., East Lansing, MI 48824

Dopamine (DA) released from tuberoinfundibular (TI) DA neurons terminating in the median eminence (ME) is transported via the hypophysial portal blood to the anterior pituitary gland where it acts to inhibit prolactin secretion. TIDA neurons have a low affinity reuptake system for released amine and, most likely, dihydroxyphenylacetic acid (DOPAC) measured in the ME predominantly reflects the intraneuronal metabolism by mitochondrial monoamine oxidase (MAO) of newly synthesized DA rather than metabolism of DA that has been released and recaptured by these neurons. Since procedures that alter the activity of TIDA neurons also alter the rate of DA synthesis, changes in TIDA activity may be reflected by corresponding changes in DA metabolism. The purpose of the present study was to examine the effects of increasing or decreasing the activity of TIDA neurons on DOPAC concentrations in the ME.

Within 5 min following the administration of the MAO inhibitor pargyline (50 mg/kg, i.v.) ME DOPAC concentrations declined to 15% of control indicating that this metabolite has a very high turnover rate and is rapidly removed from the ME. Probenecid (250 mg/kg, i.p.) produced a time-dependent increase in ME DOPAC concentrations suggesting that this metabolite is at least partially transported out of the ME via an acid transport system. Prolactin (10 μg/rat; icv; 12 h), which increases TIDA neuronal activity, produced a corresponding increase in ME DOPAC concentrations in control and probenecid-treated male rats. Restraint stress (30 min), which decreases TIDA neuronal activity, produced a corresponding decrease in ME DOPAC concentrations in diestrous female rats. ME DOPAC concentrations in diestrous female rats, whose TIDA neuronal activity is higher than in the male, were two-fold greater than that measured in male rats. The results from the present study indicate that DOPAC concentrations in the ME may be an index of TIDA neuronal activity. (Supported by USPHS Grant NS09174.)

NEUROENDOCRINE EFFECTS OF DIHYDROERGOKRYPTINE (DEKP) AND DIHYDROERGOCRISTINE (DECS): EVIDENCE FOR A DOPAMINOMIMETIC ACTION. 145

F.Mailland*, L.Fiore, M. Poli**, U.Scapagnini, P.L. Canonico.
Inst. Pharmacology, University of Catania; *Poli Research Center, Milan; **2nd Dept. Internal Medicine, S. Paolo Hospital, Milan, Italy.

Ergot alkaloids are a well known class of prolactin secretion-inhibitors, owing to their dopaminomimetic or antiserotonergic activities. We compared the effects of DEKP and DECS, two C-9,10-hydrogenated ergot alkaloids, on prolactin release either in vitro or in vivo. We also investigated their effects on cyclic AMP (cAMP) accumulation in primary cultures of anterior pituitary cells. Both DEKP and DECS inhibited in a concentration-dependent manner prolactin release and cAMP levels in these cells. The effect of DEKP started to be significant at a 10 nM-concentration and was maximal (about 50% inhibition) at 10 uM. DECS effect was present at 100 nM and maximal (30% inhibition) also at 10 uM. The specificity of action of the two ergot alkaloids at the level of dopamine receptor was shown by the fact that their effect on both prolactin release and cAMP accumulation were completely reversed by 100 nM haloperidol or pimozide. Exposure of the cells to pertussis toxin antagonized the effect of maximally effective (10 uM) concentrations of either DEKP or DECS, further supporting the involvement of the adenylate cyclase-cAMP system in the inhibitory action of the two compounds.

In healthy volunteers, DEKP and DECS produced a significant, long lasting and dose-dependent decrease of plasma prolactin levels.The two ergot alkaloids showed their effects both in conditions of hyperprolactinemia produced by the dopamine antagonist sulpiride and in TRH- or cimetidine-induced hyperprolactinemias. DEKP was twice as potent as DECS, but less potent than bromocriptine. However DEKP and DECS did not elicit any side effect, whereas equipotent doses of bromocriptine caused nausea, vomiting and postural hypotension in some subjects.

The results obtained indicate that DEKP and to a less extent DECS are strong dopaminomimetic drugs at the mammotroph. Their therapeutical efficacy appears to be relevant, also in view of the almost complete lack of side effects.

EGF RECEPTORS PRESENT IN NORMAL RAT AND HUMAN PITUITARIES ARE ABSENT IN HUMAN PRL-, GH- AND NON-SECRETING PITUITARY ADENOMAS 146

M. Michard, P. Birman, F. Peillon, D. Bression
INSERM U. 223, Faculté de Médecine Pitié-Salpétrière, 105 Boulevard de l'Hôpital, 75013 Paris, France.

The presence of EGF receptors was assessed on membranes of rat and human pituitaries with I^{125} EGF binding studies.

In normal rat and human pituitaries, a treatment of the membranes with a high ionic strength ($MgCl_2$, 0.5 M) had to be used to enhance binding of EGF which was, even though always above non specific binding, difficult to measure without any treatment. The effect of the treatment was reversible. When membranes were washed after $MgCl_2$ treatment, binding decreased to the same level as before the treatment and a second treatment had the same effect as the first one. Using this procedure, we demonstrated that EGF binds to normal pituitaries to one class of sites with high affinity (Kd ≃ 0.30 M) and low capacity (Bmax ≃ 20 fmoles/mg prot). At 25 C, total binding was in the order of 2 % of total radioactivity and specific binding generally between 25 and 40 % of total binding. Equilibrium was reached after 30 min. Binding is specific for EGF. Insulin, FGF, NGF do not compete for the binding.

No specific binding was found on adenomatous pituitary membranes whatever the nature of the adenoma was and $MgCl_2$ treatment had no effect.

These results raise several questions : 1) Why EGF receptors in normal pituitaries are in their majority not directly accessible to EGF ? $MgCl_2$ could unmask sites occupied by endogenous EGF or give access to cryptic sites. The modifications induced by $MgCl_2$ being reversible, our results favor the hypothesis of cryptic sites. 2) Why EGF receptors are absent on human adenomatous membranes ? It is known that EGF receptors are located on rat tumoral PRL- and GH-secreting cell (GH_3 cells). Their absence in the adenomatous tissue gives importance to their physiological function in the normal pituitary, function which might concern the hormonal regulation and the cellular differentiation.

PITUITARY ADENOMAS: IN VIVO STUDY WITH POSITRON EMISSION TOMOGRAPHY (PET) OF DOPAMINE RECEPTORS AND METABOLISM 147

C. Muhr, M. Bergström, P.O. Lundberg, K. Bergström, H. Lundqvist, B. Långström
Department of Neurology, Uppsala University, Akademiska sjukhuset, Uppsala, Sweden

Methods. PET enables tracer in vivo kinetic studies of metabolism and receptor binding. 15 patients with a pituitary adenoma were examined with ^{11}C-methionine and ^{11}C-labelled dopamine D_2 antagonists (N-methylspiperone and raclopride) and dopamine agonist (bromocriptine) including repeated studies after Haloperidol protection. The D_2 binding and the amino acid metabolism were analysed using kinetic models.

Results. The D_2 receptor binding was high in all the prolactinomas, reaching values higher than in the striatum. The hormonal inactive (null cell) adenomas showed low levels of receptor binding. The receptor binding of spiperone showed a continuous association. Raclopride showed slow dissociation, steady state after 20 min. Bromocriptine showed a faster dissociation. The metabolically inactive stereoisomer ^{11}C-D-methionine was rapidly distributed within the tumor with no signs of irreversible trapping, whereas ^{11}C-L-methionine showed a continuous trapping. In the prolactinomas a reduction in amino acid metabolism up to 60 % was noted after bromocriptine treatment. Also a significant decrease in receptor binding was observed after bromocriptine treatment.

IN CONCLUSION PET using ^{11}C-dopamine ligands makes it possible to detect and quantify dopamine receptor binding in pituitary adenomas. For the first time an in vivo technique has demonstrated high receptor levels in prolactinomas and low levels in null cell adenomas. PET with ^{11}C-L-methionine can reveal a decrease in amino acid metabolism as a very early sign of effect of treatment. These findings are of great importance in the classification of pituitary adenomas and in the evaluation of dopamine agonist treatment of such tumors.

MULTIPLE METASTATIC PROLACTINOMA: IN VIVO STUDIES WITH POSITRON EMISSION TOMOGRAPHY (PET) DEMONSTRATING DOPAMINE RECEPTORS AND EFFECT OF BROMOCRIPTINE TREATMENT 148

C. Muhr, M. Bergström, P.O. Lundberg, M. Hartman, K. Bergström, B. Långström, L. Pellettieri
Department of Neurology, Uppsala University, Akademiska sjukhuset, Uppsala, Sweden

Multiple metastatic adenomas are extremely rare and we have found no publication on multiple intracranial metastases of a prolactin producing adenoma earlier. A 26-year old man had at the age of 14 rapid progressive visual disturbances and was operated on for a sellar tumor, he was also substituted for pituitary insufficiency. The patient presented 12 years later with headache and CT now revealed multiple metastases located to the cerebellum and both hemispheres. Biopsy from operation showed pituitary adenoma cells with positive PRL immunoreactivity. The DNA content was abnormal. PRL/s was considerably increased, 3-4000 ug/l (N<20 ug/l). In vivo studies with PET using the dopamine antagonists ^{11}C-methylspiperone and ^{11}C-raclopride including repeated studies after Haloperidol protection to evaluate the specific D_2 binding revealed high dopamine receptor binding within the pituitary tumors, comparable to the amounts found in striatum. PET with ^{11}C-L-methionine showed irreversible trapping as signs of high amino acid metabolism. Repeated PET studies after treatment with bromocriptine retard injection showed considerable decrease in the amino acid metabolism and in the D_2 receptor binding. The patient has so far responded well to bromocriptine treatment.

Conclusion. This unique case of metastatic prolactinoma illustrates the great potentials of PET in characterization of tumor properties like dopamine receptor binding and amino acid metabolism. PET was also superior in revealing treatment effects, especially early effect on functional parameters.

EVIDENCES FOR AND AGAINST THE EXISTENCE OF A HYPOTHALAMIC PRL-INHIBITING PEPTIDE 149

R.M.G. Nair, M.A. Barnes, M. Somasundaran, P. Subramaniam, J. Sagel, P. Pritchard
VA Medical Center and Depts. of Medicine and Neurology, Medical University of South Carolina, Charleston, SC

The influence of amygdala on the tuberoinfundibular neurons which modulate anterior pituitary secretion has been shown by electrophysiological studies. Our recent reports have indicated transient elevation of PRL following complex partial seizures (CPS). Determination of levels of the inhibitory neurotransmitter amino acid GABA from the serum of CPS patients before and after seizure indicated significant decrease. The levels of phenylalanine, the dopamine precursor, also were significantly decreased. Such decrease in the inhibitory amino acids was mimicked by electrical stimulation of the amygdala using depth electrodes.

A peptide purified from bovine hypothalamic extracts inhibited the secretion of human PRL in an *in vitro* perfusion system consisting of PRL-secreting adenomatous tissue removed at transphenoidal surgery. The administration of secretagogues (K^+, 56 mM at 2 min. and Ca^{++}, 3 mM at 8 min.) together with the PIF-peptide (1 ng/ml) in the perfusate, vs. secretagogues alone indicated 75-80% inhibition of PRL release by the PIF ($p < .001$). Similar inhibition (50%, $p < .001$) of PRL secretion was observed for rat anterior pituitary tissue in the same perfusion system. This hypothalamic PIF fraction is peptide in nature and is free from dopamine or GABA as shown by chromatographic analysis and radioreceptor assay. A later chromatographic fraction from the hypothalamic extracts was also PIF-active in the same perfusion system, and was identified as GABA by microcolumn analysis. High pressure liquid chromatographic purification of porcine hypothalamic extracts by other laboratories as well, yielded a PIF-peptide active at 5 ng dose levels in *in vitro* bioassays. Pure GABA fractions which inhibited PRL-secretion frompituitaries were also isolated during such chromatographic separations.

These studies suggest the influence of dopamine, GABA and also a PIF-peptide in the neuroendocrine regulation of prolactin. This work is supported by the Veterans Administration.

SYNERGISTIC POTENTIATION OF NOXIOUS STIMULI-INDUCED PROLACTIN SECRETION BY HYPOVOLEMIA 150

T. Onaka, M. Hamamura, K, Yagi
Dept. of Physiol. Jichi Med. Sch. Tochigi, Japan

Footshocks have been shown to potentiate prolactin (PRL) secretion. Hypovolemic stimuli are known to potentiate PRL secretion. Noxious and hypovolemic stimuli are reported to potentiate corticotrophin secretion in a synergistic manner. Since PHI27 (prolactin-releasing factor) has been shown to co-exist with corticotrophin-releasing factor in parvocellular neurosecretory cells of the hypothalamic paraventricular nucleus, the possibility arises that PRL secretion after noxious stimuli is potentiated synergistically by hypovolemic stimuli. The present study aimed to discover whether noxious and hypovolemic stimuli interact with each other on prolactin secretion in conscious and anesthetized male rats.

Plasma PRL levels were elevated both after hemorrhage (1 % B.W.) and after saphenous nerve stimulation (3-mA pulses at 4 Hz and 3-min duration) in rats anesthetized with α-chloralose and urethane. Magnitude of the PRL increase after nerve stimulation was larger in hypovolemic rats than that in control animals.

An I.P. injection of dextran increased blood hemoglobin without altering plasma osmolarity. Plasma PRL levels were elevated in a dose-dependent manner by the dextran injection. Plasma PRL levels were also raised by footshocks (50 Hz, 1 min) in a stimulus intensity-dependent fashion and reached at the maximum 5 min after the onset of footshocks. The mean increase of PRL evoked by footshocks in dextran-injected rats was larger than that in saline-injected rats.

These results suggest the existence of interaction between noxious and hypovolemic stimuli with regard to PRL secretion in rats.

CHANGES IN TUBEROINFUNDIBULAR DOPAMINERGIC NEURONS ACTIVITY DURING THE RAT ESTROUS CYCLE. CORRELATION WITH THE PRL SURGE AND ALTERATION BY A MAMMARY CARCINOGEN. 151

C. Pasqualini*, F. Bojda*, E. Teissier°, B. Guibert•, V. Leviel•, R. Rips°, B. Kerdelhué*
* U. Neurobiol. Reprod., INRA-CNRS, 78350 Jouy-en-Josas; ° INSERM, U.98 Pharmacol. Chim., 17 rue Fer à Moulin, 75005 Paris ; • Lab. Physiol. Nerv., CNRS, 91190 Gif-sur-Yvette, France.

An attempt was made to correlate the physiological or the DMBA-enhanced serum PRL surge which occurs on proestrus afternoon in Sprague-Dawley (SD) female rats, with physiological or pathological changes in two biochemical estimates of the tuberoinfundibular dopaminergic (TIDA) neurons activity. Dopamine (DA) and Dihydroxyphenylacetic acid (DOPAC) concentration as well as tyrosine hydroxylase (TH) activity were measured in the median eminence (ME) of SD rats, pretreated or not with DMBA, throughout the estrous cycle, in relation to PRL secretion. In control or DMBA-pretreated females, DA and DOPAC contents, DOPAC/DA ratio and TH activity were high in the ME in diestrus I and II and remained so until morning of proestrus. At that time, in control animals, DA and DOPAC contents, DOPAC/DA ratio and TH activity showed a marked decrease. Then, on proestrus afternoon, when serum PRL levels were maximal, there was a marked and transient increase in DA and DOPAC contents as well as a brief surge in DOPAC/DA ratio and TH activity. Conversely, in DMBA-treated females, the DOPAC/DA ratio and TH activity showed a marked increase in the morning of proestrus, before decreasing dramatically after 12.00 h. No surge in DOPAC/DA ratio or in TH activity was detectable in the afternoon of proestrus. Finally, on estrus day, in both groups of rats, DA and DOPAC contents, DOPAC/DA ratio as well as TH activity increased again to reach the levels seen in diestrus. Thus, as determined by two different indexes, TIDA neurons activity fluctuates markedly throughout proestrus and DMBA pretreatment of the SD rats alters the pattern of these cyclic changes. Such altered dynamics observed prior to and after the preovulatory surge in serum PRL suggest that DMBA pretreatment could permanently induce an increased sensitivity to estradiol of TIDA neurons.

NATURE OF PATHOLOGICAL AND PHARMACOLOGICAL HYPERPROLACTINEMIA INFLUENCES OPIOID CONTROL OF LH SECRETION IN WOMEN. 152

F. Petraglia, V. DeLeo*, C. Nappi**, F. Facchinetti, A. Volpe, A.R. Genazzani.
Depts. Obstetrics and Gynecology, Univ. of Modena, *Siena and **Naples, Schools of Medicine, Italy.

In patients affected by amenorrhea opioid control of LH secretion is impaired, as shown by the lack of LH response to naloxone. Menopause is also accompanied by the unresponsiveness of LH to naloxone, and is restored by estrogen-progesterone therapy indicating a role for gonadal steroids in modulating the opioid inhibition of LH in women. However, in women with prolactin (Prl) secreting pituitary adenomas the LH increase induced by naloxone is maintained, despite the amenorrheic state and the low circulating estradiol levels. This suggests the presence of opioid inhibition on LH secretion may be a determining factor in the amenorrhea of hyperprolactinemic patients. The present study investigated whether the activity of opioid system is modified in women affected by other pathological (idiopathic) or pharmacologically-induced (metoclopramide) hyperprolactinemic states. First, we compared the LH response to naloxone hydrocloride (4 mg, iv) between amenorrheic patients affected by tumoral (n=11) or idiopathic (n=12) hyperprolactinemia. Basal Prl levels were significantly different between the two groups (97+23 ng/ml vs 33+8.5 ng/ml, mean+s.d.m.). Conversely, basal plasma LH levels were not different between and significantly increased after naloxone in both groups ($P<0.01$ at 30 and 45 minutes, vs. placebo). The maximum percent increase after naloxone was of the same order of magnitude (95+18% and 102+13.5% tumoral and idiopathic, respectively). Testing the LH response to naloxone in 10 postmenopausal women before and after 1 week of treatment with the dopamine antagonist, metoclopramide (10mg, t.i.d) we found no significant change, despite a 6-fold increase in Prl. These results suggest: 1)tumoral and idiopathic hyperprolactinemia induce functional changes in the opioid regulation of LH secretion; 2)this effect is independent of the absolute concentration of Prl; 3) 1 week exposure to high circulating Prl levels in postmenopausal subjects does not influence the opioid system.

PROLACTIN LOWERING EFFECT OF CQP201-403; A NEW DOPAMINE AGONIST 153

R. Rolland, P.F.M. van der Heijden, J. Brownell*, J. van Gennep**.
Dept. of Obstetrics and Gynecology, St. Radboud Hospital, Nijmegen, The Netherlands and *Clinical Research Dept. Sandoz, Basle, Switzerland, and**the Netherlands.

Since the introduction of the dopamine agonist bromocriptine (ParlodelR) this has become the treatment of choice in the therapy of hyperprolactinaemia. In some patients however, treatment must be discontinued due to severe side effects CQP201-403, a new dopamine agonist has in preliminary studies shown good prolactin lowering action without severe side effects. In a double blind randomized study the prolactin lowering effect of CQP was tested in three groups of hyperprolactinaemic women. Each group consisted of eight women of whom two received a placebo and six received 10, 20 or 30 ug CQP, respectively. The acute prolactin lowering effect of CQP was studied on day 1 and again in steady state after 7 day once-daily drug intake.

In group A (10ug) mean prolactin level at time zero of 3483 mU/l decreased to 2223 mU/l (-36%) after 4 hours and remained at this level for the next 4 hours. On day 7 the mean prolactin level was 2286 mU/l (34% decline as compared to time zero of day 1) and decreased further during this day to 1445 mU/l 8 hours after intake (58% decline as compared to time zero on day 1). Twenty-four hours after drug intake the mean prolactin level was still reduced to 2491 mU/l. In group B (20 ug) the decline on day 1 was 66%, on day 7 before drug intake the prolactin level was 77% below the initial value on day zero. On day 7 a further decline of 36% occurred (83% decrease as compared to time zero on day 1). In group C (30 ug) identical results were obtained as in group B. Both in group B and C some side effects were recorded 2 hours after drug intake. These were: lightheadedness, faint feeling and nausea. In general they were mild and disappeared within a few hours. Safety studies did not reveal any significant change during or after drug intake.

It is concluded that CQP shows good prolactin lowering effects in hyperprolactinaemic women. With once-daily intake, a sustained prolactin suppression lasting for 24 hours is seen in steady-state.

THE BENZODIAZEPINE RECEPTOR LIGANDS REGULATE THE CELL PROLIFERATION OF THE RAT ANTERIOR PITUITARY GLAND IN ADRENALECTOMIZED RATS 154

H. Stępień, J. Kunert-Radek, M. Pawlikowski
Institute of Endocrinology Medical Academy of Łódź, 91-425 Łódź

The stereospecific binding sites for benzodiazepines /BZD/ have been described in the central nervous system and anterior pituitary gland /APG/. Recently, several studies have established that BZDs can influence both the proliferation and the differentiation of various cell lines in vitro. Previously we have shown, that the peripheral-type BZD antagonist potentiates the stimulatory effect of estradiol on the APG DNA synthesis. We now report the effect of diazepam, peripheral /Ro 5-4864/ and central-type /Ro 15-1788/ BZD receptor ligands on APG cell replication in adrenalectomized male Sprague-Dowley rats.

Sham-operated /SO/ and adrenalectomized /AX/ rats were used in the experiment. Six days after the operation the BZD receptor ligands in the doses 5 mg/kg b.w. or wehicle were given s.c. 3 times at 12 h intervals. Twelwe, hours after the last injection the incorporation of ^{3}H-thymidine into DNA /cmp/ug DNA/ was measured after the short-term incubation with ^{3}H-thymidine. As expected AX enhanced the DNA synthesis in APG /SO - 136.2 ± 32.2, AX - 222.3 ± 41.1, p< 0.01/. A treatment with Ro 15-1788 not only reversed the effect of AX, but even decreased the APG DNA synthesis below the level in SO-rats /101.5 ± 39.5, p 0.01 vs AX/. Diazepam /177.9 ± 66.9/ and Ro 5-4864 /184.7 ± 68.8/ did not affected significantly ^{3}H-thymidine uptake in the same experimental conditions. These results suggest the possible involvement of BZD receptor in the control of the APG cell proliferation.

A NEW DOPAMINE AGONIST IN THE TREATMENT OF HYPERPROLACTINAEMIA 155

K.T. Stokke, L.E. Hanssen, S. Reinli*, S. Stray-Pedersen, J. Halse, J. Jervell
Rikshospitalet, N-0027 Oslo 1, Norway and Ullevål Hospital*, N-0407 Oslo 4, Norway

Present drugs used for hyperprolactinaemia have side effects. We wanted to study effects and side effects of a new propylergoline derivative (CQP 201-403, Sandoz). This compound has been shown effective in healthy man.

Twenty-four otherwise healthy women (21-44 years) with stable hyperprolactinaemia (35-318 µg/l), but without suprasellar extension of pituitary adenomas took part in a randomized double-blind study. They had all been without dopamin agonist for at least 4 weeks and were studied for one week, receiving either placebo, 0.005, 0.015 or 0.025 mg CQP daily at the morning meal.

Fasting prolactin levels decreased significantly (p<0.025, n=6) in all CQP groups (0.005 mg to 78%, 0.015 mg to 40% and 0.025 to 27% of premedication level) when day 7 was compared to day 1. The levels in the placebo group did not change (99%). The area under curve of the prolactin day curve (1-8 hours after drug administration) decreased significantly (p<0.025, n=6) at all CQP doses (0.005 mg to 77%, 0.015 mg to 46% and 0.025 mg to 35% when day 7 of therapy was compared to the first day of therapy. No change was seen in the placebo group (95%).

No serious side effects were seen, but 4 patients experienced a faint feeling and had to lie down when standing blood pressure was to be measured.

CQP is able to significantly lower the prolactin levels in hyperprolactinaemic patients at all doses employed. The effect is seen even the first day of treatment and lasts for at least 24 hours. The side effects are tolerable. This seems a promising new drug, but further comparison with existing drugs is needed.

THE ESTRADIOL-INDUCED INCREASE IN ANTERIOR PITUITARY DOPAMINE IS NOT MEDIATED BY PROLACTIN 156

N.Telford, Y.N.Sinha
Univ. of So. Calif., Los Angeles, CA 90089-0191

Estradiol (E2) causes an increase in serum prolactin (PRL) as well as an accumulation of dopamine (DA), a putative PRL inhibitory factor, in the anterior pituitary of C57BL/6J female mice (Telford et al., Neuroendocrinology, in press). To assess whether the increase in pituitary DA is a direct effect of E2 or is mediated by the E2-induced increase in serum PRL, ovariectomized mice were given pituitary transplants under the kidney capsule to elevate serum PRL independently of E2; half of the transplanted and control mice received two E2 implants (ca. 15 pg E2/ml serum). All mice were killed three weeks later by decapitation. Serum PRL was assayed by RIA; DA in the in situ anterior pituitary was measured by HPLC. The results are shown in the table (means ± SEM; n = 6-9 mice per group).

Group	1	2	3	4	Intact
E2 Implants	0	0	2	2	
Exogenous Pituitaries	0	2	0	2	
Pituitary DA (ng/mg protein)	0.47 ±0.09	0.99 ±0.13	2.63 ±0.22	5.98 ±0.86	0.67 ±0.16
Serum PRL (ng/ml)	7.0 ±1.0	78.9 ±17.1	9.5 ±1.8	210.2 ±85.5	13.3 ±3.2

Both E2 implants and exogenous pituitaries increased pituitary DA (p<0.05). E2 can increase pituitary DA about 5-fold without increasing serum PRL (compare groups 1 and 3). A 10-20 fold increase in serum PRL in the absence of differences in E2 treatment increases pituitary DA about 2-fold (compare group 1 vs 2 and group 3 vs 4), possibly due to PRL feedback increasing the DA output of the tuberoinfundibular neurons. There was a significant interaction between the effects of E2 implants and exogenous pituitaries (p<0.01), indicating that E2 and PRL act synergistically to increase pituitary DA. We conclude that the E2-induced increase in pituitary DA is not mediated, but is enhanced by, an increase in serum PRL.

INVESTIGATION OF THE ROLE OF DOPAMINE AS THE PROLACTIN INHIBITING FACTOR IN SHEEP. 157

G.B. Thomas, J.T. Cummins, G.A. Smythe+, R. Gleeson and I.J. Clarke
Medical Research Centre, Prince Henry's Hospital, Melbourne and +Garvan Institute of Medical Research, St. Vincent's Hospital, Sydney, Australia.

There is substantial evidence to support the notion that dopamine (DA) is a prolactin inhibiting factor (PIF) in a variety of species. We conducted experiments to assess the role of DA as a PIF in sheep.

Firstly, to determine whether or not DA could suppress PRL by a uniquely pituitary effect, we infused (i.c.) 1 µg/kg/min DA into hypothalamo-pituitary disconnected (HPD) ewes and control ewes. PRL levels in plasma fell ($P<0.01$) by 64 ± 3% in controls and by 67 ± 1% in HPD ewes. Following infusion levels rebounded to 120 ± 19% (control) and 103 ± 4% (HPD) of pre-infusion values.

Secondly, we used the combined GC/MS method for biogenic amines and metabolites with selected ion monitoring to quantify DA, norepinephrine (NE), dihydroxyphenylacetic acid (DOPAC) and dihydroxyphenylethyleneglycol (DHPG) in hypophyseal portal and peripheral blood. Serial samples were taken over 4-6h from 3 ewes. Levels of DA were similar in portal (1.1 ± 0.2pmol/l) and peripheral blood (0.6 ± 0.4), but NE was higher in portal (6.0 ± 0.9) than in peripheral. (2.3 ± 0.3) blood ($P<0.05$). Levels of DOPAC and DHPG were similar in portal and peripheral samples.

Finally, we infused 1 µg/kg/min DA and measured the above biogenic amines and metabolites in peripheral blood. During the infusion, DOPAC and DHPG levels rose but DA and NE did not. Plasma PRL levels were significantly ($P<0.01$) decreased during DA infusion.

On the grounds that in sheep 1) DA levels in hypophyseal portal blood are not distinguishable from peripheral levels and 2) DA is rapidly metabolized in blood, it seems unlikely that DA is a PIF. Thus infusion of DA may suppress PRL via a metabolite which is not DOPAC, as 10 µg/kg/min i.v. infusion of this had no effect on PRL. In view of the portal jugular differential in NA, and the ability of this amine to suppress PRL (Deaver & Dailey, 1982, Biol. Reprod. 27, 624), this is a possible PIF.

PHARMACOLOGICAL ASPECTS OF TERGURIDE AND ITS CLINICAL ROLE IN PRL SECRETION 158

Venturini P.L., Fasce V., Gorlero F., Valenzano M., Costantini S., Horowski R., Rainer E. and De Cecco L.
Clinica Ostetrica e Ginecologica, University of Genoa, V.le Benedetto XV, 16132, Genova, ITALY.

Recently a new class of drugs, 8-alpha-ergolines derived from Lisuride, has been identified. Among these Terguride (Transdihydrolisuride,TDHL) has shown a unique neuropharmacological profile combining both agonistic and antagonistic properties within its molecule and acting as a partial DA agonist.

The effect and the tolerance of Terguride have been evaluated by an acute administration (0.2 mg orally) in 12 normal women, 12 hyperPRL patients and 12 women with puerperal hyperprolactinaemia. TDHL lowered PRL levels without significative differences between the 3 groups, with a maximum suppressive effect (65% of decrement) between the 4th and the 6th hour. PRL values gradually raised to 70% of basal levels within 24 hours.

We studied the effect of a subchronic treatment (5 days) with two different dosages of TDHL in puerperal hyperprolactinaemia (0.4 and 0.8 mg daily). PRL levels were lowered in a dose dependent manner and normal range PRL levels were reached on the 3rd day during the higher dose treatment. These data indicate the 0.8 mg daily dose to be the effective one.

Finally, in order to exclude an antidopaminergic activity of Terguride on lactotropes, we have administered together Lisuride 0.2 mg and Terguride 0.4 mg to 6 hyperprolactinaemic patients comparing the results with those obtained giving to the same women Lisuride 0.2 mg and placebo. Since Terguride summed its PRL lowering effect to Lisuride we have shown that the antidopaminergic properties of Terguride do not interfere with the drug activity on DA receptors of lactotrops.

BROMOCRIPTINE AS PRIMARY TREATMENT FOR PROLACTIN SECRETING MACROADENOMAS: A RADIOLOGICAL, OPHTHALMOLOGICAL AND ENDOCRINOLOGICAL STUDY. 159

J.W. van 't Verlaat, R.J.M. Croughs, M.J. Hendriks, N.J. Bosma, J.W.R. Nortier, J.H.H. Thijssen.

Departments of Neurosurgery, Endocrinology and Radiology, University Hospital Utrecht, Utrecht, The Netherlands.

Fourteen patients, six women and eight men, with macroprolactinomas characterized by extrasellar extension and basal plasma prolactin levels 6 U/l were treated with 10-20 mg bromocriptine daily in four divided doses for a mean period of 2.5 years (range 0.5-4.0 years).

The following observations were made:

1.Plasma prolactin levels fell dramatically in all patients and values in the low normal range were obtained in twelve patients.

2.Tumor size was reduced by more than 75% in thirteen patients and by 50-75% in one patient. Tumorreduction was associated with the development of a partial empty sella in ten cases. In four cases the pituitary became visible.

3.Diminished visual acuity (four patients), bitemporal hemianopia (four patients), unilateral or bilateral central scotomas (three patients) and oculomotor palsy (two patients) restored to normal.

4.Hypogonadism (all patients), hypothyroidism (seven patients) and hypocorticism (four patients) improved or normalized in most cases.

It is concluded that in the medical treatment of macroprolactinomas 10-20 mg bromocriptine in four divided doses effectively reduces both plasma prolactin leveland tumor size.

Criteria to predict the outcome of drug therapy in patients with prolactinoma. 160

W. Winkelmann, B. Allolio, U. Deuß, D. Heesen.
Dept. Internal Med. II, Univ. of Köln, FRG

Dopamine agonists (DAG) are successfully used to normalize serum prolactin (PRL) in patients with prolactinoma. Some of them may be cured by drug therapy alone. However, no criteria are established to predict the effect of drug withdrawal on PRL. - 77 patients with prolactinoma (10 micro- , 67 macroprolactinoma) were treated with DAG for 3-10 yrs. After drug-induced normoprolactinaemia had lasted 2-3 yrs drug therapy was interrupted for 4 weeks. If hyperprolactinaemia recurred drug therapy was resumed and again interrupted after 1-2 yrs. During therapy basal and TRH stimulated PRL was measured in regular intervals. - 12 patients (5 micro-, 7 macroprolactinomas) treated between 2 and 6 yrs have persistent normoprolactinaemia (pn) for 7-57 months after withdrawal of DAG. The acute response to DAG prior therapy was similar in patients with pn compared to the remaining patients (mean PRL decrease 80.1 ± 8.1 vs 76.6 ± 14,3%). Prior to therapy all patients had a negative response to TRH (PRL increase<100%). However, during drug-induced normoprolactinaemia the negative TRH test converted into a positive PRL response in 47% of the patients. All patients, in whom this positive response to TRH became negative again, had pn after DAG withdrawal while a positive response to TRH during DAG therapy indicated recurrence of hyperprolactinaemia after DAG withdrawal. 9 out of 12 patients with pn had PRL levels below 3 ng/ml during DAG therapy compared to 21 out of 65 of the remaining patients ($p < 0.05$). Longterm therapy with DAG led to persistent normoprolactinaemia in 12 out of 77 patients with prolactinoma (16%; 5 out of 10 microprolactinomas = 50% and 7 out of 67 macroprolactinomas = 10%). The following criteria may be important to achieve pn: 1. During DAG therapy PRL should be suppressed below 3 ng/ml. 2. A positive PRL response to TRH during DAG therapy indicates recurrence of hyperprolactinaemia after drug withdrawal. 3. PRL decrease of at least 65% after acute administration of DAG seems to be a prerequisite to aim for pn.

ASSESSMENT OF THE REPRODUCTIVE AND ANTLER PERFORMANCE OF THE MALE WHITE-TAILED DEER BY GN-RH STIMULATION TEST. 161

G.A. Bubenik, D. Schams* and A.J. Sempere, Dept. of Zoology, Univ. of Guelph, Guelph, Ontario, Canada, NIG 2W1 and Dept. of Physiology, TU-Univ. Munchen-Weihenstephan, D-805 Freising, FRG.*

Reproductive success of the male deer is usually associated with a larger body size and an extraordinary capability to produce antlers. In order to examine the possible utilization of a Gn-RH stimulation test to assess the antler trophy, and sire potential of the male white-tailed deer, 12 bucks (ranging in age from 3 to 10 years) were injected with Gn-RH (100 ug/deer) during the rut (November) and in the spring (April). LH, FSH and testosterone (T) levels were determined by RIA in 3 pretreatment samples (10 min apart) and 7 posttreatment samples (30 min. apart). The deer were grouped accordingly to their body weight, antler size and the level of assertiveness. All bucks in the top score group responded to Gn-RH test in the rut with a relatively small increase of LH (below 20 ng/ml) and a profound elevation of T (reaching 30 to 50 ng/ml). The bucks at the low end of the score were found to have a high increase of LH (around 30-40/ng/ml) but a very low rise in levels of T (below 10 ng/ml). FSH levels increased only slightly after Gn-RH with an unexpectedly wide range of levels which were not related to reproductive performance. During the spring, the increase in LH levels greatly exceeded the rise of T in all bucks tested; however this time there was no relationship between hormonal levels and reproductive potential.

It can be concluded that Gn-RH (administered during the rut) might be a suitable tool to access the reproductive potential of the male deer. It appears that the pituitary-gonadal axis of the reproductively weak bucks does not mature sufficiently between the early reactivation of reproduction in the spring and the peak performance in the rut. Therefore, their LH and T patterns after Gn-RH challenge exhibit an almost inverse relationship to that observed in the group of top performers.

NPY AND GABA ACT AS α-MSH-RELEASE INHIBITING FACTORS ON FROG MELANOTROPHS 162

J.M. Danger, M. Lamacz, M.C. Tonon, E. Leneveu, S. Adjeroud, M. Tappaz*, M.E. Stoeckel**, G. Pelletier***, and H. Vaudry.
UA CNRS 650, Unité Alliée INSERM, Univ. Rouen, 76130 Mt-St-Aignan, France; *INSERM U171, Hôp. Ste Eugenie, 69001 Lyon, France; **UA CNRS 309, Univ. L. Pasteur, 67084 Strasbourg, France; ***Grp. MRC, CHU Laval Québec, Canada.

Using specific antisera to glutamic acid decarboxylase (GAD) and neuropeptide Y (NPY) we show that the frog neurointermediate lobe is supplied by rich networks of GABA-ergic and NPY-ergic fibers. These results led us to examine the possible role of GABA and NPY in the control of α-MSH secretion in amphibians. This study was conducted using the perifusion technique combined with a specific radioimmunoassay for α-MSH. GABA (10^{-6} and 10^{-4} M) caused a brief stimulation of α-MSH release followed by a marked inhibition. Picrotoxine (10^{-4} M), a Cl^- channel blocker, abolished the stimulatory effect of GABA, whereas bicuculline, a specific antagonist of $GABA_A$ receptors totally inhibited the first phase (stimulation) and reduced the inhibitory effect of GABA. The $GABA_A$ agonist muscimol mimicked the biphasic effect of GABA on α-MSH release. Administration of baclofen, a $GABA_B$ agonist (10^{-7} to 10^{-4} M) induced a dose-dependent inhibition of α-MSH secretion. In contrast to GABA or muscimol, baclofen did not cause any stimulatory effect whatever the dose. Synthetic NPY (10^{-8} to 10^{-6} M) inhibited α-MSH release in a dose-dependent manner. Since both DA and GABA are potent inhibitors of α-MSH release in frog, we have studied whether NPY could act presynaptically on dopaminergic or GABA-ergic fibers. The inhibitory effect of NPY (10^{-7} M) was not altered in the presence of haloperidol (10^{-5} M) or bicuculline (10^{-5} M) suggesting that NPY does not exert its effects via DA or GABA pathway. Taken together these results indicate that, in amphibians, α-MSH secretion is under multifactorial inhibitory control : DA, GABA (through both $GABA_A$ and $GABA_B$ receptors) and NPY inhibit α-MSH release. Since NPY was more potent than DA and GABA to reduce α-MSH secretion, it appears that NPY might be an important MSH-release inhibiting factor in the frog.

HYPOTHALAMIC AND EXTRAHYPOTHALAMIC MESOTOCIN-LIKE IMMUNOREACTIVITY IN THE BULLFROG (*RANA CATESBEIANA*) 163

G.C. Gonzalez and K. Lederis
University of Calgary, Calgary, Alberta, Canada T2N 4N1

Immunocytochemical methods were used to describe the distribution of mesotocin in the brain and spinal cord. In agreement with previous immunocytochemical studies, hypothalamic mesotocin-like immunoreactivity (MT-ir) was found in perikarya of the preoptic nucleus (PON). The distribution of perikarya and fibres were different from vasotocin immunoreactive neurons and fibres. Distinctive flask-shaped CSF-contacting MT-ir neurons were observed close to the ependyma of the third ventricle and recessus preopticus. Preterminal dendritic dilatations were found in the ependyma and ventricle terminals were seen protruding into the third ventricle.

Telencephalic MT-ir fibres were found in the superimposed (S) region of Hoffman of the lateral pallium (area of the zona limitans lateralis). Subpallium MT-ir fibres were also found in the striatum, medial septal nucleus, lateral septal nucleus, and amygdala. In the diencephalon, MT-ir fibres extended to dorsal and ventral habenula as well as to thalamic nuclei and pretectal area. Dense mesencephalic MT-ir fibres were seen projecting to nucleus posterodorsalis tegmenti mesencephali. Relatively weaker MT-stained fibres were also found in the optic tectum and torus semicircularis.

Mesotocin immunoreactive fibres were also seen along the spinal cord in the dorso-central field (close to the central canal) and the dorso-lateral funiculus (pial surface) from cervical to lumbar regions. In the filum terminale MT-ir fibres were found in the dorsal funiculus.

The results suggest that mesotocin, a naturally occurring oxytocin-like neuropeptide in amphibia, may have a role in behavioural (forebrain) and autonomic (spinal cord) functions as well as an undefined interaction with CSF, owing to the protrusion of nerve fibre terminals into the CSF (i.e. third ventricle and its preoptic recess).

(Supported by the Medical Research Council of Canada.)

GABAERGIC INNERVATION OF THE MEDIAN-EMINENCE PITUITARY COMPLEX : A COMPARATIVE IMMUNOCYTOCHEMICAL STUDY IN MAMMALS AND FISH 163a

O. Kah, C. Decavel, M. Rabhi, M.G. Martinoli, P. Dubourg, B. Onteniente, M. Geffard*, A. Calas
Lab. Physiologie des Interactions Cellulaires, UA 339 CNRS and *Lab. Neuroimmunologie, Bordeaux, France

To investigate the morphological support for the involvement of GABA in the neuroendocrine regulation of pituitary functions, the distribution and ultrastructural characterization of GABAergic terminals were studied in the median eminence (ME)-pituitary complex of rats, mice and goldfish by means of antibodies against GABA itself at the light and electron microscope levels.

In both fish and mammals, a high density of terminals was found in the intermediate lobe (IL) in direct, occasionally synaptic-like, contact with the glandular cells. These immunoreactive (ir) terminals were characterized by the presence of dense cored and synaptic vesicles. Similar ir profiles were observed in the posterior lobe where some fibers containing large neurosecretory vesicles were also positive.

In mouse and rat, no GABA ir fibers were detected in the anterior lobe. However, a heavy GABAergic innervation was present in the ME. The ultrastructural characteristics of these terminals, often found in contact with the capillaires of the primary plexus, were similar to those observed in the IL.

In goldfish, which lacks the typical portal system, the anterior lobe receives a direct innervation that represents the functional equivalent of the ME. Accordingly, numerous GABA ir profiles were observed in the pars distalis. At electron microscope level, these terminals, similar to those of the ME of mammals were observed in direct, sometimes synaptic-like, contact with all cell types.

Thus, the GABAergic innervation of the ME-pituitary complex displays similar features in remote classes of vertebrates. The direct innervation of all anterior pituitary cell types by GABAergic fibers in fish shows the interest of such comparative studies to approach the neuroendocrine functions of GABA neurons.

EFFECTS OF INSULIN-LIKE GROWTH FACTOR I (IGF-I) ON GROWTH HORMONE-RELEASING FACTOR (GRF) AND THYROTROPIN-RELEASING HORMONE (TRH) STIMULATION OF GH SECRETION IN THE DOMESTIC FOWL. 163b

F.C. Buonomo, T.J. Lauterio* C.A. Baile and W.H. Daughaday*. Monsanto Co., Anim. Sci. Div. and *Washington University School of Medicine, St. Louis, MO., USA.

Recent studies in mammalian species indicate that IGF-I may act as a negative feedback inhibitor of GH release through alteration of the secretion or sensitivity to hypothalamic regulatory factors. Although avian GH secretion may be regulated via the differential secretion of hypothalamic inhibitory (somatostatin) and stimulatory (GRF and TRH) factors, feedback effects of GH-stimulated IGF-I on GH release in birds have not been investigated. To study the effects of elevated IGF-I concentrations on GRF and TRH-stimulated GH secretion, 4-wk old chicks received an intravenous injection of recombinant human IGF-I either 10ug simultaneous (study 1) or 6ug 15 min prior (study 2) to GRF 5 ug/kg) or TRH (.5 ug/kg) administration. Radioimmunoassay analysis of plasma collected prior to and following peptide treat ment showed that circulating IGF-I concentrations were elevated 83.9%, 60.6%, 77.9% and 88.8% at the time of TRH or GRF administration in the first and second study, respectively. Peak GH secretion (mean of 5 and 15 min samples) subsequent to TRH injection was significantly ($p<.01$) depressed 45.1% and 48.2% in IGF-I-treated as compared to control chicks in study 1 and 2, respectively. GRF-stimulated GH secretion was significantly ($p<.01$) decreased by IGF-I administration in study 2 (41.3%) but not in study 1. An estimated IGF-I half-life in the chicken is less than 15 min based on the disappearance rate of the elevation produced by exogenous IGF-I injections. The effect of IGF-I treatment on TRH-stimulated T_3 elevation was also examined in study 2. The increase in plasma T_3 levels observed after TRH administration was significantly ($p<.05$) suppressed 40.9% in IGF-I-treated chicks as compared to those receiving TRH and vehicle. Thus, IGF-I may exert a negative feedback effect on pituitary hormone secretion in avian, as well as mammalian species.

CHARACTERIZATION OF UROTENSIN I AND CRF-LIKE PEPTIDES IN *CATOSTOMUS* BRAIN AND PITUITARY BY HPLC AND RADIOIMMUNOASSAY 164

D. McMaster and K. Lederis
University of Calgary, Calgary, Alberta, Canada T2N 4N1

Urotensin I (UI), a peptide with hypotensive action in mammals, and corticotropin releasing (CRF) activity in mammals and fish, is present in the caudal neurosecretory system (CNS) of teleost and elasmobranch fish. UI has been isolated and characterized from the urophysis (the neurohaemal organ of the CNS) of two species, *Catostomus commersoni* and *Cyprinus carpio*, and in both cases is a 41-residue peptide with 21 residues in common with ovine CRF (oCRF) and 24 in common in the rat/human CRF (rCRF). The presence of UI in the brain and pituitary as well as in the spinal cord of *Catostomus* has been shown by both radioimmunoassay (RIA) and immunocytochemical techniques. Using appropriately heterologously blocked and affinity purified UI and CRF antisera, the presence of a CRF-like substance other than UI (and apparently present in larger amounts than UI) has also been demonstrated by immunocytochemistry in *Catostomus* brain and pituitary (C.R. Yulis, K. Lederis, K.L. Wong and A.W.F. Fisher, Peptides, in press).

In RIA using oCRF antisera, brain and pituitary extracts showed little or no oCRF immunoreactivity (ir). In a recently developed RIA using rCRF antisera, however, a high degree of immunoreactivity was obtained, especially in pituitary extracts (~40ng/pituitary), and experiments have been initiated using high pressure liquid chromatography (HPLC) and RIA, to characterize further the UI-like and CRF-like peptides. HPLC of hypothalamus and telencephalon extracts (UI-ir levels: 1600-11000 pg/animal; 450-1900 pg/mg dry weight) followed by UI RIA has shown that the major UI-ir peak had the same retention time (R.T.) as authentic UI. HPLC of pituitary extract followed by rCRF RIA has shown essentially a single peak of rCRF-ir material, eluting close to rCRF (i.e. several minutes later than UI). Blank runs were carried out, and fractions assayed, before HPLC of the brain and pituitary extracts. Two approaches are being pursued in further studies (a) HPLC of brain extracts followed by both UI and rCRF RIA and (b) isolation of the CRF-like peptide from pituitaries with a view to further characterization.

PINEAL, RETINAL AND SERUM MELATONIN AND N-ACETYL-SEROTONIN (NAS) RHYTHMS ON LIGHT PHASE SHIFTING AND BLINDING 165

I. Nir, *S.F. Pang, *A.E. Allen
Hebrew University-Hadassah Medical School, Jerusalem
*Hong Kong University Faculty of Medicine, Hong Kong

After reversing a 12 hr light/12 hr darkness regimen of environmental illumination, the first mid-darkness serum melatonin levels of White Leghorn chicks were not much different from their original mid-light values. However, on continuing with the reversed regimen, the next mid-darkness levels were sharply increased and maximum levels were reached after a further 2 days' exposure. Light under the same experimental conditions had much more drastic effects and 6 hrs on the reversed regimen were sufficient to bring down completely the high value of the original mid-darkness period to the level of the starting mid-light nadir. Pineal and retinal melatonin levels recorded at the first mid-darkness measurement on the reversed schedule were greatly enhanced and reached the maximum levels after 3 more days; those recorded during the light periods indicate gradual decline but far from to the nadir of the original light period, even at the end of the experiment.

Retinal NAS measured simultaneously, had an identical pattern to melatonin but the pineal NAS rhythm did invert completely, albeit gradually.

Blinding did not prevent inversion of pineal and serum melatonin rhythms, which were identical in blinded and control chicks on the reversed lighting schedule. However, retinal melatonin values of the light periods were significantly less depressed in blinded than in control birds. Moreover, blinding completely prevented the retinal NAS depression under light but did not affect the pineal NAS. During darkness retinal and pineal NAS elevation was sluggish in the blinded chicks.

Different patterns appear to control pineal and retinal circadian rhythms generated by light stimuli.

ALTERNATIVES TO DOPAMINE: WHAT CONTROLS PROLACTIN SECRETION IN SOME FISHES? 166

R. S. Nishioka, H. A. Bern, K. Kelley, E. G. Grau*, R. Rivas, and G. Young. University of California, Berkeley, CA 94720 and *University of Hawaii, Honolulu, HI 96744.

In the tilapia, Oreochromis mossambicus, a teleost fish, prolactin secretion is influenced by a complex array of hypothalamic and extrahypothalamic factors. (Hypothalamic factors are delivered to the pituitary by nerve fibers in teleosts.) Nevertheless, tilapia prolactin cells show considerable independence, and high spontaneous release of prolactin occurs in vitro, similar to the typical mammalian pattern, especially under conditions of low osmotic pressure. Prolactin release is stimulated by thyroid-releasing hormone and possibly by angiotensin II. Inhibition by dopamine and other catecholamines in vitro is well documented but the prolactin cells lack demonstrable aminergic innervation by the Falck-Hillarp formaldehyde-induced fluorescence technique. However, several additional factors, including somatostatin, urotensin II, and surprisingly, vasoactive intestinal peptide, inhibit prolactin release in vitro in a dose-related fashion. Other agents are being tested.

A well-defined delivery system for somatostatin has been identified. Fibers containing somatostatin-like immunoreactivity terminate directly on or near prolactin cells in the rostral pars distalis of tilapia. These fibers emanating from the basal hypothalamus possibly originate from either the nucleus preopticus or the nucleus lateralis tuberis. Thus, prolactin secretion in tilapia, and possibly in other teleosts, may prove to be under peptidergic inhibitory control. Supported by NSF Grants PCM 84-05249 and PCM 83-14294.

THE EFFECT OF HYDROCORTISONE, VASOPRESSIN (AVP) AND CRF ADMINISTRATION ON ACTH, αMSH AND AVP PULSATILE SECRETION IN THE PITUITARY VENOUS EFFLUENT OF THE HORSE. 167

C. Redekopp, *C.H.G. Irvine, R.A. Donald, J.H. Livesey, *S.L. Alexander.
Dept. of Endocrinology, The Princess Margaret Hospital, *Dept. of Veterinary Science, Lincoln College, Christchurch, New Zealand.

In order to study the hypothalamic control of pituitary ACTH secretion it is desirable to sample the hypothalamic or hypophyseal venous effluent in the conscious, unpremedicated animal. We have previously described the close temporal relationship between pulses of ACTH and AVP secretion occurring spontaneously in the pituitary effluent of the horse. (1)

In this study we have measured the above hormones and αMSH in the Pituitary venous effluent of 5 resting conscious horses at 5 minute intervals following the intravenous infusion of 25mg hydrocortisone hemisuccinate over 1 hour, or an IV bolus of 10 units of AVP, or 500µg CRF. Peripheral jugular samples were also taken at 15 minute intervals.

A rise in plasma hydrocortisone was associated with marked suppression of plasma ACTH levels in all horses, but no demonstrable effect on AVP peaks. Administration of AVP or CRF resulted in an increase in the amplitude of ACTH peaks in pituitary portal plasma but the pulsatility of ACTH secretion was maintained. The ACTH response to CRF appeared delayed or impaired if preceeded by a rise in plasma cortisol. Plasma ACTH and αMSH secretory episodes were generally unrelated and hence are probably regulated independently.

(1) Redekopp C., Irvine C.H.G., Donald R.A., Livesey J.H., Sadler W., Nicholls M.G., Alexander S.L., Evans M.J., 1986 Endocrinology (April, In Press).

COMPARATIVE ASPECTS OF HYPOTHALAMIC α-MSH-LIKE IMMUNOREACTIVE SYSTEMS 168

M. Vallarino
Istituto Anatomia Comparata, Università di Genova, Genova Italy

α-MSH, a tridecapeptide synthetized as part of the 31K opiomelanocortin precursor in the pituitary gland, has been found in the brain of different mammal species within neuronal centers and fiber networks involved in various neuroregulatory functions. In other vertebrate groups α-MSH has been studied extensively in the pituitary, while comparative analyses of its presence in the brain are scanty, despite the very interest to know its evolutionary history and implications. So, I have recently started an immunocytochemical study on the occurrence of α-MSH-like peptide in the brain of fishes, amphibians, and reptiles using an antiserum generated against bovine synthetic α-MSH (RIA,UK).

By means indirect immunofluorescent and PAP methods reactions were performed on brains of: *Scyliorhinus canicula*, *Squalus acanthias*, *Boops boops*, *Rana esculenta*, and *Lacerta muralis*.

α-MSH-like immunoreactive neurons and fibers were found in the hypothalamus of all perfused animals, mainly located in the paraventricular region. In dogfishes a single α-MSH-like center lies in the dorsal posterior paraventricular region, while in teleosts it is distributed in the preoptic area. In the frog brain two α-MSH like immunoreactive centers were seen in the preoptic region and in the nucleus infundibularis ventralis. In lizard α-MSH-like staining occurred within preoptic, paraventricular, and supraoptic areas. From these results an α-MSH-like neuroendocrine system seems to be constantly present during evolution of lower vertebrates, anatomically related to the organization of periventricular gray matter.

EFFECTS OF [D-ALA^6, PRO^9-NEt]-LHRH AND CATECHOLAMINERGIC DRUGS ON GONADOTROPIN SECRETION AND OVULATION IN THE CHINESE LOACH 169

G. Van Der Kraak[1], H.R. Lin[2], C. Peng[2], R.E. Peter[1]
[1]Department of Zoology, University of Alberta, Edmonton, Alberta, Canada; and [2]Department of Biology, Zhongshan University, Guangzhou, China

Gonadotropin (GtH) secretion in teleosts is regulated by the stimulatory effects of a gonadotropin-releasing hormone (GnRH) and the inhibitory effects of a gonadotropin-release inhibitory factor (GRIF). Several lines of evidence indicate that dopamine functions as a GRIF by modulating spontaneous as well as GnRH-stimulated release of GtH in teleosts. In the present studies we have determined the effects of [D-Ala^6, Pro^9-NEt]-LHRH (LHRH-A) alone and in combination with drugs which influence the actions of dopamine or the synthesis of catecholamines on GtH secretion and the induction of ovulation in the Chinese loach (*Paramisgurnus dabyranus*).

LHRH-A alone stimulated an increase in serum GtH levels in the loach, but was a relatively ineffective treatment for the induction of ovulation. Injection of the dopamine receptor antagonist pimozide caused a marked potentiation of the GtH release-response to LHRH-A, and combined injections of pimozide and LHRH-A induced ovulation. Reserpine, a drug which causes depletion of catecholamines from presynaptic terminals, also caused a marked potentiation of the GtH release-response to LHRH-A and combined treatment induced ovulation. Similarly, administration of alpha-methyl-para-tyrosine to block conversion of tyrosine to L-dopa, and carbidopa to block conversion of L-dopa to dopamine, potentiated the GtH release-response to LHRH-A and induced ovulation. In contrast, the use of diethyldithiocarbamate, to block conversion of dopamine to norepinephrine, failed to augment the action of LHRH-A on GtH release and ovulation.

The present results provide further evidence that dopamine functions as a GRIF in teleosts, and demonstrate that drugs which block either the synthesis or actions of dopamine potentiate the action of LHRH-A in teleosts.

Supported by IDRC and AHFMR.

COMPARISON OF *IN VITRO* EFFECTS OF DIFFERENT SPECIES SPECIFIC GnRH AND THEIR ANALOGUES IN A DISPERSED CELL SUPERFUSION SYSTEM 170

S. Vigh,* A. Horváth, G. Kéri, T. Gulyás, V. Csernus,* K. Nikolics, I. Teplán and B. Flerkó*
1st Institute of Biochemistry, Semmelweis University Medical School, 1444 Budapest, Hungary;
and (*) Department of Anatomy, University Medical School of Pécs, 7643 Pécs, Hungary

The existence of structural variation in gonadotropin hormone releasing hormone (GnRH) in vertebrates has been known for only the last few years.

Mammalian, salmon and chicken gonadotropin-releasing hormones (mGnRH, sGnRH, cGnRH) and their analogues were synthesized in our laboratories by solid-phase methods. In the present study, their ability to stimulate *in vitro* LH and FSH release in a superfused cell-column system was tested.

Rat pituitary cells were dispersed with collagenase, mixed with Biogel P2, and perfused on a column with oxygenated Medium-199 containing 50 mg/l Gentamicin. LH and FSH levels in superfusates were measured by RIA using reagents provided by NHPP (NIADDK, NIH). With the aid of this system, we found a linear relationship between the log of the dose of synthetic mGnRH, two mGnRH analogues, sGnRH, cGnRH, two cGnRH analogues and the total amount of LH and FSH released by the perfused pituitary cells. However, the dose ranges, where linear dose-related response was observed, were different when these peptides had been administered.

We also tested the biological potencies of these peptides in a cultured rat pituitary cell system, as well as their *in vivo* effect on the artificial propagation of fishes. From these results, we found that using three of these analogues, we were able to fulfill the induced artificial propagation of several types of fishes which could not be artificially propagated before.

THE EFFECTS OF TESTOSTERONE ON METABOLIC CLEARANCE RATE OF GH IN FEMALE RATS 171

T.M. Badger, D. O'Sullivan, J. LaRovere, W.J. Millard, J.B. Martin
Massachusetts General Hospital, Boston, MA 02114

Plasma growth hormone (GH) patterns of male and female rats differ significantly. Females have increased GH pulse frequency and greater basal GH concentrations than males. Since GH pulse frequency is directly related to frequency of GRF and/or somatostatin secretion from the hypothalamus, sex-related differences in GH pulse frequency may be associated with central control of these neuropeptides. On the other hand, sex-related basal GH levels could merely be a reflection of GH pulse frequency or could be caused by differences in GH clearance. Since we have previously demonstrated that T-treated females exhibit male plasma GH patterns, we hypothesized that the MCR should be greater in T-treated females than intact females if MCR is responsible for sex-related differences in basal GH levels. MCR for GH was studied in intact (I), or ovariectomized T-treated (OVT) females by the method of constant rate infusion. Rats were sham-operated or ovariectomized, and simultaneously implanted with empty or T-filled Silastic capsules on Day 0 and fitted with a jugular and a femoral cannula on Day 7. On Day 14, GH (200 Ug/hr) was infused through the jugular cannula for 4 hr and blood was collected through the femoral every 30 min. Steady state GH concentrations were achieved and used to calculate the MCR. At 4 hr, the infusion was stopped and the disappearance of exogenous GH from the plasma was determined and the t1/2 calculated.

	MCR	t1/2
Intact	0.60 $\pm$ 0.04 ml/min/100gBW	5.7 $\pm$ 0.4 min
OVT	0.57 $\pm$ 0.03 ml/min/100gBW	5.3 $\pm$ 0.4 min

No differences were found between the MCR or t1/2 in I and OVT. These results suggest that the sex-related differences in basal plasma GH levels are not related to MCR. These data further suggest that the greater basal plasma GH levels of female rats are probably a reflection of the increased GH pulse frequency.
Supported in part by HD 14586 & AM 26252.

GROWTH HORMOME SECRETION IN ACROMEGALY: EFFECTS OF SOMATOSTATIN ANALOGUE SMS 201-995 (SANDOZ). 172

A. Barkan, R. Lloyd, W. Chandler, R. Kelch, I. Beitins, N. Hopwood. Departments of Medicine, Pathology, Neurosurgery and Pediatrics, University of Michigan, Ann Arbor, MI 48109, U.S.A.

The etiology of acromegaly is unknown, and both de novo formation of an autonomous pituitary adenoma as well as primary hypothalamic dysfunction (increased GRF or decreased somatostatin secretion) have been postulated. Pituitary surgery seldom results in cure of acromegaly, especially in patients with macroadenomas. Growth hormone secretion was studied in 9 patients with active acromegaly before and up to 6 months on SMS therapy (50-100 µg s.c. TID-QID). GH secretion was highly variable throughout the day (every 20 min. sampling for 24 hours). GH pulse frequency in patients was increased (5-10 pulses/24h; 6.3±1.3, M±SE), as compared to 1-5 pulses/24h (3.7±1.7) in healthy adult controls. The amplitude of GH pulses (8±1 ng/ml) was similar to normal controls (8.7±1.3 ng/ml), and GH responses to i.v. GRF 1-44 (1 µg/kg) were similar in patients and controls (35±12 ng/ml vs. 26±17 ng/ml). Nocturnal augmentation of GH secretion was observed in acromegalic subjects. Treatment with SMS inhibited GH secretion in all patients, and in 5 of them mean serum GH became normal (<3 ng/ml). However, spontaneous GH pulses and GH responses to TRH persisted in some patients. In 4 patients with previously untreated pituitary macroadenomas, treatment with SMS resulted in a significant (60-70%) decrease in tumor volume, and disappearance of suprasellar expansion was observed. Three of these patients underwent selective pituitary adenomectomy and postoperative GH became normal in all. Histologic examination revealed features characteristic of pituitary adenoma, but decreased cellular size, increased number of GH secretory granules per cell and perivascular fibrosis were observed. We conclude: 1. Acromegaly may be due to augmented hypothalamic GRF secretion, presumably to increased frequency of GRF pulses. 2. Long-term therapy with SMS 201-995 is effective in control of acromegaly, but does not correct the entire biochemical and morphological picture of the disease. Thus, somatostatin deficiency is an unlikely cause of acromegaly. 3. In patients with pituitary macroadenomas, pretreatment with SMS 201-995 decreases tumor size, and may improve surgical outcome.

THE PRESENCE OF NEURAL PATHWAYS INHIBITING THE EXCITEMENT OF HYPOTHALAMIC GH-RH-NEURONS IN THE RATS 173

K. Chihara, Y. Okimura, T. Kita, Y. Kashio, M. Sato, T. Fujita
Kobe University School of Medicine, Kobe, Japan

The effect of electrical stimulation of the median eminence (ME-ES) on plasma GH levels was examined under various experimental conditions in pentobarbital-anesthetized adult male rats. In intact control animals, plasma GH levels were not changed during ME-ES and markedly increased immediately after cessation of ME-ES whereas plasma somatostatin levels in hypophysial portal blood were greatly elevated during ME-ES and returned to the base-line level rapidly after ME-ES. Plasma GH rises occurring after ME-ES were completely suppressed by passive immunization with anti-rat GHRH serum. In rats immunized passively with anti-somatostatin serum (ASS), the pattern of plasma GH response to ME-ES was not different from that in normal serum (NS)-treated control rats, although plasma GH levels in ASS-treated rats were greater in all sampling points than those in NS-treated rats. In rats with either complete or anterolateral deafferentation of the basal medial hypothalamus by Halász knife, basal plasma GH levels were elevated up to the value comparable to that in ASS-treated rats, but in a striking contrast to the pattern of plasma GH response to ME-ES in ASS-treated rats, plasma GH raised immediately after the start of ME-ES with sustained increase throughout an observation period.

These findings suggest the following: first, the release of somatostatin from the hypothalamus is enhanced during ME-ES, the excitement of hypothalamic GH-RH-neuron is conversely suppressed during ME-ES by inhibitory neurons which enter anterolaterally into the basal medial hypothalamus, and consequently plasma GH levels are completely suppressed during ME-ES. Second, an abrupt stimulation of GH release is triggered immediately after cessation of ME-ES possibly by enhanced secretion of hypothalamic GH-RH. (This work was supported in part by research grants from the Japanese Ministry of Health and Welfare; the Japanese Ministry of Education, Science and Culture; and the Growth Science Foundation for 1984 and 1985).

ARCUATE hGHRF MAINLY OCCURS IN AN EXTRA-INFUNDIBULARLY PROJECTING MULTIPEPTIDERGIC NEURONAL SYSTEM 174

Ph. Ciofi and G. Tramu,
INSERM U156, place de Verdun, 59045 LILLE Cedex, France

The comparative immunohistochemical study of the hypothalamic arcuate nucleus of colchicine-treated guinea-pigs, cats and rats showed that neurons displaying human somatoliberin- (hGHRF-), gastrin/cholecystokinin- (G/CCK-) and neuropeptide Y- (NPY-) like immunoreactivities (LI) have a closely resembling distribution.

Therefore, using the elution-restaining procedure, we investigated the possible co-occurence of these three peptide-LI in the same arcuate neurons and demonstrated that : i) in all three species, about 90% of the arcuate perikarya displaying hGHRF-LI exhibited simultaneously NPY-LI, while there was no periportal NPY-LI in the external zone of the median eminence, ii) the remaining 10% arcuate hGHRF-LI neurons reacted only for hGHRF, iii) G/CCK-LI and NPY-LI were always co-localized in neurons of the cat and guinea-pig arcuate nuclei, when the G/CCK-like staining was low to undetectable in rat arcuate cells, iiii) hGHRF-LI and pro-opiomelanocortin-LI were found in discrete arcuate neuronal systems.

Taken together, these results suggest that, in the mammalian species studied here, the arcuate hGHRF-LI neuronal population is subdivided in at least two subgroups of unequal extent: a minority of neurons reacting only for hGHRF thus giving rise to the hGHRFergic-like innervation of the portal plexus, and a majority of hGHRF-NPY-LI cells also co-reacting for G/CCK having extra-infundibular projections.

FEEDBACK EFFECT OF GROWTH HORMONE ON HYPOTHALAMIC OPIOID AND GHRH PRODUCING NEURONS

175

D. Cocchi, I. Ganzetti, F. Petraglia, E.E. Müller
Department of Pharmacology, School of Medicine, University of Milan and Department of Obstetrics and Gynecology, University of Modena, ITALY.

Reportedly, most acromegalics are refractory to the growth hormone (GH)-releasing effect of central nervous system-acting stimuli. For instance, the synthetic analogue of met-enkephalin (Enk) viz. FK 33-824 fails to alter the high circulating GH levels of acromegalics. The most likely interpretation of such behavior is that circulating GH disrupts, for a negative feedback effect, hypothalamic opioid function and/or GH-releasing hormone (GHRH) producing neurons, through which opioid compounds would exert their action. We have evaluated in male rats the effect of a high-dose GH regimen on the hypothalamic stores of endogenous opioid peptides (EOPs) and GHRH. In addition, in the same animals we have determined the GH-releasing effect of FK 33-824.

Administration of human GH (250 μg b.i.d. for 4 days) to male rats reduced β-endorphin (βEP) and Enk-like immunoreactivity (LI) stores in the medial basal hypothalamus (40% and 30% decrease, respectively). In the same animals, treatment with GH resulted in a significant reduction of GHRH-LI in the median eminence (35% decrease). Despite the profound biochemical alterations induced by GH treatment, rats given GH exhibited a normal responsiveness to FK 33-824 (0.2 mg/kg iv). FK 33-824 increased also prolactin (PRL) levels to a similar extent in both groups of animals.

The following conclusions can be drawn: 1) high circulating GH levels exert directly or through somatomedins a feedback effect on hypothalamic EOP-and-GHRH-producing neurons; 2) the reduction of hypothalamic EOP stores does not affect the sensitivity of opioid receptors, as indicated by normal GH and PRL response to FK 33-824; 3) in contrast to the long-term exposure to high GH levels (acromegaly?), short-term GH exposure does not impair the ability of opioid agonists to release enough GHRH from the depleted hypothalamic stores.

Supported by Special C.N.R. project "Oncology" grant N. 85.02266.44

ETHANOL AND GROWTH HORMONE SECRETION IN THE FEMALE RAT.

176

W.L. Dees, V. Rettori and S. Kentroti
Department of Physiology, Univ of Tx Hlth Sci Ctr, Dallas, Texas 75235.

The objective of this study was to determine the effects of ethanol (ETOH) on GH secretion in the female rat following both short-term (3 days) and acute (single dose) exposure. One week prior to the experiment rats weighing 250-300 g were surgically implanted with a permanent intragastric cannula. Animals in the short-term study were administered either an ETOH or a rigidly controlled isocaloric liquid diet regimen for 3 days and killed by decapitation 1.5 hr following the last injection. Additional control animals were cannulated and maintained on Lab Chow and water, but were left untreated. Results indicated a marked reduction in serum GH levels in the ETOH-treated animals ($P<0.05$). In order to assess more closely the mechanism by which ETOH diminished GH secretion we have analyzed the pulsatile secretory pattern of the hormone following an acute intragastric injection of either saline or of various ETOH-saline solutions ranging in dose from 2.0-4.0 g/kg. GH levels were measured by RIA of jugular blood samples drawn every 10 min from freely moving conscious rats via an indwelling silastic catheter. Analysis of the areas under the individual curves of secretion indicated that ETOH significantly depressed GH levels in a dose-dependent manner ($P<0.01$ at 3 or more g/kg), with the greatest reduction being at 1.5 hrs post-injection. Also, a significant ($P<0.05$) 30% reduction in the number of GH pulses was noted in ETOH vs. saline-injected animals. Additionally, a submaximal challenge dose of GRF (200 ng) to both saline and ETOH-injected rats revealed that pituitary responsiveness was the same for both groups. Thus, these data demonstrate the detrimental effects of ETOH on GH secretion in the female rat, and suggest for the first time that the site of action for this effect is at the hypothalamic level. (Supported by Grant NIAAA-06014)

HUMAN FETAL CORTICAL NEURONES IN CULTURE: A MODEL FOR THE STUDY OF THE NEUROSECRETORY ACTIVITY OF HUMAN BRAIN.

177

R.Elli,V.Silani,A.Pizzuti,G.Toffano, G.Scarlato,G.Faglia.
Departments of Endocrinology and Neurology, School of Medicine,University of Milan,Italy.

Neurosecretion in human brain may differ to that in rodents, in particular with regard to the alterations that take place in neurodegenerative disorders as senile dementia(Alzheimer type,associated to Parkinson's disease) in wich a dicrease of brain somatostatin (SS) is proved.

We developed a tecnique to maintain dispersed fetal human cortical neurones in culture until morphological and neurosecretory maturation.

Briefly,human fetal cortical tissue was obtained after informed consent and therapeutical abortion at the 16th. week of gestation. Cells underwent to enzymatic and mechanical dispersion and plated ($2X10^6$) onto 35 mm,poly-L-Lysine coated Falcon dishes. Culture medium was DMEM 20% FCS for the first 3 days and DMEM 10% FCS afterwards. Cells were feeded every 3 days and kept up to 6 months in culture. At day 14 in vitro 5 sister cultures were exposed to Krebs solution (10 min for 4 times) and then to to Krebs containing high K concentration for 10 min. SS spontaneous release in the culture medium and in Krebs before and after high K depolarization was measured by a very sensitive RIA using an excess of antiserum 1758 (gift of Dr.Holst,Univ of Copenhagen). Detection limit was 0.4 pg/tube. Neurones reached maturation and esthablished cellular contacts at day 10 in vitro;at that time the combined lenght of all processes reached a stable plateau. The 5 cultures challeged with krebs solutions increase the release of SS from 0.6±0.1SD to 1.3±0.2SD pg/ml/min after exposure to high K concentration. We propose human cortical neurones in culture as a model to study the neurosecretory human extrahypothalamic brain,to identify and test neurotrophic factors and to get inside neurodegeneration.

AUTOINHIBITION OF HYPOTHALAMIC SOMATOSTATIN RELEASE : LOCALIZATION BY IN VITRO RELEASE EXPERIMENTS AND ULTRASTRUCTURAL EVIDENCE.

178

J. Epelbaum, L. Tapia-Arancibia*, G. Alonso*, H. Astier*, C. Kordon.
U 159 INSERM, 2ter rue d'Alésia, 75014 Paris and *ERA 85 CNRS, Montpellier, France.

Somatostatin (SRIF), like others neurotransmitters, is able to inhibit its own secretion in neuronal cell cultures. In the present work, we attempted to localize this autoinhibition by taking advantage of the spatial configuration of the tuberoinfundibular hypothalamic SRIF neurons. This was achieved by 1) measuring SRIF release from carefully dissected anterior hypothalamic structures : (AH) containing most of the SRIF perikarya or median eminence (ME) which contains only nerve terminals. 2) by ultrastructural immunocytochemistry of interconnections between SRIF neuronal elements in the two hypothalamic regions. In vitro, a biologically active, but non immunoreactive SRIF analog (DTrp 8 SRIF), inhibited 25 mM K+ induced SRIF release from AH but not ME. The effect was dose dependent and maximal at 10^{-7} M. In AH, DTrp 8 SRIF was ineffective on the release of LHRH, another peptide measured in order to check selectivity of the effect. In the periventricular nucleus, perikarya and dendrites of labelled SRIF neurons showed frequent apposition of their limiting membranes. Classical synapses were also observed between SRIF containing axonal processes and labelled perikarya or dendrites. Although membrane appositions between neighbouring SRIF axons frequently occurred in the median eminence, no synaptic like SRIF-SRIF connection could be detected at that level.

The data demonstrate a direct inhibitory action of a SRIF agonist on the anterior periventricular hypothalamic release of the peptide. The effect is consistant with the occurrence of SRIF-SRIF synapses in this region ; taken together, the data suggest that SRIF can exert a negative feedback on its own release, presumably through autoreceptors located on the perikarya or dendrites of SRIF containing neurons.

IMPACT OF INTENSIVE VENOUS SAMPLING ON DETECTION OF GROWTH HORMONE PULSES IN NORMAL MEN 179

W.S. Evans, A.C.S. Faria, E. Christiansen, K.Y. Ho, J. Weiss, A.D. Rogol, M.L. Johnson, R.M. Blizzard, J.D. Veldhuis, M.O. Thorner
University of Virginia Medical Center, Charlottesville, Virginia 22908

Recent studies in the human (JCEM 59:96, 1984) and rat (AJP 247 [Endocrinol Metab] 10:E130, 1984) have shown that the number of LH pulses identified using computer assisted pulse detection algorithms is influenced remarkably by the frequency with which samples are obtained. To test the importance of this phenomenon in studies of growth hormone (GH) secretion, 7 normal young men (ages 21-27) were sampled at 5 minute intervals for 24 hours in the fed state. GH pulses were identified and characterized using an objective, multiple point, statistically based pulse detection algorithm (Cluster; AJP, in press, 1986) which defines significant hormone excursions in relation to internal measurement error within the actual experimental data series at any given false-positive rate. The parent 5-minute data set and the constituent (10-, 15-, 20-, 30- and 60-minute) data series were analyzed to define the numbers of pulses detected per 24 hours (mean ± SEM) as a function of sampling rate and the results shown in the Table.

	Sampling Interval (minutes)						
	5	10	15	20	30	45	60
Pulses /24h	5.9 ±0.6	3.4 ±0.3	2.8 ±0.3	2.9 ±0.6	2.5 ±0.4	2.2 ±0.2	1.9 ±0.2

Analysis of variance of the log-transformed pulse frequencies revealed that significantly more pulses were detected at a 5 minute sampling rate than at any other ($p < 0.0001$). No differences in the number of pulses detected was demonstrated among 10, 15, 20, or 30 minute sampling frequences.

These results indicate that analysis of GH data obtained by sampling less often than every 5 minutes will fail to enumerate an appreciable number of GH pulses. We conclude that the phenomenon of GH pulsatility in health and disease requires redefinition using optimal sampling paradigms.

THE GHRH-INDUCED GH RELEASE IS MODULATED BY THE CHOLINERGIC SYSTEM. 180

E. Ghigo, E. Mazza, V. Locatelli*, E.E. Müller*, F. Camanni, F. Massara
Department of Biomedicine, University of Turin and Department of Pharmacology, University of Milan*, Italy.

The effects of a muscarinic receptor antagonist (pirenzepine, PIRE) and of an acetylcholinesterase inhibitor (pyridostigmine, PD) on the GH response to GHRH (1 µg/kg iv bolus)-induced GH release were studied in normals, short children and acromegalics in order to verify the role of the cholinergic system in the neuroregulation of GH secretion.

In normals (n=9) PIRE (0.6 mg/kg iv bolus 5 min before GHRH) blunted the GHRH-induced GH release (integrated areas, mean ± SEM: 81 ± 17 vs 481 ± 211 ng/ml/hr; $p < 0.01$)while conversely PD (120 mg os 30 min before GHRH) markedly potentiated it (1045 ± 245 vs 481 ± 211 ng/ml/hr; $p < 0.01$). PD was also able to abolish the well known somatotrope refractoriness to repeated (50 µg iv every 120 min) GHRH boli when administered 30 min before the second GHRH bolus. In children with short stature (n=13, age 5-16 yrs, pubertal stage I-II) with insulin (ITT)-induced GH peak repeatedly lower than 8 ng/ml (mean ± SEM 4.2 ± 0.7 ng/ml) the GH response to GHRH was clerly higher (14.6 ± 3.9 ng/ml; $p < 0.05$ vs ITT) though overlapping ITT in 7/13 cases. PD (60 mg os 60 min before GHRH) potentiated the GH response to GHRH (28.5 ± 5.7 ng/ml; $p < 0.005$ vs GHRH) in all but 2 children, who were not responder to both ITT and GHRH. In 8 PD + GHRH responsive children, PD alone induced a GH rise always higher than ITT (15.0 ± 3.9 vs 5.3 ± 0.7 ng/ml; $p < 0.025$). In acromegalics (n=5) PIRE variably inhibited the GHRH-induced GH response, but was unable to modify either basal and TRH-induced GH levels.

In conclusion, our data show that cholinergic system plays an important role in the modulation of GHRH effects. The marked GH responsivity to cholinergic enhancement, even in children who could be defined as GH deficient based upon auxologic evaluation (predicted height lower than midparental height), ITT and GHRH test, suggest that a functional hypothalamic alteration involving cholinergic system may sometimes underlie hyposomatotropinism. Moreover, PD may be useful for a better diagnostic evaluation of short stature. The cholinergic muscarinic blockade does not seem promising in the medical treatment of acromegaly.

This work was partially supported by a grant from M.P.I.

RAPID PROGRESSION OF A GROWTH HORMONE PRODUCING TUMOR DURING BROMOCRIPTINE TREATMENT 180a

A-L Hulting, K. Heidvall, B. Isberg, L. Fredstorp, S. Werner
Dept. of Endocrinology, Karolinska Hospital, Stockholm

Dopamine agonists have been used as medical treatment in patients with acromegaly, especially those with concomitant hyperprolactinemia. However, the results are not uniform - some studies claim reduced hormone levels and tumor size, whereas in other studies no clinical, biochemical or roentgenological effect has been reported.

Case report: A 40-year old man with symptoms of acromegaly for 12 years; acral enlargement, thickening of the soft tissue of the face and lips, hyperhidrosis and headache. Radiographical examination revealed an intrasellar pituitary tumor with supra- and parasellar extension. Plasma growth hormone (GH) was 4ug/l (ref <9ug/l) and serum prolatin (Prl) 150ug/l (ref <25ug/l) .

Bromocriptine treatment was tried as first therapy because of the "low" GH- and "high" Prl levels in this patient compared to others with acromegaly.

Four months after the onset of bromocriptine treatment (10mg/day) GH levels had increased to 75ug/l with a concomitant decreace in Prl to 30ug/l and another four months later GH was 360ug/l and Prl 20ug/l. Progression of tumor size and appearance of visual field defects were noticed.

Conclusion:

1. Hyperprolactinemia can reduce synthesis and release of dopamine from the hypothalamus.
2. A reduction of dopamine tone can increase somatostatin release and inhibit the release of GH releasing factor (GRF).
3. GH secretion is inhibited by somatostatin and stimulated by GRF also in most patients with acromegaly. The rapid increment in GH levels with a concomitant inhibition of Prl levels and the enlargement of the pituitary tumor in our patient during bromocriptine treatment might thus be explained by increased dopamine content in the hypothalamus leading to reduced somatostatin and increased GRF release.

OPIOID AND ADRENERGIC RECEPTORS INVOLVING IN THE NEURAL REGULATION OF GROWTH HORMONE SECRETION ARE CHANGED BY GLUCOCORTICOIDS 181

B. Kanyicska, B. Kacsoh*, M.I.K. Fekete, E. Stark
Inst.Exptl.Med., Hung.Acad.Sci., Semmelweis Univ., Med. School, 2nd Dept.Anatomy, Budapest, Hungary

Long term exposure to glucocorticoids cause a decrease of growth hormone (GH) secretion and leads to the retardation of somatic growth. While the direct action of the glucocorticoids on the somatotrophs is stimulatory,their effects on the central nervous systems probably inhibitory in nature concerning the GH secretion. Normal secretion of GH also requires intact adrenergic and opioid systems. The question arised whether the central effects of glucocorticoids are involved an attack of the adrenergic or opioid system,or both? Therefore, in the present study the effect of chronic glucocorticoid treatment (cortisol, 25 mg/kg, s.c., daily for 14 days) on the effectiveness of morphine and an alpha-2 adrenergic agonist, clonidine have been investigated. Moreover, the spontaneous bursts of GH secretion and the responsiveness of somatotrophs to exogeneous GRF after cortisol treatment have been studied.

The cortisol markedly decreased the potency of morphine and completely eliminated clonidine's increase of GH secretion. Surprisingly, clonidine caused a decrease of plasma GH level in steroid pretreated group. This latter effect of clonidine could be blocked by an alpha-2 antagonist, yohimbine. These results suggest that glucocorticoids diminished the sensitivity of stimulatory alpha-2 receptors and so the inhibitory alpha-2 receptors ,which normally are subsidiary, became much more prominent.

The episodic bursts of GH secretion were still present following cortisol treatment, and the alpha-2 antagonists yohimbine or idazoxane, which completely blocked the pulsatile secretion of GH in normal animals, failed to do so after steroid treatment. The existing pulses of GH secretion suggest that the GRF-cells have retained their responsiveness, and that the neural circuits commanding the pulsatile rhythm may be functionally reorganized (in spite of that those alpha-2 adrenergic receptors which normally are necessary for the mediation of stimulatory messages to GRF-neurons are masked by cortisol).

DISTRIBUTION OF GASTRIN-RELEASING PEPTIDE (GRP) IN THE RAT BRAIN CONCURS WITH ITS PROPOSED MECHANISM OF ACTION ON GH RELEASE. 182

S. Kentroti and L. Dees
Department of Physiology, Univ of Tx Hlth Sci Ctr, Dallas, Texas 75235

We have previously demonstrated the potent ability of GRP to inhibit both basal and GRF-induced GH release via a somatostatinergic mechanism. We have also shown that incubation of somatotrophs in medium containing GRP results in an increase in GH release. Other investigators have reported the presence of GRP 1-27-like immunoreactivity (GRP-LIR) in various hypothalamic extracts. We have shown that a highly specific antiserum generated against the GRP 1-27 molecule produces an increase ($P<0.001$) in plasma GH levels when given intraventricularlly to conscious rats. Using this same antiserum we have immunocytochemically examined the preoptic area (POA) and the rostro-caudal extent of the hypothalamus and median eminence (ME) for GRP immunoreactivity using the immunoperoxidase technique. No fibers or terminals were observed in the POA. Conversely, most of the immunoreactivity was confined to the rostral hypothalamic area (RHA), specifically within the SCN, the area lateral to SCN, and dorsally, in the region of the periventricular nucleus (PeVN). Additionally a sparse population of fibers was observed in the PeVN region of the intermediate hypothalamus. GRP-positive perikarya were found in the rostral region of PeVN and in the ventral portion of PVN. Of particular importance is the absence of GRP-LIR in other areas, especially the ME. All positive staining was eliminated by immunoabsorption of the primary antiserum with GRP 1-27. In a previous study using immunofluorescence, a more restricted localization was reported. In conclusion, GRP-LIR in somatostatin-rich areas of the RHA, as well as its absence in the ME concurs with our physiological findings. Supported by NIH grants HD 09988 and AA 06874.

GROWTH HORMONE RELEASE INDUCED BY ELECTRICAL STIMULATION OF THE BASOLATERAL AMYGDALA, OBSERVED IN PENTOBARBITAL ANESTHETIZED RATS 183

N.Koibuchi, M.Kato, T.Kakegawa, M.Suzuki
Department of Physiology, Institute of Endocrinology, Gunma University, Maebashi, Japan

Electrical stimulation of basolateral amygdala (ABL) is known to increase plasma growth hormone (GH). The aim of this study was to clarify the neural mechanism leading to the GH release induced by the elctrical stimulation of the ABL. Concentric bipolar stimulating electrode was implanted in the unilateral ABL and blood samples were taken from a cannula implanted into the right atrium via the right external jugular vein. Under pentobarbital anesthesia, electrical stimulation for 10 min caused a significant increase in plasma GH level from resting value 27.25±5.7 ng/ml (mean±SE) to 62.5±7.5 ng/ml at the termination of stimulation. This effect was markedly augmented to 152.0±23.0 ng/ml after lesion of the periventricular hypothalamic nucleus (Pe), where somatostatinergic neurons project to the median eminence. On the other hand, lesion of the stria terminalis (st) fully or partly abolished GH release induced by ABL stimulation. These results suggest that GH release induced by ABL stimulation should not be due to the inhibition of SRIF neurons in the Pe but to the exitation of GRF neurons and that st is essential pathway for the effect. Futhermore, electrical stimulation of medial amygdala (AME) causes an inhibitory effect on GRF-induced GH secretion by the exitation of SRIF neurons in the Pe and its pathway is st (1). In conclusion, amygdala has both stimulatory and inhibitory effect on GH secretion. ABL is stimulatory and AME is inhibitory. And the essential pathways are st in either case.

Reference

(1) Kato, M.; Kakegawa, T.; Suzuki, M.; Electrical stimulation of several limbic areas suppressed the growth hormone (GH) release induced by human pancreatic GH releasing factor in pentobarbital anesthetized rats. Endocrinology 118/3 (1986).

LONG-LASTING DOPAMINERGIC STIMULATION OF PITUITARY SECRETION 184

Ioana Lancranjan, L. Portmann, C. Felley and J.P. Felber
Department of Endocrinology, University Hospital, Lausanne, Switzerland

Important evidence has been accumulated showing that the dopaminergic system is involved in the control of pituitary secretion in man. A long-acting injectable form of bromocriptine which produces a sustained dopaminergic stimulation was used to reassess in man the timing and amplitude of changes in PRL, GH, TSH, LH and ACTH secretion.

The 24 hour profile of PRL, GH, LH, TSH and ACTH was investigated in 10 young normal volunteers by hourly blood collection before, the first day, 14 and 28 days after a 50 mg dose of bromocriptine long-acting injected deep i.m.

The plasma concentrations of bromocriptine were 1.5 ± 0.6 ng/ml (2 hours after the injection), 1.0 ± 0.2 ng/ml one day after, 0.6 ± 0.1 ng/ml 14 days and 0.3 ± 0.1 ng/ml 28 days following the injection.

A suppression of basal and sleep related PRL peak occurred in all volunteers throughout the 28 day study period. Nocturnal PRL peak decreased from 10.7 ± 4.3 ng/ml to 0.9 ± 0.3 ng/ml on day 1 to 0.8 ± 0.3 ng/ml the 14th day and to 1.3 ± 0.9 ng/ml the 28th day after injection. GH secretion was stimulated within 4 hours after the injection of bromocriptine from 0.4 ± 0.3 ng/ml to 6.2 ± 5.0 ng/ml with enhancement in the number and amplitude of subsequent GH pulses only throughout the 12-hour period following the injection. The mean and 24 hour profile of plasma LH and ACTH secretion remained unchanged during the dopaminergic stimulation. Conversely, a significant decrease of TSH secretion associated with a reduction in pulsatile activity occurred the day of injection. The reduction in mean level was more pronunced during the night time than during the day-time. On days 14 and 28 after the injection TSH levels were still lower that prior to the dopaminergic stimulation.

In conclusion, the long-term dopaminergic stimulation leads in man to a marked, prompt and prolonged reduction of PRL secretion, to a significant and prolonged reduction of TSH and to a short lasting stimulation of GH secretion.

INFLUENCE OF THEOPHYLLINE ADMINISTRATION ON BASAL AND GHRH STIMULATED GH SECRETION IN ACROMEGALY. 185

Losa M, Schopohl J, Alba-Lopez J, Sobieszczyk S, Spiess Y, Müller OA, von Werder K.
Med. Klin. Innenstadt, University of Munich, FRG

Theophylline (T) modulates the intracellular concentration of cAMP through either inhibition of phosphodiesterase or, at more therapeutic dosage, competition with the adenosine receptor. We have previously shown that in 6 normal subjects the GH released after acute and continuous GHRH administration was significantly lower after T pretreatment (1966.2 ± 494.3 ng min/ml vs. 590.7 ± 283.9 ng min/ml, $p<0.05$). We report now the influence of T administration on GH secretion in acromegaly.

Five patients with untreated acromegaly were subjected to: a) 2 hours basal sampling followed by a 100 µg GHRH bolus dose with further blood sampling over 2 hours. b) a T infusion (3.56 mg/min) over 4 hours started 2 hours before the administration of 100 µg GHRH. GH, PRL, and GHRH were measured by standard double antibody RIAs.

Basal GH secretion remained constant over the 2 hours of basal sampling (51.9 ± 26.6 ng/ml at 0 min and 51.8 ± 23.6 ng/ml at 120 min) and was not influenced by T (48.8 ± 24.1 ng/ml at 0 min and 49.0 ± 21.6 ng/ml at 120 min). GHRH led to prompt GH release in all but one patient who had a minimal GH increase (< 100% of basal value) at the end of the test. T administration blunted the GH response to GHRH as demonstrated by the lower amount of GH released (53.2 ± 20.8% of the control GHRH test). However, this effect was not homogeneous since it occurred only in 4 of 5 patients and was very variable in magnitude. Plasma GHRH levels were not different in the two studies, so excluding an interference of T with GHRH metabolism. GHRH caused a small PRL increase in 3 patients (171.0 ± 11.5% of basal value), which was not influnced by T (158.0 ± 13.2% of basal value).

In conclusion, T pretreatment is able to blunt the GH response to GHRH in most acromegalic patients, though in contrast to normal subjects this effect is not always seen and presents a greater variability in magnitude. The abnormal PRL response to GHRH occurring in some patients is not influenced by T pretreatment.

THE MANNER OF GHRH INVOLVEMENT IN GH STIMULATION TESTS IN MAN

186

A.Masuda, T.Shibasaki, T.Imaki, H.Demura and K.Shizume
Dept. of Medicine, Tokyo Women's Medical College, Tokyo 162, Japan

Growth hormone releasing hormone (GHRH) is a potent stimulator of growth hormone (GH) secretion from pituitary. In order to clarify the manner of GHRH involvement in GH stimulation tests such as insulin tolerance test (ITT), L-dopa test and arginine infusion test in man, we measured GHRH in peripheral plasma during these tests with a specific radioimmunoassay for GHRH (Shibasaki et al J Clin Endocrinol Metab 59:263, 1984). Plasma IR-GHRH increased in ITT and L-dopa test, the peaks of which were found somewhat prior to or simultaneously with those of GH (ITT:basal GH 1.1±0.4 ng/ml, basal IR-GHRH 8.1±3.0 pg/ml, peak GH 18.2±4.7 ng/ml, peak IR-GHRH 26.8±5.3 pg/ml, L-dopa test:basal GH 0.3±0.2 ng/ml, basal IR-GHRH 9.4±3.3 pg/ml, peak GH 11.5±2.3 ng/ml,peak IR-GHRH 35.5±6.3 pg/ml). However, no significant change of plasma IR-GHRH was observed in arginine infusion test in spite of increase in plasma GH levels (peak GH 15.4±3.9 ng/ml). These results indicate that GHRH is not involved in the mechanism by which GH secretion is stimulated in arginine infusion test.

An intravenous (iv) administration of 200 µg synthetic human GHRH(1-44)NH_2 120 min after first iv injection of 200 µg of GHRH(1-44)NH_2 did not induce a significant plasma GH peak, whereas ITT 120 min after iv injection of 200 µg GHRH(1-44)NH_2 induced a plasma GH peak as reported previously (Shibasaki et al J Clin Endocrinol Metab 60:1265, 1985). Plasma GH peaks induced by L-dopa test and arginine infusion test were not affected by prior injection of GHRH(1-44)NH_2. Furthermore, we measured plasma TSH levels in these tests by immunoradiometic assay to monitor somatostatin release from hypothalamus, since the secretion of TSH is suppressed by somatostatin. When 200 µg GHRH(1-44)NH_2 was injected, plasma TSH levels were significantly lowered in ITT and L-dopa test but not in arginine infusion test. These results, therefore, suggest that some factor(s) in addition to GHRH is involved in the mechanisms by which GH secretion is stimulated in ITT, L-dopa test and arginine infusion test.

THE HYPOTHALAMO-INFUNDIBULAR GROWTH HORMONE RELEASING FACTOR (GRF) SYSTEM OF THE RAT

187

I. Merchenthaler, A. Arimura, P. Petrusz,
University Medical School, Pécs, Hungary; Tulane University, New Orleans, Louisiana, U.S.A.; University of North Carolina, Chapel Hill, North Carolina, U.S.A.

It is generally assumed that the perikarya of GRF-producing neurons that project to the median eminence (ME) are located in the medial-basal hypothalamus (MBH). This view is based on physiological and morphological evidence obtained after surgical isolation of the MBH or selective destruction of the neurons of the arcuate nucleus (ARC) by neonatal treatment with monosodium glutamate (MSG). In colchicine-treated rats, however, GRF-containing perikarya are also seen in the ventral perifornical region, the lateral-basal hypothalamus, and the dorsomedial and paraventricular nuclei. The present studies were designed to evaluate whether perikarya located outside of the MBH also contribute GRF afferents to the ME.

Two to ten days after complete unilateral surgical isolation of the MBH or three months following neonatal MSG treatment, the distribution of GRF-immunoreactive neuronal structures was studied in vibratome sections of rat brains by PAP immunocytochemistry with an antiserum to rat GRF. After neonatal MSG treatment, the number of GRF-immunoreactive fibers and terminals in the ME became substantially reduced; however, these structures did not disappear completely as reported earlier. The reduction was greater in the rostral portion of the ME than in its caudal portion. Complete unilateral deafferentation of the MBH caused only a slight decrease in GRF immunostaining in the posterior regions of the ipsilateral ME. At this level, GRF accumulation was observed in scattered transected fibers lateral to the cut, outside of the MBH.

These results indicate that, although the ARC is the major source of the hypothalamo-infundibular GRF system in the rat, neurons located in other areas such as the ventral perifornical region and the lateral-basal hypothalamus may also send GRF-containing fibers to the ME, especially to its posterior regions.

Supported in part by USPHS Grant No. AM 09094.

GROWTH HORMONE (GH) SECRETION DURING A CONTINUOUS 6-HOUR INFUSION OF GH-RELEASING FACTOR (GRF) IN MONOSODIUM GLUTAMATE (MSG) TREATED RATS

188

S. MINAMI, I. WAKABAYASHI, H. SUGIHARA, S. AKIRA, F. TAKAHASHI, A. MOTOYAMA, N. LING*
Nippon Medical School, Tokyo, Japan and *The Salk Institute, San Diego, California, U.S.A.

To evaluate altered GH regulation in MSG rats, we have observed plasma GH profiles in unrestrained adult male MSG rats given continuous infusion of human GRF [1-44] NH_2.

Male Wistar rats were treated with MSG (4 mg/g BW, sc) as neonates and were used for the study on 150-173 days of life. All rats were provided with two indwelling cannulae 4 to 5 days previously; one in the right atrium for undisturbed blood collection and the other in the inferior vena cava for vehicle or GRF infusion. Vehicle or human GRF was administered by infusion pump (0.6 ml/h) for 6 h at a dose of 50 or 200 ng/kg BW/min. Serial blood samples were obtained every 20 min.

During 6-h vehicle infusion, plasma GH levels in MSG rats were maintained low with occasional small fluctuations while pulsatile GH secretion was observed every 3.2 h in controls. During low dose GRF (50 ng/kg BW/min) infusion, pulsatile GH secretion appeared at irregular intervals among MSG rats while the amplitude of naturally occurring pulsatile GH secretion was augmented in controls. During high dose GRF (200 ng/kg BW/min) infusion, plasma GH levels rose steadily in MSG rats while pulsatile GH secretion was observed in controls. When goat anti-somatostatin serum and low dose GRF infusion were given, plasma GH levels increased without pulsatile secretion in both groups of rats. The amount of GH released during 6-h in response to two doses of GRF infusion increased significantly in a dose dependent manner in both groups of rats, but it was significantly less in MSG rats than controls.

Results show that in adult male MSG rats, the capability of the pituitary gland to secrete GH in response to continuous GRF infusion is reduced and the release of somatostatin which exerts the intermittent tonic inhibition on GH secretion during GRF infusion is compromised.

CHOLINERGIC MUSCARINIC RECEPTOR BLOCKADE WITH PIRENZEPINE ABOLISHES SLOW WAVE SLEEP-RELATED GH RELEASE IN NORMAL AND INSULIN DEPENDENT DIABETIC SUBJECTS

189

M.D. Page, H.P.F. Koppeschaar, C. Dieguez, J.R. Peters, M.F. Scanlon
Neuroendocrine Unit,
University of Wales College of Medicine, Cardiff

Cholinergic pathways play an important role in the regulation of GH secretion from the anterior pituitary gland and cholinergic muscarinic receptor blockade reduces or abolishes the GH response to several known stimuli. In this study we have investigated whether cholinergic muscarinic receptor blockade with pirenzepine, a drug which is safe, long-acting and widely used in the treatment of peptic ulcer disease, displayed any inhibitory action on slow wave sleep (SWS)-related GH release in normal and diabetic subjects.

Six normal males (24-37 yrs) and 5 patients with insulin dependent diabetes mellitus (IDDM) (3 M, 2F; 20-27 yrs) were studied in randomised order. All subjects fasted from 18.00 hrs on the study days and rested from 21.00 hours. Pirenzepine (100 mg p.o.) or placebo was administered at 22.00 and again at 24.00 hrs. Blood was sampled from 24.00 hrs at 15' intervals until 01.00 hrs and at 10' intervals thereafter until 03.00 hrs. At 12.00 hrs, lights were switched off and the subjects allowed to sleep. The portable EEG tape recorders were switched on and blood sampling proceeded without disturbing the subjects.

All subjects showed episodes of SWS on each study day and on each occasion this was followed by peaks of GH release with considerable interindividual variation when placebo alone was administered (range of GH peaks; normal 4-50 mU/l; diabetic 6-115 mU/l). Pirenzepine treatment completely abolished SWS-related GH release in each individual without altering the occurrence of SWS. Because of the total abolition of GH peaks during pirenzepine treatment, statistical analysis was neither possible nor necessary. Mean plasma glucose levels did not differ significantly throughout each study period in diabetic subjects and there were no episodes of clinical or biochemical hypoglycaemia.

Cholinergic muscarinic receptor blockade with pirenzepine completely abolishes SWS-related GH release in normals and in patients with IDDM. Cholinergic pathways may play an important intermediary role in the generation of SWS-related GH release although the level and mechanism of action are presently unknown. This approach may be useful in studying the relationship between GH neuroregulation and the pathophysiology of IDDM.

IN VITRO SIMULTANEOUS RELEASE OF ENDOGENOUS SOMATOSTATIN AND GROWTH HORMONE FROM HUMAN ADENOMATOUS PITUITARY CELLS

190

F. Peillon*, C. Liapi**, P. Garnier***, A.M. Brandi*, D. Evain-Brion**, D. Bression*, H. Scherrer****, M. Donnadieu**
*INSERM U. 223, **INSERM U. 188, ***Fondation de Recherches en Hormonologie, ****Service d'Endocrinologie la Pitié, Paris, France.

It is well known that SRIF is the physiological inhibitor of GH release and acts directly in vitro on pituitary somatotrophs. Recent studies indicate that in normal rat pituitaries, SRIF is internalized in its target cells. Although the same finding has not been yet described in human pituitary, we demonstrate here that SRIF is contained in GH-secreting pituitary adenomatous cells and released in vitro with GH by the same cells.

Dispersed GH adenomatous cells obtained from fragments of 10 GH-secreting adenomas were studied in vitro using dynamic studies in perifusion columns. The cells were perifused in a Krebs Ringer buffer. Fractions were collected each 5 min (2.5 ml) for 2-5 hours and assayed by RIA for their GH and SRIF content. Basal in vitro GH varied from one adenoma to another (from 10 to 94 ng/ml/10^6 cells). Within the first 15 minutes of the perifusion SRIF was detected in five cases (from 5 to 41 pg/ml/10^6 cells). However in five cases where SRIF was undetectable at the beginning of the perifusion, there was a great release of SRIF after 90 minutes or more (from 7 to 75 pg/ml/10^6 cells). In two cases during the perifusion, the variations of GH and SRIF levels were significantly negatively correlated ($p < 0.001$).

We can conclude from these studies 1) SRIF is released in vitro from human pituitary GH-secreting cells, 2) the sometimes high level of SRIF release raises the question of its origine : internalization or endogenous synthesis ? 3) the inverse correlation found in two cases between SRIF and GH levels could be in favour of the involvement of the intracellular SRIF in the regulation of GH secretion.

PREVENTION BY SOMATOSTATIN OF THE DESENSITIZATION OF hpGRF-INDUCED GH RELEASE FROM RAT ANTERIOR PITUITARY *in vitro*

191

H. Soya, M. Suzuki
Department of Physiology, Institute of Endocrinology, Gunma University, Maebashi 371, Japan

In order to study the role of somatostatin (SRIF) on GH secretion, the hormone release profiles were examined in an *in vitro* system.

When whole anterior pituitaries of rats were perifused with hpGRF (0.1 μM), an increase in GH level in the effluents peaked within 20 - 30 min. Two hr after the 1st hpGRF stimulation, 2nd application of hpGRF caused a blunted response as low as 10 % of that of control level. Integrated amounts of increased GH release over the basal level for 1hr were 18.49 ± 3.08 μg by the 1st application of hpGRF and 1.89 ± 2.38 μg by the 2nd application respectively.

On the other hand, a high KCl (50 mM) stimulation could induce a similar response as the 1st hpGRF did, and a repetitive application of the high KCl caused a similar increase in GH release. When the 2nd hpGRF application was substituted for high KCl (50 mM) stimulation, there was no decrease in the release response in the 2nd phase. Moreover the pituitary response to hpGRF stimulation did not change even after 2hr, when the 1st hpGRF stimulation was omitted, or replaced by the high KCl. Thus it appears that the cause of the desensitization to hpGRF is not due to a depletion in a putative releasable pool of the pituitary somatotrophs.

However when SRIF (0.1 μM) applied to the pituitaries for 50 min after the 1st hpGRF stimulation, the decreased response to the 2nd hpGRF was not observed. When SRIF concentration was increased to 1.0 μM, the effect was less than that of 0.1 μM (36.5 % of the 1st GH response). In the present study however, no off response was observed in GH release after SRIF withdrawal.

These data suggest that SRIF not only suppresses the basal GH release, but also prevents the desensitization by repetitive stimulation of hpGRF.

INTERACTION OF GROWTH HORMONE (GH) RELEASING FACTOR (GRF) AND SOMATOSTATIN (SS) TO ESTABLISH PULSATILE GH RELEASE in vitro

192

J. Weiss, M.O. Thorner, M.J. Cronin
University of Virginia, Charlottesville, Virginia 22908

Growth hormone is secreted as pulses in vivo. To establish an equivalent model of pulsatile GH secretion in vitro requires a perifusion system. Accordingly, we dispersed male rat anterior pituitaries and perifused them (RPMI-1640 medium, dexamethasone, T_3, BSA, antibiotics) with pulses of human GRF-40, with or without a SS tonus, at concentrations reflecting pituitary portal blood levels (Science 230: 461, 1985). An experiment consisted of a 1 hr baseline collection, followed by 4 pulse cycles for a total of 13 hr. Each cycle consisted of a 10 min infusion of 3 nM GRF [confirmed in our system to be maximally effective in releasing GH] followed by vehicle for the remainder of the 3 hr period. In SS experiments, the protocol was identical except that 0.3 nM SS was added 30 min into the initial baseline period, and was then continued throughout the remainder of the study. All data are reported as ng/min/10 million cells and represent "n" independent experiments (i.e., different days). Peaks of GH release are expressed as the mean of the 2 highest release rate points following the addition of GRF. Interpeak baselines are assessed by sampling midway between successive release peaks. The effect of SS was immediate, reducing unstimulated GH release from 25 to 9 within 10 min ($P < 0.05$, n = 5). These SS-inhibited baselines remained depressed for the duration of the experiment, residing at -36%, -36% and -49% of control between GH peaks 1 & 2, 2 & 3, and 3 & 4, respectively (n = 3-5). GRF-induced peak GH responses were from 200-500, and were not significantly changed in the presence of SS-altered baselines ($P > 0.2$, n = 3-6). There was, however, a 40-45% loss of peak response between pulses 2 and 4 in all studies. We conclude that this is a valid system for exploring the dynamic interactions of GRF and SS in vitro.

(Supported by AM32632 & RCDA 1K04NS00601)

SECRETION OF GHRH IN PATIENTS WITH HYPERSOMATOTROPISM

193

R.Yamasaki, S.Saito, H.Saito, K.Kameyama, S.Mitsuhashi, E.Hosoi, T.Sano
School of Medicine, The University of Tokushima, Tokushima, Japan

Plasma growth hormone releasing hormone (GHRH) was measured in patients with hypersomatotropism by radioimmunoassay to clarify the pathophysiological role of GHRH.

Plasma immunoreactive (IR)-GHRH in normal adults was 10.4+4.1(SD) pg/ml and there was no sex difference in the level. Fourteen patients with acromegaly and one with giantism showed values within or below the normal range. The acromegalics showed no response of plasma IR-GHRH even when their plasma growth hormone (GH) levels were increased after TRH administration and during arginine infusion. A high level of plasma IR-GHRH(average,300pg/ml) was found in a case of MEN type I with symptoms of acromegaly. In this patients, gel-chromatographic analysis of the plasma showed that about 80% of total IR-GHRH was eluted in the same position as synthetic GHRH. His plasma IR-GHRH levels did not significantly change after oral administration of L-Dopa or bromocriptine. Insulin hypoglycemia, arginine infusion and TRH administration induced a marked GH release, but no apparent fluctuation of plasma IR-GHRH concentration was observed. Somatostatin infusion failed to suppress the plasma level of IR-GHRH but suppressed the plasma GH level. The circulating plasma IR-GHRH level fell to normal range after resection of his pancreatic tumor. Many IR-GHRH positive cells were demonstrated in the tumor.

These results indicate the usefulness of plasma GHRH determination to clarify the pathophysiological role of GHRH in acromegaly and GHRH-producing tumor.

MOLECULAR CHARACTERIZATION OF A NEUROPHYSIN-COPEPTIN PRECURSOR FROM GUINEA PIG NEURO-INTERMEDIATE PITUITARY 194

R. Acher, J. Chauvet, M.T. Chauvet, D. Sunde[+] and A.N. Thorn[+]
Lab. of Biol. Chemistry, Univ. of Paris VI (France) and Inst. Med. Physiol., Univ. of Copenhagen (Denmark)

From the guinea pig neuro-intermediate pituitary, have been isolated and sequenced, on one hand vasopressin (9 residues), MSEL-neurophysin (93 residues) and copeptin (a 38-residue glycopeptide), on the other hand a glycoprotein precursor (132 residues) comprising both MSEL-neurophysin and copeptin. Paper chromatoelectrophoresis of the precursor tryptic peptides shows a map identical with a cumulative map including MSEL-neurophysin and copeptin trypsic peptides, except that the C-terminal tryptic peptide of MSEL-neurophysin (T_6) is displaced and extended by an arginine residue. Microsequencing of the precursor and characterization of its tryptic fragments give the complete sequence. About 20% of the putative initial precursor vasopressin–MSEL-neurophysin–copeptin remain in this partially processed form.

The ternary precursor vasopressin–MSEL-neurophysin–copeptin seems to be subjected to a two-step processing involving two enzymic systems. The first system cleaves off vasopressin from the N-terminal end of the precursor, apparently completely. This cleavage likely implies an endopeptidase splitting at the level of a base pair, a carboxypeptidase B removing the two basic residues and a glycine dehydrogenase making the amide group of the peptide hormone.

The second system probably involves a trypsin-like endopeptidase splitting between neurophysin and copeptin at the level of a single basic residue. The second cleavage may not have a physiological significance since it may be incomplete. The guinea pig slow processing might be due to a species variation either in precursor sequence or in specificity of the trypsin-like endopeptidase.

CONCOMITANT DOPAMINERGIC AND GLUCOCORTICOID CONTROL OF ANTERIOR AND INTERMEDIATE LOBE β-ENDORPHIN. 195

D.J. Autelitano, I. Nikolaidis, J.A. Clements, J.W. Funder
Medical Research Centre, Prince Henry's Hospital, Melbourne, Australia 3004.

Glucocorticoids and CRF regulate POMC synthesis and ACTH/βEP release in the anterior pituitary (AP); in contrast dopamine (DA) is the major factor controlling POMC synthesis and β-endorphin (βEP) release in the intermediate lobe. In the present study, we have given dexamethasone (DM) and/or haloperidol or bromocriptine to intact male Sprague-Dawley rats for 14 days.

In the AP, DM reduced ir-βEP content to <half that in controls; neither dopaminergic agent alone had any effect. In rats treated with both DM and haloperidol, however, AP ir-βEP content was elevated ($P < 0.05$) compared with DM alone rats, but lower ($P < 0.01$) than control or haloperidol alone rats. Northern blot analysis of AP RNA showed similar but not identical changes in POMC mRNA. DM lowered POMC mRNA, which was partially restored towards control levels in DM/haloperidol rats. Bromocriptine had no effect on AP POMC mRNA levels; haloperidol, however, increased POMC mRNA compared with levels in control rats.

Bromocriptine (1 mg/kg) caused a 50% reduction in neuro- intermediate lobe (N-IL) levels of ir-βEP, while haloperidol (1 mg/kg) caused a 2-3 fold increase; treatment with DM alone (20 μg/day) did not affect N-IL content. In contrast, rats treated with both haloperidol (1 mg/kg) and DM showed levels of ir-βEP reduced to 50% of those in rats treated with haloperidol alone ($P < 0.01$). There was insufficient N-IL to determine POMC mRNA in this study.

We interpret these data to suggest that dopaminergic antagonists and glucocorticoids can both modulate POMC synthesis and/or ir-βEP levels in both AP and N-IL. In the AP, haloperidol may affect synthesis and release in parallel, giving essentially unaltered tissue levels, except in DM-treated rats. In the N-IL the DM effect is seen only in animals withdrawn from tonic dopaminergic inhibition. The hypothalamo-pituitary mechanisms involved in this difference in primary and secondary control are currently under investigation.

GLUCOCORTICOID REGULATION OF PRO-OPIOMELANOCORTIN (POMC) mRNA CONTENT OF RAT HYPOTHALAMUS AND AMYGDALA 196

S. Beaulieu, B. Gagné, N. Barden
MRC Group in Molecular Endocrinology, CHUL, Laval University, Quebec, Canada, G1V 4G2

The presence of neurons containing POMC-related peptides in the hypothalamus (HYPO) and amygdaloid complex (AMYG) raises the question as to whether or not the POMC gene in these tissues is regulated by glucocorticoids as in the anterior pituitary gland (AP). Resolution of this question will aid our understanding of the limbic-hypothalamic mechanisms regulating ACTH secretion, particularly in view of the ACTH and CRF hypersecretion observed in patients suffering from endogenous depressive illness.

Animals (male or female rats) were divided into four groups: adrenalectomized (ADX) (receiving vehicle), sham-ADX (vehicle), ADX + corticosterone (2.5 mg per 100 g, B.W.) and ADX + dexamethasone (0.2 mg per 100 B.W.). Rats were decapitated on the seventh day of treatment and trunk blood was collected in order to measure plasma ACTH. The AP, the neurointermediate lobe (NIL), the HYP and AMYG were rapidly dissected and their RNA content isolated by the guanidinium-thiocyanate-cesium chloride method. Total RNA was dot-blotted on nitrocellulose or analyzed by formaldehyde gel electrophoresis followed by transfer to nitrocellulose (Northern). The filters were hybridized with a rat POMC cDNA probe (750 bp corresponding to most of the exon 3) labelled by nick translation, or the corresponding POMC RNA probe labelled by T7 polymerase run-off transcription of the cDNA inserted into the plasmid p-GEM-1.

As expected, plasma ACTH levels were greatly increased by adrenalectomy and returned to normal levels by treatment with corticosterone or dexamethasone. Adrenalectomy did not influence the concentration of POMC mRNA of the NIL but increased it in the AP, HYP and AMYG. Corticosterone and dexamethasone reversed the effect of adrenalectomy in these three structures.

These results reinforce the hypothesis of the involvement of the POMC-related peptides of limbic origin in the control of ACTH secretion, particularly in the phenomenon of glucocorticoid negative feedback.

HORMONAL REGULATION OF POMC GENE TRANSCRIPTION IN INDIVIDUAL CELL NUCLEI OF THE RAT PITUITARY 197

R.T. Fremeau, Jr., J. Lundblad, D. Pritchett, J. Wilcox, J.L. Roberts
Columbia Univ. College of Physicians & Surgeons, NY, NY

Previous studies of the regulation of proopiomelanocortin (POMC) gene transcription following pharmacologic manipulation of the secretory activity of POMC expressing cells have suggested that transcription of the POMC gene is coupled to secretion of POMC peptides. In many instances individual cells from tissues thought to be homogeneous in their regulation of expression of a specific gene show heterogeneous responses to specific secretagogues. Therefore, to directly examine the apparent coregulation of the physiological secretion of POMC peptides and transcription of the POMC gene it is necessary to analyze POMC gene transcription at the level of the individual cell.

In this study we have used a unique sequence single-stranded RNA probe complementary to intron A of the POMC gene primary transcript to analyze by in situ hybridization histochemistry the hormonal regulation of POMC gene transcription in individual cell nuclei in the rat pituitary. This probe recognized only the primary full-length POMC hnRNA transcripts in the nucleus when analyzed by Northern blots of pituitary RNA. Adrenalectomy (Adx) resulted in a three fold increase in the number of cells actively transcribing the POMC gene in the anterior pituitary as evidenced by an increased percentage of cells with silver grains over their nucleus (Ctr 3.3± 0.9%; Adx 9.9±2.0%), and an increased rate of transcription of the POMC gene in some of the corticotrophs seen as an increase in grain density over some of the corticotrph nuclei. Dexamethasone administration to intact or Adx rats resulted in a rapid (within 30') disappearance of silver grains over the nuclei of corticotrphs in the anterior lobe, suggesting that POMC gene transcription had been inhibited. The silver grain density over intermediate lobe melanotrophs was not altered by Adx or dexamethasone administration. Thus the POMC IVS A specific in situ hybridization assay can measure physiological changes in POMC gene transcription in individual cell nuclei.

THE PROHORMONE FOR UROTENSIN II FROM THE CAUDAL NEUROSECRETORY COMPLEX OF THE GOBY 198

D.Pearson[1], Y.Cheers[1], D.Atmani[1], I.Ishida[2], T.Deguchi[2], R.S.Nishioka[3] and H.A.Bern[3]
[1]. Calif. State Univ., L.A.; [2]. Tokyo Metropol. Inst. Neurosci.; 3. Univ. Calif., Berkeley.

The caudal neurosecretory complex (CNC) of the goby, Gillichthys mirabilis, consists of an array of neurons in the posterior spinal cord which project axons posteriorly into a morphologically well defined neurohemal organ, the urophysis. Among the biologically active peptides produced in the CNC is urotensin II (UII) which has smooth muscle contracting activity in fish and exerts a variety of osmoregulatory effects in these animals. Urotensin II from the goby is a dodecapeptide with the sequence Ala-Gly-Thr-Ala-Asp-Cys-Phe-Trp-Lys-Tyr-Cys-Val. In an effort to define the UII prohormone as well as that of other caudal-specific products we have prepared a cDNA library from poly(A)RNA isolated from the posterior spinal cord of the goby. The library was screened using mixed synthetic oligonucleotide probes (14 bases) based on the UII amino acid sequence and on the sequence of a caudal-specific peptide, the caudal neurosecretory peptide (CNP). Of 11,500 recombinant clones 32 were found to hybridize with both the UII and CNP probes, indicating that they had a common prohormone. Analysis of several of the clones indicated that they had identical inserts. A detailed restriction map of one of these was prepared, the insert was subcloned and sequenced. The insert was 755 nucleotides long. It encoded a 20 amino acid signal sequence at the N-terminus. A 79 amino acid sequence including the partially characterized CNP was adjacent to the signal. Separated from CNP by Arg-Lys was a dipeptide (His-Phe), and separated from it by Arg-Lys-Arg was the UII sequence at the C terminus.
Supported in part by PCM-84-05249 to H.A.B. and SO6RRO-8101-14 to D.P.

OXYTOCIN AND UROKINASE SPECIFIC mRNA IN GRANULOSA CELLS 198a

K.H.Scheit, R.Einspanier
Max-Planck-Institut für Biophysikalische Chemie, 3400 Göttingen, W.Germany

The detection as well as the quantitation of particular mRNA's by hybridisation to specific DNA probes is well established. Principally two techniques, namely dot blot or solution hybridisation respectively are employed. The latter case represents a true equilibrium method, because hybridisation is carried out in solution and the excess of non-hybridised DNA probe is removed by the single strand specific S1 nuclease; the remaining hybrid is precipitated and quantitated. Whereas dot blot hybridisation is usually carried out with cloned cDNA, specific for the respective mRNA, solution hybridisation requires single stranded DNA, complementary to the mRNA to be measured. Preparation of the single stranded DNA probe is rather laborious. A further drawback is the species specificity of cDNA probes which limits their applicability. Since chemical synthesis of DNA of chain lenghts between 30 and 100 nucleotides became feasible due to automatisation, we synthesised DNA, complementary to mRNA's specific for bovine oxytocin and human urokinase respectively.

5'CCAGGGGGCAGTTCTGAATGTAGA 3' (OXYTOCIN)
5'GCAGGAATCTGTTTTCCATTGGGGGT 3' (UROKINASE)

The DNA's were phosphorylated at their 5'-termini with (32P)-phosphate at a specific activity of 3Ci/µmole. Total poly(rA^+)-RNA was isolated from bovine, porcine and human granulosa cells. The functionality of these preparations was examined by cell-free translation. The synthetic DNA's proved suitable both in dot blot as well as in solution hybridisation for detection and quantitation of oxytocin and urokinase specific mRNA's in granulosa cells. Furthermore, the above described synthetic DNA's were used in primer-extension experiments employing poly(rA^+)-RNA and reverse transcriptase. Examination of the formed RNA-DNA hybrid structures by poly acrylamide gel electrophoresis revealed in the case of bovine granulosa cells three populations of urokinase-specific mRNA's with approx. 600 bp, 1200 bp and 2400 bp respectively.

This is the first time that oxytocin and urokinase specific mRNA's have been characterised in granulosa cells. At present, this approach is extended to other mRNA species corresponding to other neuroactive proteins, like the recently characterised follicular inhibin.

β-ENDORPHIN PROCESSING: DIFFERENCES BETWEEN SLAUGHTERHOUSE AND UNSTRESSED SHEEP 199

A.I. Smith, C.A. Wallace, I.J. Clarke, J.W. Funder
Medical Research Centre, Prince Henry's Hospital, Melbourne, Australia 3004.

Synthesis and release of proopiomelanocortin derived peptides in the anterior pituitary (AP) are under inhibitory glucocorticoid control, and are stimulated by corticotropin releasing factor and arginine vasopressin; little, however, is known about control of post-translational processing. In the anterior pituitary (AP) of the sheep, a significant proportion (∿25%) of β-endorphin is N-acetylated, in contrast with the rat (<5%). In a study to determine the precise molecular species of this immunoreactive N-acetyl-endorphin (ir-NacEP), we noted a marked difference in the HPLC profile between sheep taken directly from the field and age-, sex- and strain-matched slaughterhouse animals. The immunoreactive profile, determined by HPLC and radioimmunoassay specific for the α-N-acetylated NH_2 terminus of β-endorphin and its shorter congeners, showed NacαEP (∿30%), NacγEP (∿30%) and NacβEP_{1-27} (∿35%) to be the major forms in field animals, with NacβEP_{1-31} (∿5%) a minor component. The profile from slaughterhouse animals was markedly different, with NacαEP (∿65%) the only major immunoreactive form, and much lower levels of NacγEP (∿8%), NacβEP_{1-27} (∿12%) and NacβEP_{1-31} (∿6%). In other studies, AP taken from farm animals chronically treated with dexamethasone showed a similar profile to slaughterhouse animals. We interpret these changes in slaughterhouse animals as a chronic stress effect due to herding, transport and penning prior to slaughter. The intermediate lobe ir-NacβEP HPLC profile was identical in all groups.

As total AP ir-NacEP content is essentially unaltered between groups these data suggest a processing change rather than a selective release of longer NacEP forms. Secondly, the equivalent ir-NacEP profiles in slaughterhouse and dexamethasone-treated sheep suggests that the effect is glucocorticoid mediated; whether the effects are direct or centrally mediated remains to be established. Finally, these studies suggest that slaughterhouse material may reflect the stressed rather than the physiological baseline state.

CIRCULATION OF NEURALLY DERIVED CALCITONIN GENE-RELATED PEPTIDE 200

Zaidi M, Bevis PJR, Diez Guerra J, Lynch C, Wimalawansa SJ, Emson PC, MacIntyre I
Endocrine Unit, Department of Chemical Pathology, Royal Postgraduate Medical School, London W12 and MRC Neurochemical Pharmacology Unit, Babraham, Cambridge (UK).

Besides the calcitonin (CT) precursor, the CT gene also encodes another peptide, calcitonin gene-related peptide (CGRP). CGRP has been shown to be the major product of the CT gene in man and a potent vasodilator in four species (Brain et al, 1985: Nature 313, 54). In the present study we have tested the hypothesis that the circulating peptide in the rat comes mainly from perivascular nerve terminals.

We have measured CGRP in extracts of rat plasma by a sensitive (detection limit 250 amol/tube) and specific radioimmunoassay. Plasma CGRP levels ranged between 3.9 and 94 pmol/l (mean ± sem 24.9 ± 3.7 pmol/l). The major immunorective peak of the extract co-eluted with synthetic rCGRP on HPLC. Administration of a nerve terminal depolariser, capsaicin, to adult rats caused a 15-fold increase in plasma CGRP levels. When the transport of the peptide along the perivascular nerve axons was blocked by colchicine, plasma CGRP levels were significantly ($p < 0.005$) reduced. There was also a significant decline of plasma CGRP when the dorsal root ganglia were lesioned by administering capsaicin neonatally. In a separate experiment capsaicin administered acutely either to neonatal capsaicin-treated or colchicine-pretreated rats was followed by a smaller (5-6 fold) rise of plasma CGRP. The levels following acute administration of capsaicin to adult rats significantly correlated ($r = 0.81$, $p < 0.005$) with those prior to treatment.

This study indicates that circulating CGRP is derived from the perivascular nerves. We have recently suggested that circulating CGRP may be an important regulator of blood flow in man. Release of CGRP from the perivascular nerves may be the mechanism by which this postulated regulatory role is exercised.

GnRH ACTIVATES A RAPID Ca^{2+}-INDEPENDENT PHOSPHODIESTER HYDROLYSIS OF POLYPHOSPHOINOSITIDES IN PITUITARY GONADOTROPHS 201

Zvi Naor
Department of Hormone Research, The Weizmann Institute of Science, Rehovot 76100, Israel

Addition of gonadotropin releasing hormone (GnRH) to cultured rat pituitary cells prelabeled with [^{32}]Pi or with myo-[2-^{3}H]inositol, resulted in a rapid decrease (~10 s) in the level of [^{32}P]phosphatidylinositol 4,5 bisphosphate (PIP_2), and a slower decrease (~ 1 min) in [^{32}P] phosphatidylinositol 4-phosphate (PIP). A transient decrease in [^{32}P]phosphatidylinositol (PI, 30 s) was followed by increased labeling of PI (1 min), and phosphatidic acid (PA, 1 min). No significant effect on the labeling of phosphatidylcholine or phosphatidylethanolamine was noticed. Concomitant with the rapid hydrolysis of the polyphosphoinositides, GnRH stimulated the appearance of [^{3}H]-myo-inositol 1,4,5-trisphosphate (IP_3, 10 s), [^{3}H]-myo-inositol 1,4-bisphosphate (IP_2, 15 s), and [^{3}H]-myo-inositol 1-phosphate (IP_1, 1 min). The stimulatory effect of GnRH on inositol phosphates (Ins-P) production was dose-related, and was blocked by a potent antagonist. Elevation of cytosolic free Ca^{2+} levels ($[Ca^{2+}]_i$), by ionomycin and A23187 from intracellular or extracellular Ca^{2+} pools respectively, had no significant effect on [^{3}H] Ins-P production. GnRH-induced [^{3}H]Ins-P production was not dependent on extracellular Ca^{2+}, and was noticed also after extracellular or intracellular Ca^{2+} mobilization by A23187 or ionomycin respectively. The stimulatory effect of GnRH on [^{3}H]Ins-P accumulation was not affected significantly by prior treatment of the cells with the tumor promoter phorbol ester 12-O-tetradecanoylphorbol 13-acetate (TPA) or with islet activating protein (IAP), pertussis toxin. These results indicate that GnRH stimulates a rapid phosphodiester hydrolysis of polyphosphoinositides. The stimulatory effect is not mediated via an IAP-substrate, is not dependent on elevation of $[Ca^{2+}]_i$, neither is it negatively regulated by TPA which activates Ca^{2+}/phospholipid-dependent protein kinase (C-kinase). The results are consistent with the hypothesis that GnRH-induced phosphoinositide turnover is responsible for Ca^{2+} mobilization followed by gonadotropin release.

PROTEIN KINASE C ACTIVATION ATTENUATES SECRETAGOGUE-INDUCED INOSITOL PHOSPHATE GENERATION IN NORMAL PITUITARY AND 7315a TUMOR CELLS 202

A.M. Judd, W.D. Jarvis, R.M. MacLeod
Dept. of Internal Medicine, University of Virginia School of Medicine, Charlottesville, Virginia 22908

The activation of protein kinase C by diacylglycerol (DAG) may play a role in the stimulation of anterior pituitary hormone release by secretagogues that promote the hydrolysis of phosphatidylinositol 4,5-bisphosphate (PIP_2) to inositol trisphosphate and DAG. However, DAG also exerts a negative feedback effect on PIP_2 hydrolysis in some tissues. To investigate the effects of protein kinase C activation on PIP_2 hydrolysis in the pituitary, primary cultures of female rat anterior pituitary cells or prolactin-secreting 7315a tumor cells were labeled with [^{3}H]-inositol for 24 hours; the cells were then exposed to secretagogue in the presence or absence of protein kinase C activators, and the production of total inositol phosphates (IP_x) was measured as an index of PIP_2 hydrolysis. TRH (1 to 100 nM) significantly increases IP_x generation in normal pituitary and 7315a cells. Phorbol myristate acetate (PMA), a protein kinase C activator, has no effect on basal IP_x production, but inhibits TRH-stimulated IP_x production in normal pituitary and 7315a cells. The inhibition by PMA of 100 nM TRH-induced IP_x production is concentration-related, with 1 nM having no significant effect while 10 nM (28%), 100 nM (33%), and 1 uM (40%) decrease (p < .01) IP_x production by the indicated amounts. 100 nM neurotensin (170%), angiotensin II (400%), bombesin (380%), and gonadotropin releasing hormone (215%) increase IP_x production as indicated and 100 nM PMA decreases each of these values by 40 to 60%. Synthetic diglyceride, 1,2-dioleoylglycerol, at 250 uM decreases by 30% (p < .01) the IP_x production elicited by 0.01 to 100 nM TRH. In summary, protein kinase C activators decrease secretagogue-induced IP generation in pituitary cells, and therefore, in addition to a stimulatory effect on pituitary hormone release, DAG appears to have a negative feedback effect on secretagogue-induced PIP_2 hydrolysis. (Supported by Am. Cancer Soc. Institutional Grant 149B and NIH grant CA-07535).

EFFECTS OF ESTRADIOL ON RECEPTORS COUPLED TO ADENYLATE CYCLASE AND ON PHOSPHOLIPID METHYLATION OF ANTERIOR PITUITARY CELLS. 203

A. Enjalbert, S.V. Drouva, P. Bertrand, S. Krantic, J. Epelbaum, E. Laplante, E. Rerat and C. Kordon
INSERM U. 159, 2ter rue d'Alésia, 75014 PARIS, France.

Estradiol modulates the sensitivity of anterior pituitary cells to various neurohormones. In order to further analyse the mechanisms underlying that modulation, we studied in parallel effects of 17 β-estradiol on hormone secretion, specific neurohormone sensitive adenylate cyclase (AC), DA and SRIF binding sites and phospholipid methylation on rat anterior pituitary cells. Treatment with 17 β-estradiol (10^{-9} M) did not affect basal adenylate cyclase activity ; however it resulted in a 80 % suppression of the DA inhibition of AC as well as in a 50 % decrease of the DA inhibition of prolactin secretion. DA binding sites however, as labelled by ^{3}H-spiroperidol, were not affected. In contrast 17 β-estradiol treatment increased SRIF inhibition of prolactin secretion as well as of AC activity (80 %). Furthermore ^{125}I Tyr DTrp 8 SRIF binding sites were increased (114 %) by the steroid without modification of their apparent affinity. Under the same experimental conditions, phospholipid methylation was also affected by 17 β-estradiol in a dose and time (from 15 to 120 hours) dependent manner. The increase in methyltransferase activity shows kinetic and pharmacological properties similar to those of AC. In addition, both parameters are insensitive to the inactive isomer 17 α-estradiol. We conclude that 1) estradiol affects pituitary sensitivity to both agonists by different mechanisms : a decrease of DA receptors coupling efficiency and an increase in the number of SRIF receptors. 2) A concomitant estradiol effect is observed on methyltransferase activity and on DA and SRIF sensitive AC. Methylation of phospholipid has been shown to induce changes in membrane viscosity, a process which could be involved in modulation of pituitary AC sensitivity to neurohormones.

A NOVEL SERINE PROTEASE FROM HUMAN AND PORCINE PITUITARY CLEAVING AT PAIRS OF BASIC RESIDUES IN PRO-OPIOMELANOCORTIN AND PRO-ATRIAL NATRIURETIC FACTOR RELATED PEPTIDES: A CANDIDATE PROCESSING ENZYME? 204

N.G. Seidah, J.A. Cromlish, G. Thibault, M. Chrétien
Clinical Research Institute of Montreal, Montreal, Quebec, Canada

A novel Serine Protease, which we have called IRCM-Serine Protease #1 (IRCM-SP#1), was purified from whole human pituitaries and from both anterior and neurointermediate porcine pituitary lobes. This proteinase displayed "trypsin-like" specificity toward a number of tripeptide coumarin containing substrates, with kcat/Km values ranging from 10^4-10^6 $M^{-1}s^{-1}$. In both species IRCM-SP#1 behaves as a dimer of Mr 160-190 K on gel filtration and gel electrophoresis and as a monomer of Mr 88-90 K on SDS/PAGE. The enzyme is composed of two subunits held together by disulfide bond(s). The catalytic subunit migrates on SDS with an apparent Mr of 38 K. IRCM-SP#1 cleaves various synthetic and natural substrates related to the POMC and ANF precursors either C-terminal or in-between all pairs of basic residues known to be cleaved in vivo. Many other potential tryptic-like cleavage sites not cleaved in vivo were also not touched by IRCM-SP#1. In porcine anterior pituitaries, differential centrifugation demonstrated that the majority of active IRCM-SP#1 is found in small vesicles sedimenting at 100,000 xg. An activatable form was also found in the mature secretory granule fraction, sedimenting at 27,000 xg. The active enzyme displays identical architecture as the one obtained from frozen tissue.

If IRCM-SP#1 participates in pro-hormone maturation in vivo, we propose a model in which this protease is present in an enzymatically active form in small vesicles, possibly within clathrin-coated structures (pro-secretory granules), which are then transformed to mature secretory granules by a process which would also inactivate most of the enzyme.

MECHANISM OF ACTION OF GROWTH HORMONE-RELEASING FACTOR (GHRF): ROLE OF CYCLIC AMP AND CALCIUM ION 205

J. Kraicer, B. Lussier, M.S. Sheppard, B. Moor, N. Narayanan
Department of Physiology, University of Western Ontario, London, Ontario

We continue to use a purified preparation of dispersed rat somatotrophs, obtained by a two-stage discontinuous density gradient procedure, to investigate the mechanisms by which rGHRF stimulates the release of GH. We use both static incubation and a perifusion system. Our data supporting a role for cAMP as a second messenger include a) rGHRF increases adenylate cyclase activity in a somatotroph plasma membrane preparation in a dose-related manner, b) this precedes, or is concurrent with, a dose-related increase in cAMP accumulation in the somatotrophs, c) which is followed by a dose-related increase in GH release. This, taken with previous observations that a) cAMP analogues stimulate GH release and b) the phosphodiesterase inhibitor, IBMX, potentiates the increase in GH release and cAMP accumulation induced by rGHRF, establishes an essential role for cAMP.

Ca^{++} also plays an essential role in the release process, since a) rGHRF does not stimulate GH release if Ca^{++} is removed from the incubating medium and b) the Ca^{++}-channel blockers, diltiazem and nifedipine inhibit basal GH release, increase basal cAMP accumulation, and block rGHRF-induced GH release. Ca^{++} is essential at a step subsequent to cAMP accumulation, since when Ca^{++} is removed from the incubation medium, a) cAMP analogues no longer stimulate GH release and b) the accumulation of cAMP in response to rGHRF is not reduced. In fact, the rGHRF-induced increase in cAMP accumulation is further increased 5-7 fold in the Ca^{++}-free medium.

We conclude that cAMP is an intracellular mediator in the action of GHRF and that Ca^{++} is essential in order for cAMP to express its action. (Supported by Medical Research Council of Canada).

COPPER-AMPLIFIED PGE_2 STIMULATION OF LHRH RELEASE FROM MEDIAN EMINENCE (ME) EXPLANTS: A POST-RECEPTOR EVENT AT THE LEVEL OF THE ADENYLATE CYCLASE SYSTEM 206

Ayalla Barnea, Gloria Cho
Depts Ob-Gyn & Physiol, Green Ctr. Reprod. Biol, Univ. of Texas Health Sci. Ctr., Dallas TX 75235

We have previously shown that copper amplifies PGE_2 stimulation of LHRH release from ME explants 3-4 folds. Since cAMP has been implicated in PGE_2 action, in this study we wished to ascertain if amplification of PGE_2 action by copper occurs at the level of the PGE_2 receptor or at a post-receptor step, i.e., the adenylate cyclase or cAMP action. ME of adult male rats were incubated for 5 min with Cu(II) complexed to histidine (CuHis; 200 μM) and then for 15 min with either PGE_2 (10 μM; Cu/PGE_2), forskolin (100 μM; Cu/F), or 8-Br-cAMP (1 mM; Cu/cAMP). Controls were incubated without CuHis or with CuHis alone. LHRH release during the 15 min period of incubation was evaluated by RIA. Basal release of LHRH was 4.6 ± 0.45 pg/15min per ME (m ± SE; n=15). Net-stimulated release after exposure to PGE_2, F, or cAMP was 3.6 ± 0.52 (n=11), 3.1 ± 0.39 (n=16) and 1.6 ± 0.42 (n=10) pg, respectively. Net-stimulated release after exposure to Cu/PGE_2, Cu/F, or Cu/cAMP was 12.7 ± 2.25 (n=15), 9.9 ± 1.46 (n=19), and 1.4 ± 1.9 (n=8) pg, respectively. When ME were incubated with a mixture of PGE_2 and F, the effect on LHRH release was not additive, regardless of whether the ME were pretreated with CuHis. Moreover, when calcium was omitted from the incubation buffer, PGE_2- and F-stimulated release as well as Cu/PGE_2- and Cu/F-stimulated release was each reduced by about 50%. In summary: 1) copper amplifies PGE_2 as well as F stimulation of LHRH release 3-4 folds; 2) copper does not amplify cAMP action; 3) PGE_2 and F action (amplified and non-amplified) has a partial requirement for calcium; 4) PGE_2 and F appear to operate by a common mechanism in both untreated and copper-treated ME. These results are consistent with PGE_2 stimulation of LHRH release mediated by an increase in the formation of cAMP and with copper enhancing the functional state of the adenylate cyclase system.

CYCLIC AMP AND PROSTAGLANDIN F2α STIMULATE GnRH SECRETION BY HUMAN PLACENTAL CELL CULTURES. 207

F. Petraglia, A.T.W. Lim and W. Vale.
The Clayton Foundation Laboratories for Peptide Biology, The Salk Institute, La Jolla, CA.

The recent cloning of human placental GnRH identical to those of hypothalamic origin strongly suggests that the decapeptide is expressed in placental tissue. Employing rabbit antiserum raised against the N-terminal of synthetic [Lys 8]-GnRH, we have explored the production, secretion and localization of GnRH like-immunoreactivity (LI) in long term monolayer cell cultures of human placenta. Trophoblasts of placental specimens, obtained from subjects undergoing elective caesarean section, were enzimatically dispersed yielding $2x10^6$ cells per gm of tissue and the cells were plated at $1.5x10^6$ cells per 35mm well in 10% fetal calf serum enriched B-PJ culture medium. After an attachment period of 48 h, the cultures were washed and stimulated by high K+[59mM] in HEPES buffered Krebs-Ringer bicarbonate solution every two days for 10 days. Basal secretion of GnRH-LI from the cultures was 10+2.5 pg/well/3 h and the release rates were consistently doubled in the presence of high K^+ at all times. The stimulatory effect of high K^+ was abolished in the absence of Ca^{++} or in the presence of Ca^{++} channel blocker, cobalt chloride (1mM). GnRH-LI content of the cultures, determined following acid extraction and C-18 octadecyl column elution was 33.5+3.7 pg/well. GnRH-LI extracted from media of non-stimulated cultures or from cell content was further characterized with high pressure liquid chromatography and in both instances elution profiles similar to that of synthetic GnRH were observed. Immunoperoxidase staining revealed that 10-15% of the cultured cells were positive for GnRH. Furthermore, dibutyryl cyclic AMP or forskolin appeared to double GnRH-LI release in a dose-related manner (from 10^{-7} to 10^{-4}). Prostaglandin F2 stimulation showed a biphasic GnRH-LI release with maximal effect at 10^{-6} (24+3.4 pg/well/3h). We thus conclude that (i) GnRH-LI is produced and secreted by a subpopulation of human trophoblast cells and that (ii) its secretion is modulated by prostaglandin F2 and forskolin, probably mediated by adenylate cyclase-cyclic AMP system.

ARACHIDONATE EPOXIDES ARE POTENT STIMULATORS OF PROLACTIN SECRETION IN NORMAL RAT PITUITARY CELLS 208

D. Grandsaert, J.R. Cashman, R.I. Weiner
University of California San Francisco, San Francisco, California

Arachidonic acid metabolites have been proposed as second messengers in Prolactin (PRL) release from lactotrophs after stimulation by Thyrotropin Releasing Hormone (TRH). In GH3 rat tumor pituitary cells, we have determined that an arachidonate metabolite of the Cytochrome P-450 epoxygenase system, 5,6-epoxyeicosatrienoic acid (5,6-EET), may also contribute to the process of PRL release, and is more biologically potent than cyclooxygenase or lipoxygenase (hydroxyeicosatetraenoic acid) metabolites. We have extended our studies to normal rat anterior pituitary cell dispersions where we found that 5,6-EET causes a dramatic and sex-related increase in PRL release.

Normal rat anterior pituitary cells were isolated, dispersed and grown for 24 hours in wells coated with corneal extracellular matrix. Cells were determined to be viable before and after challenge experiments by observing the exclusion of trypan blue dye. PRL was quantitated from each sample with a double antibody radioimmunoassay. Cells from male rats treated with 50 μM 5,6-EET produced 54.7±3.6 compared to basal 25.3±1.8 ng PRL/10^6 cells/20 mins. Cells from female rats treated with 50 μM 5,6-EET produced 1075±56 compared to basal 56±12 ng PRL/10^6 cells/20 mins. PRL release from female anterior pituitary cells was time and dose dependent, with apparent maximal values at 8 mins and 75 μM 5,6-EET, respectively.

Taken together, these data suggest that (1) 5,6-EET selectively stimulates the release of PRL in normal pituitary cells, (2) 5,6-EET may be one of the most potent intracellular mediators for PRL release known, and (3) P-450 epoxygenase may provide a point of regulation for PRL release in vivo.

IDENTIFICATION AND SORTING OF ANTERIOR PITUITARY CELLS THAT BIND CORTICOTROPIN-RELEASING FACTOR; ABSENCE OF ADRENOCORTICOTROPIN RESPONSE TO VASOPRESSIN IN SORTED CELLS 209

J. Schwartz, J. Trotter, J. Rivier and W. Vale The Clayton Foundation Laboratories for Peptide Biology and Flow Cytometry Laboratory, The Salk Institute, La Jolla, CA 93037.

In order to study the interaction of corticotropin-releasing factor (CRF) and vasopressin on adrenocorticotropin (ACTH) secretion, a fluorescent bioactive analog of CRF, [fluorescein-Ser^1,$Nle^{21,38}$,Arg^{36}]-rCRF, was synthesized. This analog was found to be 37% as potent as oCRF in stimulating ACTH secretion in cultured bovine anterior pituitary cells. It was also found to label 6.1±0.6% of dissociated bovine anterior pituitary cells, visualized by fluorescence microscopy. This labelling was receptor-specific, being abolished by co-incubation with 200 fold molar excess of unlabelled [$Nle^{21,38}$,Arg^{36}]-rCRF or oCRF but not by vasopressin, GRF or a biologically inactive analog of CRF.

Dissociated bovine anterior pituitary cells, labelled by incubation with the fluorescent CRF analog, were also sorted by fluorescence-activated cell sorting. Populations of sorted and unsorted cells were cultured for 3 to 11 d in medium containing 2% fetal calf serum. Experiments were performed following repeated washing of the cells and an incubation in serum-free medium. Experiments consisted of a 3h control incubation followed by a second 3h incubation in the presence of 100 nM vasopressin or 2.5 nM oCRF. Aliquots of medium from both incubations were assayed for ACTH by radioimmunoassay. In unsorted cells, vasopresin produced a four fold increase in ACTH secretion (1.30±0.42 to 5.70±2.93 ng/ml per 3h,$P<0.05$). In contrast, in sorted cells vasopressin had no effect on ACTH secretion, despite stimulation of ACTH secretion by CRF (1.24±0.48 to 9.29±1.93, ng/ml per 3h,$P<0.001$). These results demonstrate the specific labelling of CRF target cells in the anterior pituitary by the fluorescent analog, and are consistent with CRF and vasopressin acting on different populations of anterior pituitary cells to stimulate ACTH secretion. Supported by NIH grants AM26741 and HL06808.

ULTRASTRUCTURAL ANALYSIS OF THE CATECHOLAMINERGIC INNERVATION OF THE HYPOTHALAMIC PARAVENTRICULAR NUCLEUS WITH SPECIAL REFERENCE TO CORTICOTROPIN RELEASING FACTOR SYNTHESIZING NEURONS 210

Zs. Liposits, C. Phelix, W.K. Paull
Department of Anatomy, University of Missouri-Columbia, Columbia, Mo.

Catecholamine synthesizing enzymes were detected in the hypothalamic paraventricular nucleus (PVN) of intact and colchicine treated rats by preembedding immunocytochemical methods. Phenylethanolamine-N-methyltransferase (PNMT) and dopamine-ß-hydroxylase (DBH)-immunoreactivities were exclusively found in axons and their terminals, establishing asymmetric synapses with dendrites, dendritic spines, somata and somatic appendages of both parvo- and magnocellular neurons in the PVN. Tyrosine hydroxylase (TH) immunoreactivity - in addition to axons - was also present in dendrites and perikarya. The paraventricular TH-positive neurons were fusiform and multipolar in shape and exhibited somatic and dendritic spines. TH-immunoreactive axons terminated on both non-labeled and TH-immunopositive neurons of PVN. The latter indicates an intrinsic organization of the catecholaminergic system.

These ultrastructural data support the concept that catecholamines modulate the function of paraventricular neurons.

In order to elucidate, whether corticotropin releasing factor (CRF)-synthesizing neurons are targets for terminating catecholaminergic axons, catecholamine-synthesizing enzymes and CRF were simultaneously visualized in sections of PVN. The preembedding dual localization technique utilized silver-gold intensified diaminobenzidine (DAB) and natural DAB endproducts as tracers. The juxtaposition of PNMT, DBH and TH-immunoreactive axons with dendrites and perikarya of CRF neurons was characteristic of the light microscopic picture. The ultrastructural analysis revealed that the catecholaminergic terminals established asymmetric synaptic specializations with dendrites, somata and spinous structures of CRF-synthesizing neurons.

This finding indicates that the central catecholaminergic system can directly influence the function of CRF-producing neurons in the PVN and via this system the activity of the hypophyseal-adrenal unit.

CHARACTERIZATION OF HUMAN PLACENTAL CORTICOTROPIN RELEASING HORMONE 211

G.K. Stalla, H. Bost, T. Kaliebe, M. Huber
J. Stalla, K. von Werder, O.A. Müller
Med. Klinik Innenstadt, Univ. of Munich, FRG

After demonstrating CRH-IR with a heterologous oCRH system in serum of pregnant females, we have compared immunological, physicochemical and biological properties of placental CRH with the hCRH-standard.

Placental CRH was measured with C- and N-terminal specific hCRH-RIA. The extracts from sera and placenta were chromatographed on Sephadex G 50 column and reversed phase HPLC. The biological activity was investigated using rat pituitary fragments and pituitary cells in culture. Extracts of pregnant sera and CRH standard were added to the incubation medium and resulting ACTH, rPRL and rGH secretion was measured.

In 149 females in the last trimenon elevated endogenous CRH-levels were measured up to 20 ng/ml. Post partum CRH-levels were not detectable. Dilution curves of pregnant serum and placental extracts were parallel with the C- and N-terminal hCRH standard curve. The elution pattern of serum CRH from pregnant females and placental extracts were identical with the hCRF standard in gel permeation chromatography and reversed phase HPLC. Estimated CRH concentration was 0.2 ng/g wet weight of human placenta. The incubation with fragments or cells from rat pituitaries revealed significant ACTH stimulation after adding extracts from pregnant serum and placental extract. The ACTH increases were dose related and within the same range compared to hCRH standard extracted from pooled normal serum. rGH and rPRL secretion was unchanged.

In conclusion, circulating CRH in pregnant females is of placental origin. Though placental CRH is physicochemically undistinguishable from hypothalamic CRH and as biologically active as hCRH standard, the biological significance of placental CRH remains unclear.

INHIBITION OF CRF RELEASE IN HYPOPHYSIAL PORTAL BLOOD AFTER 6-OHDA-LESION OF THE VENTRAL NORADRENERGIC BUNDLE. 212

V. Guillaume, B. Conte-Devolx, A. Szafarczyk, N. Pares-Herbute, M. Grino, I. Assenmacher, C. Oliver

Lab. Neuroendoc. INSERM U 297 Fac. Med. Nord F. 13326 Marseilles and CNRS UA 639 Univ. Montpellier F. 34060 Montpellier France.

It has been recently shown by Szafarczyk et al (Amer. J. Physiol. 294, E219, 1985) that ACTH secretion decreases after neurotoxic lesion of the ventral noradrenergic bundle (VNAB) by 6-hydroxydopamine (6-OHDA), suggesting that central catecholamines stimulate anterior pituitary ACTH release.

In order to study the possible involvement of hypothalamic CRF in the catecholamine induced ACTH secretion, we have measured CRF levels in rat hypophysial portal blood (HPB) one-week after bilateral stereotaxical injection of 6-OHDA into the VNAB. Rat CRF levels in HPB was measured with an homologous RIA. The effects of 6-OHDA injection were controled by determination of catecholamine contents (Dopamine DA, Norepinephrine NE and Epinephrine E) in total hypothalamus using HPLC followed by electrochemical detection.

After the VNAB lesion, there was an 81% and 91,8% decrease in the hypothalamic content of NE and E respectively. No significant changes in DA content was observed. Concomitantly, CRF levels in HPB were significantly reduced (17.4 ± 2.9 pg/ml, n=6) as compared to controls (641 ± 75.9, n=11).

These results suggest that the stimulating effect of central catecholamines on ACTH secretion occurs through the release of CRF at the level of the hypothalamus.

Grants form INSERM 83 40 07

HISTAMINERGIC MODULATION OF THE NEUROENDOCRINE SYSTEM 213

R. Cacabelos, H. Niigawa, A. Miyake*, S. Hariguchi, T. Nishimura.
Departments of Neuropsychiatry and Gynecology*, Osaka University Medical School, Osaka 553, Japan.

Recent research of the histaminergic neuronal system has revealed that histamine (HA) neurons are located primarily in the posterior hypothalamic region (PHR). In an attempt to further clarify the role of HA in the neuroendocrine system (NES), we have studied the effects of HA, H_1- and H_2-antagonists and alpha-fluoromethylhistidine (FMH), a K_{cat} inhibitor of histidine decarboxylase, on the adenohypophyseal function. We have also studied the effect of GRF and peripheral endocrine manipulation on brain HA.

Neuronal HA seems to be essential to the normal functioning of the corticotropinergic system. When the synthesis of HA is inhibited by the action of FMH (100 mg/Kg/day), the ACTH release in response to bilateral adrenalectomy was abolished. Furthermore, HA (0.6 mmol/Kg) decreased the CRF-induced ACTH release by about 10% and the concentration of ACTH in the adenohypophysis (Ah) by about 30%. Mepyramine (Mep; 0.3 mmol/Kg) enhanced the ACTH response to CRF (5 µg/Kg) while famotidine (Fam; 0.4 mmol/Kg) abolished the response. On the other hand, HA alone increased the plasma ACTH levels from 33.5 ± 8.5 to 103 ± 15 pg/ml.

GRF (5 µg/Kg; i.c.v.) elicited a significant increase ($p<0.005$) of HA in four different parts of the hypothalamo-hypophyseal system. HA produced a rise in the plasma GH levels from 29.3 ± 5.2 to 174.5 ± 25.6 ng/ml while HA + Mep effected a rise to 210.5 ± 50.6 ng/ml. Fam suppressed the HA-induced GH release.

L-histidine loads (200 mg/day; i.p.) and HA alone did not modify the basal levels of plasma LH. When administered together with LHRH, HA reduced the LHRH-induced LH response by 45% with LH retained in the Ah. In addition, a 3 month-castration of rats resulted in an age- and sex-related increase of HA in the anterior and posterior hypothalamic regions and neurohypophysis, along with a decrease of HA in the median eminence.

All these data together suggest that HA plays an important role as a modulator of the NES. Most HA actions seem to be hormone- and area-specific.

REEVALUATION OF THE ROLE OF DIRECT beta-ADRENERGIC STIMULATION OF ACTH RELEASE FROM THE ANTERIOR PITUITARY 214

G.B. Makara[1], K. Kovács[1], I. Kakucska,[1] D. Ježova,[2] R. Kvetnansky[2]
[1] Institute of Experimental Medicine, Hung. Acad. Sci., Budapest, Hungary,
[2] Institute of Experimental Endocrinology, Slovak Acad. Sci., Bratislava, Czechoslovakia

There are conflicting reports in the literature whether direct β-adrenoreceptor stimulation of the anterior pituitary may represent an important mechanism of ACTH release in the rat during stress. The effect of two strong stimuli releasing large amounts of epinephrine (E), norepinephrine (NE), ACTH and corticosterone (B) were studied after disabling hypothalamic CRF and AVP mediated control of ACTH release by an anterolateral cut (ALC) around the medial basal hypothalamus (MBH) or a knife lesion of the MBH (MBHL). Immobilization (IMO) for 20 min elicited a marked rise of plasma E and NE in both MBHL and ALC rats while the plasma ACTH response normally following IMO was inhibited by ALC or MBHL. The small response to IMO after ALC was not decreased by either propranolol (2.5 mg/kg, i.p.) or phentolamine (2.5 mg/kg i.p.) pretreatment. It has been suggested (Mezey et al.,1984) that insulin hypoglycemia stimulated ACTH release via a propranolol sensitive mechanism which was present also after pituitary stalk section or MBHL. In our studies propranolol failed to markedly depress the plasma ACTH or B response to insulin (2.5 U/kg, i.p.)-induced hypoglycemia in rats bearing tail artery cannulas. The plasma E rise normally induced by insulin hypoglycemia was unchanged 7 days after MBHL but the plasma ACTH response was inhibited strongly by MBHL. In non-cannulated MBHL rats there was only a small rise of plasma ACTH 45 min after insulin and this rise was not significantly decreased by propranolol given 15 min before insulin.

We suggest that marked peripheral plasma E and NE rises induced by insulin hypoglycemia or IMO are not releasing ACTH directly from the anterior pituitary. A CRF and/or AVP dependent mechanism appear to dominate stress-induced ACTH release in the rat.

EVIDENCE THAT CHRONIC PREDNISOLONE TREATMENT INHIBITS PITUITARY RESPONSIVENESS BY A DUAL MECHANISM 215

S.A. Nicholson, Division of Physiology, United Medical and Dental Schools (Guy's), London SE1 9RT, U.K.

Groups of male rats were treated for 14 days with prednisolone (500 µg/ml in their drinking water) and the drug was then withdrawn for various lengths of time (up to 9 days). Pituitary responsiveness was assessed by exposure of pituitary fragments from such animals to various ACTH secretagogues in vitro, ACTH release being measured by radioimmunoassay.

The response to all secretagogues tested was significantly reduced after prednisolone treatment, in most cases being completely prevented. The effect of hypothalamic extract was only reduced by 50% and recovery was achieved earliest (by 3 days after withdrawal), supporting the idea that the extract contains several factors acting in concert to produce a very potent stimulus.

The responses to three "specific" stimuli to ACTH release, CRF-41, vasopressin and oxytocin, were only fully recovered by 7, 7 and 9 days after withdrawal respectively. "Non-specific" stimuli used were low and high doses of 8-bromo-cAMP (a stable analogue of cAMP) and putrescine (one of the polyamines; a putative "third messenger" in hormone secretion). The high dose of 8-bromo-cAMP still produced a significant stimulation of ACTH release immediately after prednisolone treatment. The response to these stimuli was restored by 7 days after withdrawal. In contrast to the specific stimuli, 8-bromo-cAMP and putrescine were capable of producing ACTH release significantly in excess of basal as early as 3 days after withdrawal.

These results suggest that in the long-term, prednisolone exerts its action in two ways. One, by reducing the number or affinity of pituitary membrane receptors for the specific ACTH secretagogues, and two, by alterations in the intracellular mechanisms normally triggered by changes in second or "third" messengers. It appears that the former of these two actions is the most long-lived after withdrawal of the drug.

This work was supported by the Nuffield Foundation.

DIFFERENCES IN RNA ABUNDANCE IN RAT HIPPOCAMPUS IN RESPONSE TO ENDOGENOUS AND HIGH DOSE ADMINISTERED CORTICOSTERONE 216

N.R. Nichols, J.N. Masters, P.C. May, S.L. Millar, C.E. Finch
University of Southern California, Los Angeles, California

Genomic mechanisms of the adrenocortical stress response are not well understood for either acute or chronic stress. Therefore, we have investigated rat hippocampal gene expression in response to high dose administered corticosterone (CORT). Previously, we have demonstrated consistent changes in the abundance of specific hippocampal RNAs in response to acutely administered CORT. In the present study we compare responses in adrenalectomized (Adx) and intact Fisher 344 rats which were injected for 3d with 10 ug/d CORT or oil vehicle (n = 10 rats per group). Hippocampal total RNA from each group was isolated by the guanidinium-thiocyanate/CsCl method; 10 ug RNA samples were translated in vitro at 30°C using reticulocyte lysates and ^{35}S-methionine. Protein patterns from 100,000 cpm (TCA-precipitable), were visually compared following 2-dimensional gel electrophoresis and fluorography. Both CORT-treated groups showed a mol wt 50K species which decreased in density and 35K, 33K and 20K species which increased in density when compared to Adx and intact controls. Two of these products (50K and 33K) respond to endogenous CORT levels and two (35K and 20K) do not differ in abundance between Adx and intact groups. Therefore, two classes of response have been identified which may reflect differences in circulating hormone levels.

Supported by the Office of Naval Research Grant No. N00014-85-K-0770 and a grant from the John D. and Catherine T. MacArthur Foundation.

LIGHT AND MOTOR ACTIVITY IN THE FERRET 217

B. T. Donovan
Department of Physiology, Institute of Psychiatry, De Crespigny Park, London SE5 8AF, England

When female ferrets are given access to an activity wheel differing patterns of motor activity between oestrus and anoestrus, and night and day become evident. The animals show more activity (run further) during oestrus, and their activity extends outside the hours of illumination. Anoestrous females run only when the lights are on (Donovan, 1985, Physiol. Behav., 34, 825). Subsequently, the total activity of ferrets kept in cages mounted on balanced rocking platforms has been followed, with divergent results. Comparison of the patterns of activity of 14 oestrous females studied over a total of 876 long days with that of 18 anoestrous ferrets similarly exposed to extended hours of illumination over 1034 days showed marked parallelism. The oestrous females were not generally more active than anoestrous ferrets, while some activity was detected during the night in both sexual states. Likewise, 16 instances of the development of oestrus under constant lighting conditions were studied. Significant changes were observed in three females, with the mean level of activity being greater during anoestrus than oestrus in one, and activity being increased during oestrus in the other two. Over the whole group there was no change in activity. Similar findings emerged from five animals studied over the transition from oestrus to anoestrus. The effect of extending the daylength was examined in 13 females over a period covering 30 days before and 30 days after the hours of lighting were increased from 8 to 16 daily. No change in the pattern of activity was seen. These measures of activity have been used in other species as an index of hypothalamic cyclicity, but it seems that they are not very helpful in the ferret.

EFFECT OF LOCAL PHARMACOLOGICAL DESTRUCTION OF THE SEROTONINERGIC INNERVATION OF THE HYPOTHALAMIC SUPRACHIASMATIC REGION OF YOUNG RATS ON CIRCADIAN HORMONE RHYTHMS 218

B. Halász, Zs. Bánky
2nd Department of Anatomy, Semmelweis Medical University, Budapest, Hungary

The suprachiasmatic nucleus plays a key role in the organization of circadian fluctuations in plasma corticosterone levels. The cell group is very rich in serotoninergic (5-HT) innervation. In our previous studies we found that selective destruction (using 5,7-dihydroxytryptamine, 5,7-DHT) of the 5-HT fibers and terminals in the suprachiasmatic region of 16-day-old rats interfered with the onset of the diurnal corticosterone rhythm.

In the present investigations we observed that the corticosterone rhythm still failed in three-month-old rats treated with 5,7-DHT at the age of 16 days. Such rats exhibited fluctuations in plasma prolactin, growth hormone and testosterone levels. Several rats injected with 5,7-DHT on day 16 of life did show a diurnal corticosterone rhythm when tested at the age of four months. A fairly intense network of 5-HT immunoreactive fibers was evident in the suprachiasmatic nucleus of four-month-old rats, but such network could not be demonstrated in younger animals having no corticosterone rhythm.- The data suggest that 5-HT innervation of the suprachiasmatic region is essential for the onset of the diurnal corticosterone rhythm.

NYCTOHEMERAL INCREASE IN THE SENSITIVITY OF THE PINEAL GLAND OF THE SYRIAN HAMSTER TO NOREPINEPHRINE 219

R.J. Reiter, G.M. Vaughan, S. Oaknin, M.E. Troiani
Department of Cellular and Structural Biology, University of Texas Health Science Center, San Antonio, Texas 78284

In the rat, the administration of norepinephrine (NE) (especially when given in conjunction with a NE re-uptake inhibitor, e.g., desmethylimipramine or DMI) or isoproterenal, a NE agonist, during the day readily stimulates pineal N-acetyltransferase (NAT) activity and melatonin production. In contrast, similar injections into either Syrian hamsters or humans fail to promote either pineal melatonin production or plasma levels of the indoleamine, respectively. The series of studies described below reveals that the hamster pineal gland is only sensitive to NE at a restricted period during the latter half of the dark phase of the light:dark cycle. In these studies, NE was injected either during the day or at night into adult male Syrian hamsters. NE (1mg/kg) was given ip and was always preceded (by 10 minutes) with an ip injection of DMI (5mg/kg). Groups of animals were then killed at 0, 1, 2 or 3 hours after the NE injection. The hamsters were kept under 14:10 light:dark cycles with lights off at 2000 h. When hamsters were treated with DMI plus NE at night they were acutely exposed to light ($50 \mu W/cm^2$) 30 min before NE to depress high nighttime melatonin values to daytime levels. The injection of NE (preceded by DMI) either during the light (at 0800 or 1600 h) or in the early dark phase (at 2200 h) failed to stimulate either pineal NAT or melatonin during the post injection period. When the drugs were administered either at 2400 or 0200 h, pineal melatonin levels (but not NAT activity) were slightly increased ($p < 0.05$) at one point during the post injection period. However, when NE was injected at 0400h (8 h after darkness onset) pineal melatonin levels increased 4-fold ($p < 0.001$) 2 hours after drug injection while NAT activity doubled. When animals were either exposed to light at night (rather than 7.5 h of darkness) or superior cervical ganglionectomized the pineal response to combined DMI and NE was severely blunted. The results indicate that the hamster pineal is maximally sensitive to NE in the latter half of the dark phase and both darkness and an intact sympathetic innervation are required for the development of maximal sensitivity. Thus, the normal nocturnal rise in pineal melatonin in the Syrian hamster appears to be determined by not only the release of NE but an increased sensitivity of the β-receptors on the pinealocyte membrane to the catecholamine. Since in the human, the pineal does not respond to isopraterenol during the day, perhaps it is like the hamster and would exhibit a sensitivity at night. Research supported by NSF grant # PCM 8410592.

HYPOTHALAMIC SITE OF ACTION OF MELATONIN IN RATS 220

F. Gibbs, J. Corcoran, L. Petterborg, and K. Rudeen
Dept. of Anatomy, Univ. of Missouri, Columbia, MO 65212

Following olfactory bulbectomy (Bx) rats will undergo gonadal involution due to properly timed melatonin (MEL) injections, short photoperiod, or blinding (Bl). To localize the brain site of action of MEL in the rat we utilized the ability of an implant of continuously available MEL to block the antigonadotropic effect of blinding in the Bx rat. We started with 62 male Sprague-Dawley rats divided into the following groups (N per group): Intact (8), Bl-Bx (8), Bl-Bx+2 mg MEL in beeswax placed subcutaneously (Bl-Bx 2 mg MEL SC)(8), Bl-Bx+10 ug MEL in beeswax in the anterior basal hypothalamus (Bl-Bx-MEL-Hypo) (15), Bl-Bx+wax in the anterior basal hypothalamus (Bl-Bx-Wax-Hypo) (15), and Bl-Bx+10 ug MEL in the cerebral cortex (Bl-Bx-MEL-Cor) (8). Surgery and implants were done on 22 day old rats, and the animals were sacrificed five weeks later. Blood and pituitaries were assayed for reproductive hormones, and pituitaries, seminal vesicles, and testes were weighed. Fifty animals survived to sacrifice and their relative testicular masses were: [Mean±SEM(N)] Intact = 1.1±0.04 g/100g body weight (8), Bl-Bx = 0.43±0.05 (5), Bl-Bx 2 mg MEL SC=1.37±0.03 (7), Bl-Bx Wax Hypo = 0.79±0.09 (13), Bl- Bx-MEL-Hypo = 1.18±0.09 (10), Bl-Bx-MEL-Cor = 1.01±0.10 (7). The testes data as well as body mass, seminal vesicle and hormonal levels are consistent with the idea that the systemically ineffective MEL implants in the hypothalamus were as effective as the large subcutaneous implants, whereas wax in the hypothalamus or MEL in the cortex did not prevent a diminution of testis size and apparent reproductive capability ($p < 0.05$ Duncan Multiple Range Test).

We conclude that there may be a site in the anterior medial basal hypothalamus at which MEL can exert an effect on the neuroendocrine-reproductive axis of the rat. Since the hypothalamic implants were close to the third cerebral ventricle, an alternative interpretation is that MEL acts at another circumventricular locus. Supported by NIH grant #HD17658 (LP) and NIAAA grant #AA05893 (KR).

THYROXINE ACTIVATION AND ITS CIRCADIAN RHYTHMICITY IN RAT PINEAL GLAND 221

K. Tanaka, M. Murakami, M.A. Greer Section of Endocrinology, Oregon Health Sciences University, Portland, Oregon 97201

Thyroxine (T_4) must be enzymatically converted by iodothyronine 5'-deiodinase (5'-D) to 3,5,3'-triiodothyronine (T_3) for its full biological activity. There are two 5'-D isozymes: Type-I is present in liver, kidney and many other organs and has an important role in maintaining serum T_3 levels; Type-II is found in only a small number of tissues including anterior pituitary and brain. Type II 5'-D is believed important in mediating local thyroid hormone action by generating an adequate intracellular concentration of T_3. We have found Type-II 5'-D in high concentration in rat pineal gland. Radioactive iodide release from ^{125}I-T_4, which represents T_4 5'-deiodination, was dependent on tissue quantity, incubation time, pH and temperature, indicating its enzymatic nature. Kinetic parameters were calculated from double reciprocal plots: Km=1.6 nM and Vmax=136 fmoles I^-/release/min/mg protein.

This enzyme fulfilled all the criteria establishing it as Type-II rather than Type-I 5'-D: 1) insensitivity to propylthiouracil; 2) preference of T_4 as a substrate over 3,3',5'-triiodothyronine; 3) increased activity in hypothyroidism.

The pineal enzyme activity had a striking nycthemeral rhythm corresponding to melatonin secretory activity. With rats in a 0600 to 1800 h light cycle, it reached a zenith at midnight 10-20 fold higher than during daylight. Subcutaneous isoproterenol (100 µg/100 g BW) caused a 2.5 fold increase in pineal Type-II 5'-D activity within 4 hours.

Conclusions: 1) Type-II 5'-D is present in the pineal and its concentration parallels melatonin secretory activity. 2) It is stimulated by a beta adrenergic agonist. 3) These data suggest that thyroid hormone may have a previously unrecognized role in rhythmic pineal function.

THE PRESENCE OF BIOLOGICALLY ACTIVE DOPAMINE RECEPTORS IN THE PITUITARIES OF LONG AND SHORT PHOTOPERIOD-EXPOSED MALE HAMSTERS. 222

D.M. Burns, C.A. Leadem and B. Benson, Department of Anatomy, University of Arizona, Tucson, AZ

We have previously reported the presence of dopamine binding sites in the anterior pituitary of long photoperiod (14:10 light:dark cycle) -exposed male golden hamsters. It was therefore of interest to investigate whether these binding sites are associated with functional inhibition of prolactin (PRL) release, and possible changes that might accompany short photoperiod(10:14 light:dark cycle) -induced PRL inhibition. To do this, pituitaries from long photoperiod-exposed animals were removed and hemisected and the resulting halves were incubated for three hours at 37 ° C in medium containing 10^{-9}M, 10^{-8}M, 10^{-7}M, 10^{-6}M or 10^{-5}M dopamine and 5.6 x 10^{-4}M ascorbic acid or medium containing 5.6 x 10^{-4}M ascorbic acid alone. Thus the hemipituitary of one animal served as the vehicle-treated control for its corresponding half incubated with one of the doses of dopamine. At the end of the incubation period, media were removed and saved for subsequent PRL radioimmunoassay. Dose response curves were analyzed and compared with dose response curves for animals housed for 15 weeks in short photoperiod from the same experiment. PRL release was significantly inhibited by 10^{-5}M, 10^{-6}M and 10^{-7}M dopamine but not by 10^{-8}M or 10^{-9}M dopamine in long photoperiod animals. The response to dopamine was identical in short photoperiod animals while the basal release of PRL in this group was an order of magnitude lower than in the long photoperiod group. These results indicate that: 1) the dopamine binding sites in the pituitaries of long photoperiod exposed male hamsters are associated with a functional dopamine receptor complex; 2) at 15 weeks, short phtoperiod exposure results in a reduction in basal prolactin release but no change in pituitary sensitivity to dopamine. (Supported by NIH Grants HD 18570 and HD 19965)

THE EFFECT OF PINEALECTOMY AND LIGHT CYCLE ON SPONTANEOUS AND PROSTAGLANDIN E_2-INDUCED RELEASE OF LH IN PROESTROUS RATS 223

J. Warberg, L.D. Wogensen, M. Møller
Departments of Medical Physiology C and Medical Anatomy B, University of Copenhagen, Copenhagen, Denmark

Diurnal alterations in the LH response to PGE_2 has been observed throughout the estrous cycle - especially at proestrus. In the present investigation we have studied the influence of pinealectomy (PX) and light cycles on the spontaneous release of LH and its fluctuating responsiveness to PGE_2 at proestrus.

PX or a sham operation (SH) was performed on female rats which were then kept for 3 weeks in light/dark cylles of either 12/12 h or 10/14 h. To determine the spontaneous secretion of LH one group of rats were decapitated on each day of the estrous cycle and the concentration of LH was measured in trunk blood. Another group of rats were anesthetized with sodium pentobarbital and 2µg of PGE_2 was infused into a lateral ventricle of the brain at 09.00 or 13.00 h on the day of proestrus and the concentration of LH in arterial plasma was determined during a 90 min. period.

When kept in a 12/12 h light cycle PX and SH rats showed normal cyclic variations in the secretion of LH but the preovulatory LH surge (17.00 h at proestrus) was reduced compared to that of intact animals. When the rats were kept in a 10/14 h light cycle the proestrus LH peak was absent in PX and SH rats while it persisted in intact animals.

In intact rats the LH response to PGE_2 was increased at 09.00 as well as at 13.00 h when the photoperiod was shortened from 12 to 10 hours but the diurnal alteration in the response was less pronounced. A further increase in the LH responsiveness was observed following PX and SH. However, PX and SH rats kept in a 12/12 as well as a 10/14 light cycle showed no diurnal variation in PGE_2-induced LH release.

It is concluded that PX or disturbances in the pineal area as caused by a sham operation diminish or eliminate the proestrous LH surge depending on the light cycle. Furthermore, the LH response to PGE_2 and its diurnal variation appears to be dependent on the pineal body.

PINEALECTOMY-INDUCED NUMERICAL INCREASE IN MITOCHONDRIA AND EXOCYTOSIS IN PERIVASCULAR COMPARTMENTS IN ADRENOMEDULLARY ADRENALINE CELLS. 224

T. Kachi, T.K. Banerji, W.B. Quay
Asahikawa Medical College, Asahikawa 078, Japan,
Univ. of Texas Medical Branch, Galveston, Texas,
Univ. of California, Berkeley, California

We previously reported that the number of exocytotic figures in perivascular-space-facing (PF) plasma membranes increases following pinealectomy and changes in relation to time-of-day, rising in early dark phase, in adrenomedullary adrenaline cells of Golden Hamsters. The present study was carried out to examine whether the number of mitochondria changes in correlation with such changes in the frequency of exocytosis.

Animals acclimated to a standardized light-dark (LD) 12:12 photoperiod were sacrificed at 11h after the onset of light (L-11h) and 1h after the onset of darkness (D-1h) (7 animals/group/time) at 28 days postoperation and at 100 days of age. The adrenal medullas were examined and analyzed morphometrically by electron microscopy. Mitochondrial profiles, which lay at least partially in a zone between the PF plasma membrane and the plane up to 2 µm from the PF plasma membrane, were counted. Mitochondrial numbers in the zone per unit length (1µm) of the PF plasma membrane showed no statistically significant differences due to experimental treatment and time-of-day by ANOVA, but tended to show higher values in PX ($\bar{X}\pm SE$:0.37±0.03)compared to NO(0.29 ±0.01)(t-test:$P<0.05$)and SPX (0.26±0.01)($P<0.01$) animals at D-1h. Relative mitochondrial number in the zone per cell showed statistically significant changes due to both experimental treatment (L-11h+D-1h:NO,3.96±0.23; SPX,3.58±0.14; PX,4.80±0.34)(ANOVA:$P<0.01$) and time of day ($P<0.01$), showing decreases at D-1h in NO and PX but no apparent time-of-day change in SPX animals. Thus mitochondrial numbers in the zone per cell at both time points showed a higher value in PX than in SPX or SPX and NO animals (t-test:$P<0.005$). From these and other related data, it appears possible that the observed increase in mitochondria is related to the increase in the frequency of exocytosis in this plasma membrane compartment following pinealectomy, but not in early dark phase, supplying more energy (ATP) and Ca^{++}.

PATHWAYS INVOLVED IN THE STIMULATION BY THYROLIBERIN OF PROLACTIN RELEASE AND OF PROLACTIN GENE TRANSCRIPTION IN GH3 CELLS 225

A. Tixier-Vidal, C. Tougard, J.N. Laverrière and D. Gourdji
Groupe de Neuroendocrinologie Cellulaire et Moléculaire C.N.R.S., Collège de France, 75231 Paris Cedex 05

Thyroliberin (TRH) has been shown to induce a dual stimulating effect on prolactin (PRL) secretion by GH3 cells : 1° a rapid biphasic release of stored PRL. 2° a delayed and sustained increase of PRL synthesis which is the consequence of a rapid stimulation of PRL gene transcription (Laverrière J.N. et al, EMBO J., 1983, 2, 1493).

The cascade of events induced by the interaction of TRH with its receptors on GH_3 cells - formation of IP3, increase of intracellular Ca^{2+}, activation of protein kinase C (PKC) - has been coupled to the acute releasing effects of TRH (Martin, T.F.J., 1983, J. Biol. Chem., 258, 14816 ; Rebecchi, M.J. et al, 1983, J. Biol. Chem., 258, 227 ; Albert, P.R. and Tashjian A.H., J. Biol. Chem., 259, 5827 ; Drust, D.S. and Martin, J.F.J., 1984, J. Biol. Chem., 259, 14520).We have shown that it is associated with the exocytosis of vesicles, in addition to that of very few secretory granules, arising from a post Golgi derived regulated route as revealed by the subcellular localization of PRL and of Golgi membrane antigens, using electron microscope immunocytochemistry (Tougard, C. et al. Biol. of the Cell, 1982, 43, 89 - J. Cell Biol., 1983, 96, 1197).

We have attempted to determine whether same messengers might be also responsible for the rapid stimulation of PRL gene transcription. We have tested by run-on assay the separate and combined effects of TRH, the calcium ionophore A 23 187 and TPA, an activator of PKC. The results indicate that increase in intracellular calcium and PKC activation participate in the regulation of PRL gene transcription but cannot account for the complete response to TRH (Laverrière, J.N. et al, this meeting). Thus the stimulating effect of TRH on PRL synthesis seems only partially coupled to its effect on PRL release.

REGULATED PHOSPHOLIPID HYDROLYSIS AS A TRANSDUCTION MECHANISM FOR NEUROPEPTIDES AND PEPTIDE HORMONES 226

T.F.J. Martin, University of Wisconsin, Madison, Wis.

Peptide hormones exert many of their actions on target cells by interaction with cell-surface receptors which couple to a transduction system capable of generating intracellular second messengers. Recently. phospho lipid hydrolysis products, DG(diacylglycerol) and IP_3 (inositol trisphosphate), have been demonstrated to serve a second messenger function for numerous receptors known not to be coupled to adenylate cyclase. Studies of thyrotropin-releasing hormone(TRH) action in clonal pituitary cells(GH_3) have provided a model system for investigating receptor-associated polyphosphoinositide hydrolysis.

TRH exerts a number of well-characterized effects on pituitary cells including the acute regulation of secretion. TRH rapidly stimulates the hydrolysis of phosphatidylinositol 4,5-bisphosphate to DG and IP_3. Evidence for the involvement of DG(activator of protein kinase C) and IP_3(mobilization of intracellular Ca^{2+}) as mediators of TRH stimulation of secretion has been obtained.

If TRH receptors are coupled to phosphoinositide hydrolysis, it should be possible to demonstrate direct effects of the hormone on hydrolysis in isolated membranes. In recent studies, TRH was found to stimulate the generation of IP_3 and DG by purified plasma membrane from GH_3 cells. Hormonal stimulation was half-maximal at the receptor K_D and was found to require GTP. Stimulation by TRH was fully antagonized by a stable GDP analog(GDP-β-S). Stable GTP analogs(GTP-γ-S) and fluoride ion were also found to stimulate hydrolysis to an extent similar to TRH+GTP. Stimulation by TRH was also found to require Ca^{2+} with optimal stimulation evident at 10^{-7}M, the resting cytosolic [Ca^{2+}] in GH_3 cells. Pretreatment of cells with cholera or pertussis toxin did not influence basal or stimulated hydrolysis in membranes.

These results demonstrate direct in vitro effects of a hormone on phospholipid hydrolysis in plasma membranes. TRH receptor-mediated activation may involve a GTP-binding factor analogous to N_s and N_i involved in receptor-regulated adenylate cyclase; however, the GTP-binding factor appears to be distinct from these.

ENZYMATIC DEGRADATION AND BIOLOGICAL INACTIVATION OF NEUROPEPTIDES 227

K. Bauer, Institut für Biochemie, TU Berlin, Franklinstr. 29, D-1000 Berlin 10, Germany

For neuropeptides, the rapid inactivation seems to be a mandatory process and a prerequisite to their functions as neuronal communication factors. This is especially true for neuropeptides with very short duration of action and high frequency of release. Present evidence strongly suggests that these substances are not removed through energy dependent uptake processes but inactivated by enzymatic hydrolysis.

So far, various peptidases capable of degrading TRH, LH-RH, Neurotensin, Substance P and the enkephalins have been identified and characterized. Based on these studies specific tests could be developed for the selective determination of the individual peptidasic activities and thus the subcellular localization of these enzymes as well as the distribution of the plasma-membrane bound enzymes between neuronal and glial cells in primary culture as well as cultured pituitary cells could be determined. These studies demonstrated that certain plasma-membrane bound peptidases are heterogeneously distributed between different cell types, thus reflecting specialized functions. The physiological role of these enzymes, however, remains to be elucidated. Primarily dependent on their strategic localization in relation to a given peptidergic pathway, some neuronal peptidases (e.g. the membrane bound TRH-degrading enzyme which exhibits high substrate specifity or the bestatin-sensitive aminopeptidase on nerve cells) might be involved in turning off peptidergic signals while other peptidases more likely serve general scavenger functions (e.g. the "enkephalinase", E.C. 3.4. 21.11, which is primarily associated with glial cells). The synthesis of selective enzyme inhibitors and the availability of enzyme-specific antibodies will provide the tools to define more precisely the specific localization of these peptidases and thus their functions for the inactivation of peptidic communication factors at specific sites.

For the neuropeptide synthesizing cells, the biological function of intracellular peptidases for the regulation of intracellular peptide concentrations will also be discussed. (Supported by Deutsche Forschungsgemeinschaft)

HORMONE-RECEPTOR COUPLING MECHANISM IN THE ANTERIOR PITUITARY: MODULATION BY PROTEIN KINASE C ACTIVATORS AND CYCLIC AMP (cAMP). 228

P.L. Canonico.
Department of Pharmacology, University of Catania, School of Medicine, Catania, Italy.

Receptors for several neurotransmitters and neuropeptides at the pituitary act to either stimulate (GRF, CRF, VIP) or inhibit (dopamine, somatostatin) adenylate cyclase leading to an increase or decrease in the intracellular cAMP concentration. Other receptors cause the accumulation of multiple intracellular second messengers. For example, a primary post-receptor event for different prolactin stimulating factors, such as TRH, angiotensin II (AII) and neurotensin, seems to be the hydrolysis of phosphatidylinositol-4,5-bisphosphate to diacylglycerol (DG) which activates protein kinase C (PKC) and inositoltriphosphate (IP3), an intracellular messenger tightly linked to the release of Ca^{2+} from intracellular stores. As a secondary event in such a cascade, these peptides stimulate the hydrolysis of arachidonate from membrane phospholipids with subsequent generation of active metabolites. We investigated whether these systems are in some way interrelated and controlled by internal feedback mechanisms. Phorbol esters bind to and activate pituitary PKC. Preincubation of hypophyseal cells with these tumor promoters, or with the synthetic DG, OAG, produces a significant inhibition of TRH-, AII- or neurotensin-stimulated IP3 accumulation, suggesting a potential operational mode of self-control of the phosphoinositide-PKC cascade. The same PKC activators amplify the ability of GRF, VIP, and PGE_1 to increase pituitary cAMP levels in short-time preincubations. However, they markedly reduce GRF-stimulated cAMP concentration after 24h and 12h pretreatments. On the other hand, in cells preincubated for 24 h (but not for 30 min, 1 or 3 h) with 8-Br-cAMP, dibutyryl cAMP, or cholera toxin, the accumulation of IP3 produced by TRH, AII or neurotensin is significantly inhibited. These results indicate that, subsequent to the activation of a pituitary receptor by a specific hypothalamic factor only one of the transducing signals seems to function initially, but it seems that both may interact during later stages of hormone release. They may function in concert providing sinergistic effects, but they may also interact each other, regulating also receptor number and function.

GROWTH HORMONE RELEASING HORMONE (GHRH)

M.O. Thorner, M.L. Vance, W.S. Evans, C. Brook, P. Smith, G.J. Klingensmith, J. Chitwood, R. Furlanetto, J. Rivier, W. Vale, A.D. Rogol, R.M. Blizzard, University of Virginia School of Medicine, Charlottesville, VA; Middlesex Hospital, London, England; Children's Hospital, Denver, CO; Children's Hospital of Philadelphia, Philadelphia, PA; and Salk Institute, San Diego, CA 229

GHRH exists as 40 and 44 amino acid hypothalamic peptides; full biological activity is retained in the first 29 amino acids. GHRH is secreted at the median eminence from hypothalamic infundibular neurons. Pulses of GH secretion results from simultaneous GHRH secretion and diminished somatostatin. GH secretion in man is pulsatile and varies with age, sex, and development. Twenty-four hour secretory profiles of GH reveal that plasma estradiol correlates positively with GH secretion. Administration of GHRH in man selectively stimulates GH secretion. Studies in GH deficient children suggest that many suffer from a hypothalamic neurosecretory disturbance rather than a somatotrope defect. Preliminary studies of GHRH therapy for GH deficient children with subcutaneous administration and various treatment schedules have been performed. Fourteen children have received GHRH for at least 6 months. Three children received twice daily injections of 4 ug/kg/dose; 11 were given the peptide via a peristaltic pump (Pulsamat; Ferring) as a dose every 3 h either only overnight (1-3 ug/kg/dose; n=6), or throughout the 24 hour period (n=5). Two children were withdrawn from the study at 6 and 7 months because of poor response and non-compliance, respectively. Eleven of 14 children had an increase in growth rate during GHRH therapy. Since continuous administration of GHRH produces pulsatile GH secretion, GHRH was administered i.v. for 14 days to 5 normal men. GH levels were measured every 20 minutes before, after 14 days of GHRH and 14 days later. GH secretion before and during GHRH administration was pulsatile and there was augmentation by GHRH of GH pulses. Serum IGF1 levels increased on day 14 of GHRH and fell 14 days after withdrawal. These findings indicate that the somatotrope remains responsive to GHRH during continuous exposure for a prolonged period of time and establishes a rationale for the development of a long-acting GHRH preparation for treatment of GH deficient children.

PATHOLOGY OF PITUITARY ADENOMAS

K. Kovacs
Department of Pathology, St. Michael's Hospital, University of Toronto, Toronto, Ontario, Canada 230

Pituitary adenomas are frequent neoplasms originating in and consisting of adenohypophysial cells. On the grounds of histologic, immunohistochemical and electron microscopic studies, they can be classified into the following morphologically distinct entities: 1) densely or sparsely granulated somatotroph adenoma; 2) densely or sparsely granulated lactotroph adenoma; 3) densely or sparsely granulated corticotroph adenoma; 4) thyrotroph adenoma; 5) gonadotroph adenoma; 6) null cell adenoma; 7) oncocytoma; 8) plurihormonal adenoma.

All known cell types of the human pituitary can give rise to adenoma and all established adenohypophysial hormones can be synthesized and released from adenoma cells. Prolactin-producing adenomas represent the most common adenoma type in the human pituitary. Thyrotroph adenomas are seen most often in patients with long-standing primary hypothyroidism. Gonadotroph adenomas in men differ in morphologic appearance from those of women. Null cell adenomas are unassociated with clinical or biochemical evidence of hormone excess. Although these tumors fail to possess morphologic markers which would reveal their cytogenesis, they invariably have secretory granules and all cytoplasmic organelles required for hormone secretion. Oncocytomas are endocrinologically inactive tumors characterized by abundance of mitochondria. Silent pituitary adenomas contain immunoreactive hormones, mainly ACTH but are unaccompanied by hormone oversecretion indicating that the stored hormones are not discharged, or they lack bioactivity. Plurihormonal adenomas produce more than one hormone, each differing in chemical composition, immunoreactivity and biologic action. They can be monomorphous or plurimorphous, i.e. composed of one or more than one cell type. In monomorphous adenomas, two or more hormones are produced in the same cell, whereas in plurimorphous adenomas, each hormone is produced in one morphologically distinct cell type. The cytogenesis of plurihormonal adenomas cannot be explained on the basis of the one cell- one hormone theory which dominates current thinking on pituitary cytopathology. (Supported in part by Grant MT-6349 awarded by the Medical Research Council of Canada)

COMBINATION THERAPY WITH FLUTAMIDE AND AN LHRH AGONIST IN ADVANCED PROSTATE CANCER. 232

F. Labrie, A. Dupont, M. Giguère, J.P. Borsanyi, A. Bélanger and Y. Lacourcière, Laval Univ. Med. Center, Quebec, Canada G1V 4G2

In order to achieve a more complete blockade of androgens of both testicular and adrenal origin at the start of treatment, we have administered the pure antiandrogen Flutamide in association with orchiectomy (13 patients) or the LHRH agonist [D-Trp^6] LHRH ethylamide (128 patients) to previously untreated patients having clinical stage D_2 prostate cancer. The main duration of treatment is 610 days (88 to 1367 days). Complete, partial and stable responses assessed according to the criteria of the U.S. NPCP have been observed in 26, 38 and 32% of patients, respectively, for a total objective response rate of 96% while progression has occurred in 4% of patients. The probability of continuing response (calculated according to Kaplan and Meier) after 2½ years of treatment is 42.5% while the probability of survival at the same time is 71%. The beneficial effect on survival becomes significant after 1 year of treatment. Two hundred and four patients showing relapse after orchiectomy, estrogens or LHRH agonists alone received the same combination therapy. Complete, partial and stable objective responses were observed in 5.4, 8.3 and 19.1% of patients, respectively, for a total objective response rate of 32.8%. The present data show that combination therapy applied at the start of treatment increases the rate of objective response, the length of the remission period and prolongs survival as compared to previous therapies. In relapsing patients, one third of them can still benefit from the combination therapy while, otherwise, progression would have continued. It is concluded that the combination therapy should be administered to all patients having advanced prostate cancer and continued for life without interruption in all cases. The beneficial effects of the combination therapy on response and survival are obtained with an excellent quality of life, the side effects being limited to hot flashes and a decrease or loss of libido.

CATECHOLAMINES AND ACTH RELEASE

E. Mezey, W.S. Young, R.E. Siegel
1st Dept. Anatomy, Budapest and LCB, NIMH, Bethesda 233

Catecholamines are known to induce ACTH release, but it has not yet been established whether they act directly on the pituitary or indirectly via a central mechenism. We showed earlier that β-adrenergic agonists may regulate pituitary ACTH cells. To determine whether this works through a peripheral or central route the pituitary was disconnected from the hypothalamus in a group of rats. In these as well as in controls ip. administered isoproterenol (25 µg) increased plasma ACTH levels. This increase could be blocked by propranolol (500 µg), a β-receptor antagonist. Further experiments showed that insulin (0.5U) also stimulates ACTH release in stalk transected rats and this increase can partially be blocked by propranolol. Since insulin itself does not affect ACTH release, the high adrenaline levels that accompany insulin induced hypoglycaemia may be responsible for the elevated ACTH levels. We concluded that there is a β-adrenergic receptor system in the pituitary corticotrophs and both peripheral and central ACTH secretagogues may release ACTH directly through these receptors.

The neurons that regulate ACTH release are located in the hypothalamic paraventricular nucleus (PVN). The same area receives a dense adrenergic innervation. To test the possible functional significance of this topographical overlap we used an inhibitor of the final enzyme in adrenaline biosynthesis (PNMT) to prevent the production of adrenaline in the CNS. There was a significant increase in the number of CRF immunopositive neurons in PVNs that were deprived of the adrenergic input. We also used in situ hybridization hystochemistry to measure the amount of CRF mRNA in these treated and control rats. We used an S^{35} labeled synthetic cDNA probe to localize CRF mRNA by autoradiography, and then compared the number of silver grains over the PVN in both groups. Our preliminary results indicate that the adrenergic innervation may have an inhibitory effect on CRF biosynthesis at the level of transcription of the CRF gene.

INVOLVEMENT OF GABA IN THE NEUROENDOCRINOLOGY OF REPRODUCTION 234

W. Wuttke
Div. Clin. Exp. Endocr.,Dept. ObGyn.,Univ. Göttingen,FRG

Recently we demonstrated that the great majority of estrogen receptive neurons in the rat preoptic anterior and mediobasal hypothalamic area use GABA as neurotransmitter. GABA turnover studies as well as pharmacological experiments utilizing GABA agonists indicated that this aminoacid neurotransmitter is inhibitory to LH release. Both, the pulsatile pattern in ovariectomized rats as well as the proestrous preovulatory LH surge can be blocked by the GABA agonist muscimol. GABA turnover and GABA release rates in the preoptic area as measured by the push-pull cannula technique are high in animals under the negative feedback action of estradiol and low in ovariectomized animals and in animals in which estrogen exerts a positive feedback action on LH. Furthermore, release rates correlate excellently in an inverse manner with LH pulses in the blood. Each LH episode is preceded by a drop of preoptic GABA release rates.

Involvement of GABAergic neurons in regulating prolactin release is also suggested by results from push-pull cannula experiments performed in the mediobasal hypothalamus. GABA release rates in the MBH of ovariectomized rats fluctuate largely whereas a few GABA release episodes are observed in estrogen primed rats. The latter animals have therefore similar mean GABA release rates as ovx non-primed rats but significantly less variance of the mean. They have also significantly increased blood prolactin levels in the afternoon as an expression of the positive feedback action of estradiol. These results suggest that pulsatile GABA release may have signal character for pituitary prolactin release. In summary, GABAergic neurons in the preoptic area seem to be involved in regulating pulsatility of the LHRH neurons. Other GABAergic neurons located in the MBH appear to be involved in the regulation of pituitary prolactin release. Whether the estrogen receptive GABAergic neurons in these structures are the predominant release sources of GABA remains to be determined.

CHANGING HYPOTHALAMIC FUNCTION AND ITS ROLE IN AGING OF THE FEMALE REPRODUCTIVE SYSTEM 235

P.M. Wise, I.R. Cohen-Becker, N.G. Weiland
Department of Physiology, University of Maryland School of Medicine, Baltimore, MD 21201, U.S.A.

Age-related deterioration of the female reproductive system is apparent in many mammalian species during middle age. In young sexually mature mammals, normal cyclic gonadotropin release depends upon complex interactions between the hypothalamus, anterior pituitary and ovaries. Evidence suggests that changes in each component of this axis contribute to declining reproductive capacity during middle-age. Our research has focused on alterations in hypothalamic neurotransmitter function that occur as rats enter the middle-age transition from regular to irregular estrous cycles. We have found that proestrous and estradiol-induced LH surges are attenuated in amplitude and delayed in timing in middle-aged rats. To determine whether altered patterns of gonadotropin release may be due to altered neurotransmitter activity, norepinephrine, dopamine and serotonin activity was analysed in several brain nuclei known to be involved in the regulation of cyclic gonadotropin release. Young (3-4 month old) and middle-aged (8-11 month old) rats that were ovariectomized and treated with Silastic capsules containing estradiol dissolved in oil were used. Turnover rates were assessed during the morning, the afternoon and the evening, prior to, during and after the LH surge, respectively. Marked changes in the diurnal rhythm of norepinephrine and serotonin were detected particularly in anterior hypothalamic areas. The integrity of these brain areas is critical to the maintenance of multiple biological rhythms, including cyclic reproductive function. Therefore, these data suggest that changes in the maintenance of neurotransmitter rhythms occur early in the aging process and may affect the ability of middle-aged rats to maintain regular estrous cycles.

Supported by NIH AG-02224 and HD-15955 to PMW, AG-05351 to IRC-B and AG05357 to NGW

CONTROL OF LUTEINIZING HORMONE SECRETION BY OVARIAN HORMONE-MONOAMINE-NEUROPEPTIDE INTERACTIONS 236

W.R. Crowley, The University of Tennessee, Memphis, TN

In female rats, the secretion of LH is under feedback regulation by the ovarian hormones, and there is increasing evidence that these controls are exerted via changes in the activity of monoaminergic and peptidergic systems that control the neurosecretion of LHRH. Results of pharmacological and neurochemical studies suggest that the adrenergic and noradrenergic systems innervating the medial preoptic area and medial basal hypothalamus are activated by the ovarian hormones to regulate the processing and the release of LHRH from the median eminence. In addition, the serotonergic innervation to the medial preoptic area appears to provide a stimulatory influence on LH secretion that can be activated specifically by progesterone. The targets of ovarian hormone feedback may be intrahypothalamic systems that regulate the release of monoamines, and therefore, gate the synaptic input to the LHRH neurosecretory cells. Agonists at GABA B and endogenous opioid peptide receptors block ovarian hormone-induced LH surges and the associated increases in NE and EPI turnover. Conversely, opiate antagonists mimic the stimulatory actions of steroids on LH and LHRH release and on catecholaminergic activity. Thus, a mechanism of ovarian hormone positive feedback may be the removal of inhibitory GABAergic and endogenous opioid influences on the release of catecholamines and LHRH. In addition to these interactions, neuropeptide Y(NPY) may serve as a co-transmitter with and/or may act in concert with central catecholamines in the control of LH secretion. After central administration, NPY produces norepinephrine-like effects on LH release that are not due simply to release of catecholamines. Ovarian hormone treatment produces parallel changes in NPY and LHRH in the median eminence, suggesting an interaction of these two peptides. Similar to norepinephrine and epinephrine, NPY stimulates the release of LHRH from the median eminence in vitro, and, in addition, NPY appears to exert a second effect to enhance the response of the pituitary gland to LHRH.

LOCALIZATION OF β-ENDORPHIN (β-END), MET-ENKEPHALIN (MET-ENK) AND NEUROTENSIN (NT) IN THE RAT HYPOTHALAMUS: AN IMMUNOHISTOCHEMICAL STUDY. 237

K.Ajika, K.Arai, S.Okinaga
Teikyo University School of Medicine, Tokyo, Japan

The distribution of β-END, MET-ENK and NT in the hypothalamus were investigated using the Avidin-Biotin immunoperoxidase technique. Sprague-Dawley rats were intraventricularly treated with colchicine 24 hours before sacrifice. The animals were fixed by cardiac perfusion with 4% paraformaldehyde. Hypothalamic sections were cut in a cryostat and serially incubated in normal goat serum, β-END (or MET-ENK or NT) antiserum, goat anti-rabbit IgG, Avidin-Biotin complex and 3,3'-diaminobenzidine-H_2O_2.

A distinctive group of β-END, MET-ENK or NT immunoreactive cell bodies was observed within the paraventricular, supraoptic and arcuate nucleus. The distribution pattern of these three neurohormone immunoreactive cells, however, were apparently different. The MET-ENK immunoreactive cell group were also found in the ventromedial nucleus and NT positive cells were found in the lateral hypothalamus. A small number of β-END immunoreactive nerve terminals were found in the internal and external layer of the median eminence. Two weeks after hypophysectomy, a number of β-END immunoreactive nerve terminals appeared in the external and internal layer of the median eminence. In the median eminence of the normal control rat, a dense meshwork of the MET-ENK and NT immunoreactive nerve terminals was observed exclusively in the external layer abutting on the portal vessels. The elution-restaining technique did not show any co-existence of these three neurohormones in the same neuron of the hypothalamus, although the abovementioned two or three neurohormones have been reported to co-exist in various combination in the same cell of the anterior or medial lobe of the hypophysis.

The present findings suggest that β-END, MET-ENK and NT have distinct neuronal system in the hypothalamus and that β-END as well as MET-ENK and NT is released into the portal vessels of the median eminence to modulate the anterior pituitary function.

SUBSTANCE P- BUT NOT CHOLECYSTOKININ-IMMUNOREACTIVE HYPOTHALAMIC CELLS CONCENTRATE ESTROGEN 238

T.R. Akesson, A. Coquelin, P.E. Micevych
Dept. of Anatomy, CHS-UCLA, Los Angeles, CA 90024

Recent evidence indicates that gonadal steroids exert both organizational and activational effects on neuropeptide systems. In rats, sexual differences in distributions of substance P (SP) and cholecystokinin (CCK) have been reported and both peptides have been shown to vary in discrete hypothalamic areas during the estrous cycle. SP and CCK, in turn, are capable of releasing pituitary hormones. Intraventricular injection of SP stimulates, while CCK inhibits secretion of luteinizing hormone (LH) in female rats. In the case of CCK, the effect on LH secretion has been shown to be site specific because implants in the medial preoptic area stimulate release of LH. We have combined the techniques of steroid autoradiography and immunohistochemistry to test the possibility that some of these observations may be explained by a direct effect of estrogen on SP- and CCK-immunoreactive cells in the hypothalamus.

Autoradiograms were prepared according to the method of Morrell and Pfaff (1983, Meth. Enzymol. 103:639). They were postfixed in Bouin's solution, developed in D-170 (Kodak), photofixed in 10% sodium thiosulfate, and tissues were incubated with primary antiserum at room temperature for 48 h. Location of primary antibodies was visualized with the ABC method (Vector). Estrogen (E) concentrating cells were identified using a computer-assisted grain counter. Distribution of SP-, CCK-, and E-labeled neurons appeared to be comparable to results we have obtained from tissue optimally processed for immunohistochemistry or autoradiography separately.

While numerous cases of CCK- and E-labeled cells were found in close proximity in the anterior paraventricular and periventricular nuclei, no cases of coexistence were observed. In contrast, SP neurons which concentrate E were found in the lateral hypothalamus and arcuate nucleus, but the majority of cases were located in a posterolateral part of the ventromedial nucleus. Supported by NS21220 to P.E.M.

ADENOSINE 3',5'-CYCLIC MONOPHOSPHATE STIMULATES DOPAMINE SYNTHESIS IN THE MEDIAN EMINENCE OF RAT HYPOTHALAMIC SLICES 239

J. Arita, F. Kimura
Yokohama City University School of Medicine, Yokohama

The regulation of dopamine synthesis in tuberoinfundibular dopaminergic (TIDA) neurons by adenosine 3',5'-cyclic monophosphate (cAMP) was investigated. Dopamine synthesis in TIDA neurons was estimated by the rate of in vitro DOPA accumulation in the median eminence of rat hypothalamic slices after incubation with a DOPA decarboxylase inhibitor. Addition of dibutyryl cAMP (db-cAMP) into medium caused an increase in the rate of DOPA accumulation in the median eminence in a dose- and time-dependent manner. 8-Bromo-cAMP also increased the rate of DOPA accumulation in the median eminence and c-AMP was less effective than db-cAMP whereas neither adenosine nor sodium butyrate altered the rate of DOPA accumulation. An increase in the concentration of endogeneous cAMP achieved by addition into medium of isobutylmethylxanthine or forskolin was associated with an increase in the rate of DOPA accumulation in the median eminence. However, db-cAMP had almost negligible effect on the secretion of dopamine from the median eminence. The stimulatory effect of db-cAMP on DOPA accumulation in the median eminence was not dependent upon the presence of extracellular Ca^{2+} and was not blocked by tetrodotoxin. Furthermore, the stimulation of DOPA accumulation induced by db-cAMP was additive with that induced by high potassium depolarization, suggesting that dopamine synthesis in TIDA neurons is distinctly regulated by Ca^{2+} and c-AMP.

REGIONALIZATION OF THE DIRECT ARTERIAL BLOOD SUPPLY AND PRL CONTENT OF THE ANTERIOR PITUITARY OF RABBITS 240

M. Bamat, G. Martinez-Escalera, R. Weiner
Reprod. Endo. Center, UCSF, San Francisco, CA 94143

In most mammalian species the blood supply of the anterior pituitary (AP) is exclusively via the hypophyseal portal system. Conflicting evidence exists that a portion of the AP blood supply in rabbits is via a direct arterial source. Regions of the AP receiving arterial blood would presumably escape tonic hypothalamic inhibition of PRL secretion. Therefore, we have determined whether (1) a direct arterial blood supply exists in regions of the AP in female New Zealand white rabbits; and (2) there are regional differences in PRL content in the gland. Fourteen µm microspheres when injected into the left ventricle of the heart can only reach the AP via a direct arterial supply. Microspheres reached the AP of rabbits and were found in largest numbers in the rostral-lateral regions. Vascular cast studies showed the source of these vessels to be from branches of the internal carotid or posterior communicating arteries. To describe the regionalization of PRL content the AP gland was frozen and sectioned at 300 µm rostro-caudal or latero-medial. PRL was measured by a homologous radioimmunoassay (A. Parlow). In 10 of 11 AP from intact, ovariectomized (OVX) or OVX-E_2 treated rabbits a steadily increasing rostral-caudal gradient in (PRL) was observed rising 3-100 fold. In 3 intact rabbits no gradient was seen latero-medially. Treatment of OVX rabbits for 2 weeks with a 4 cm silastic implant of E_2 increased mean AP (PRL) from 115.9 ± 41 µg/mg prot. (n=4) to 262 ± 49 µg/mg prot. (n=3). Serum levels of PRL in conscious, undisturbed animals sampled through indwelling left ventricular catheters were also significantly elevated in OVX-E_2 vs OVX rabbits: 14.3 ± 3.1 ng/ml vs 1.98 ± 1.12, respectively. In summary, in female NZW rabbits we observed 1) A direct arterial supply to the rostro-lateral AP; and 2) Regional differences in (PRL) with an increasing rostral-caudal gradient. Future studies will determine the relationship of the regionalized arterial blood supply to the secretion of PRL. This work was supported by NIH grant HD 08935.

PITUITARY-ADRENAL AXIS RESPONSE TO NALOXONE IN NORMALS AND IN PATIENTS WITH DEXAMETHASONE SUPPRESSIBLE HYPERALDOSTERONISM 240a

M.Boscaro, F.Fallo, N.Sonino, A.Rampazzo, F.Mantero
Institute of Semeiotica Medica, University of Padua, Italy

There is evidence that adrenal steroid secretion is modulated by opioid compounds via a pituitary dependent mechanism. However, a role of opiates in the direct control of adrenal steroidogenesis has not been ruled out as yet. We tested the response of the pitutary-adrenal axis to high-dose naloxone (NL) compared to placebo in 8 normal volunteers and in 2 patients with Dexamethasone-Suppressible Hyperaldosteronsim (DSH). 10 mg NL were injected as a bolus iv at 09.00 h in all subjects, maintained in recumbent position. Blood samples were drawn at 0,15,30,45,60, 90 min. Data are given as mean±SEM and analyzed by 2 way ANOVA with repeated measures. In normals NL caused a significant ($P < 0.01$; ANOVA F 35.5) increase of pl.cortisol from 8.76±0.97 to 16.36±1.83 µg/dl at 45 min, a slight but not significant increase of ACTH and no change in PRA and aldosterone (Aldo). In DSH patients there was a slight increase of cortisol, no change in ACTH and PRA and a marked rise of Aldo, from 10.9 to 28.7 and from 12.0 to 57.5 ng/dl at 15 min. Five normal subjects and the DSH patients were retested after dexamethasone (dex) 2 mg: baseline ACTH and cortisol were reduced and no response to NL was observed to NL alone. After dex, Aldo levels were suppressed in DSH patients and unchanged in normals, and did not respond to naloxone in any case. Conclusions: NL may increase the responsiveness of adrenal zona fasciculata to physiological levels of ACTH, since the slight increase in ACTH seems to be inadequate per se to explain the cortisol elevation after NL. ACTH levels after dex were probably too low to allow cortisol response to NL. Alternatively, NL might stimulate the release of dex-suppressible unknown pituitary factors with steroidogenic properties. Aldo response to NL supports the hypothesis of abnormal adrenocortical zonation of steroid biosynthesis in DSH.

EFFECTS OF CYSTEAMINE ON THE IN VIVO INCORPORATION OF [^{35}S]-CYSTEINE INTO SOMATOSTATIN-14, SOMATOSTATIN-28, ARGININE VASOPRESSIN, AND OXYTOCIN IN RAT HYPOTHALAMUS. 241

J.L. Cameron, J.D. Fernstrom
Department of Psychiatry and Center for Neuroscience, University of Pittsburgh, Pittsburgh PA 15213.

The effect of cysteamine injection was studied on the *in vivo* incorporation of [^{35}S]-cysteine into somatostatin-14, somatostatin-28, arginine vasopressin, and oxytocin in rat hypothalamus. [^{35}S]-cysteine was injected into the third ventricle 1hr, 4hr, or 1 week after cysteamine (300 mg/kg sc) injection. Animals were killed 4 hr later, and hypothalami were removed and homogenized, and the resulting supernatants either subjected to radioimmunoassay, or run over two sequential HPLC separations (Van Itallie and Fernstrom, Brain Research 249: 177, 1982; Fisher and Fernstrom, Life Sciences 28: 1471, 1981). Fractions were collected and counted for ^{35}S radioactivity; labeling of individual peptides was identified as radioactive peaks with the same retention times as the standard peptides. Cysteamine was observed to reduce substantially immunoreactive levels of somatostatin, but not of oxytocin or vasopressin, 4 hr after its injection. The drug also caused large reductions in label incorporation into somatostatin-14, somatostatin-28, and oxytocin 1 hr and 4 hr after its injection. However, [^{35}S]-cysteine incorporation into vasopressin was increased substantially at these timepoints, while that into acid-precipitable protein was normal. One week after cysteamine injection, label incorporation into all hypothalamic peptides was normal. Cysteine specific activity was also measured after [^{35}S]-cysteine injection, and was found to be comparable in treatment and control groups. These results suggest that cysteamine injection inhibits the syntheses of SRIF-14, SRIF-28, and OXT, and stimulates that of AVP.

POSSIBLE PHYSIOLOGICAL SIGNIFICANCE OF GLUCOCORTICOID INDUCED CHANGES OF OPIATE SENSITIVITY 241a

M.I.K. Fekete, Do Tanh Kiem, B. Kanyicska, E. Stark
Inst. Exptl. Med., Hung. Acad. Sci. Budapest, Hungary.

Glucocorticoids induce a characteristic decrease of the opiate sensitivity as it was shown formerly. Opiate peptides of different receptor specificities were given icv to rats and changes of prolactin, corticosterone and growth hormone levels were measured. Serial blood samples were taken via chronic catheter in jugular vein. It has been found that chronic treatment with glucocorticoids inhibited opiate induced prolactin, growth hormone and prolactin secretion. A 24 h pretreatment with hydrocortisone was also effective to inhibit the prolactin secretion, this effect could be inhibited by actinomycine D. Estradiol, progesterone and testosterone were ineffective to influence this opiate reaction. There was a daily rythm in the opiate induced hormonal responses. The prolactin response evoked by kappa agonists, as well as the growth hormone response caused by a delta agonist were higher in the afternoon than in the morning. Neither opiate agonist could increase the corticosterone secretion in the afternoon. These daily alterations were not demonstrable in adrenalectomized rats. It is concluded that the glucocorticoid induced changes in opiate sensitivity play an important role in physiological regulation of the release of hormones.

ANGIOTENSIN II SPECIFIC BINDING IN THE SUBCOMMISSURAL ORGAN OF NEWBORN MALE RATS 242

P.GHIANI and B.UVA
Istituto di Anatomia Comparata, Università di Genova, 16126 GENOVA ITALY

Previous researches (Uva et al., 1984, Gen. Comp. Endocrinol., 53, 448) showed that osmotic stress resulted in modifications of the secretory activity of the subcommissural organ (SCO) both in mammals and in reptiles suggesting a close correlation between renin activity and the secretion of the SCO.

Preliminary data carried out by RIA reported the presence of specific receptors for Ang II.

In the present investigation these data have been confirmed: specific and high affinity binding sites for Ang II were demonstrated in the membranes of the SCO of male rats by binding studies with iodinated Ang II. Only one type of angiotensin receptors was found (Scatchard analysis of the data: Kd = 24.6 ± 3.0 10^{-11}M;RT =15 ± 1 10^{-11} M).Affinity and capacity were reduced after sodium depletion (Kd = 20.0 ± 0.2 10^{-11} M; RT = 1.0 ± 0.01 10^{-11} M).
Affinity increased after sodium loading (Kd = 65.0 ± 4 10^{-11} M).

Autoradiographic analysis (stripping method) showed localization of 125 I Ang II (NEN 1.5 µCi) in the cells of the SCO and the immunohistochemical analysis (Coons and PAP meyhods, anserum anti Ile 5 Ang II) confirmed the localizations obtained by autoradiography.

From our data it may be suggested that besides other circumventricular organs as Subfornical organ, also the subcommissural organ is involved in water regulation.

UROTENSIN II IS VASODEPRESSOR IN RATS 243

A. Gibson, M. Ginsburg, H.A. Bern
Kings College, University of London, UK and University of California, Berkeley, USA.

Until recently urotensin II, a fish urophyseal peptide, has been considered devoid of significant activity in mammals. However, the recent demonstration of a smooth muscle relaxant effect of synthetic Gillichthys urotensin II (GUII) in mice prompted us to study its effect in other mammalian systems. We report here that GUII is vasodepressor in rats.

GUII (1.5 - 150 nmol/kg) caused a dose-dependent decrease in diastolic, and to a lesser extent systolic,pressure in urethane-anaesthetised rats. The response was slow in onset, reaching a peak 4 - 5 min after GUII administration, and long-lasting (up to 60 min). Heart rate was elevated ; this effect of GUII, but not the hypotension, was blocked by the β-adrenoceptor antagonist propranolol (1 µmol/kg). The histamine (H1) receptor antagonist mepyramine (1 µmol/kg) affected neither the hypotension nor the tachycardia.

In pithed rats, 150 nmol/kg GUII reduced (by 50%) pressor responses to sympathetic nerve stimulation (10 Hz stimulation of spinal outflows T7 - T13), but had no effect on heart rate. Pressor responses to noradrenaline (500 pmol/kg) and Arg-vasopressin (8 mU/kg) were also reduced by about 50%. GUII shows partial sequence homology with somatostatin. However, somatostatin (150 nmol/kg) produced different effects in the pithed rat, having no effect on sympathetic pressor responses but reducing basal heart rate.

Thus, the results of this study confirm that GUII possesses significant activity in mammals. In rats, it causes a slow, long-lasting hypotension associated with reflex tachycardia. This action is not somatostatin like and probably results from GUII-induced vasodilatation. The mechanism of the vasodilatation and the vascular beds involved are under study.

HYPOTHALAMIC REGULATION OF PLASMA RENIN ACTIVITY: EFFERENT PATHWAYS 244

E. Gotoh, K. Murakami, R. Golin and W.F. Ganong
Department of Physiology, University of California, San Francisco, California 94143, U.S.A.

In previous studies (Karteszi, et al., Neuroendo. 34: 233, 1982; Gotoh, et al., Physiologist 28:313, 1985) we demonstrated that the mediobasal hypothalamus and particularly the paraventricular nuclei were involved in the regulation of plasma renin activity (PRA). To determine whether vasopressin-secreting and oxytocin-secreting neurons projecting from the hypothalamus to the brain stem or spinal cord are involved, we have studied (1) the effects of various stimuli on PRA in Brattleboro rats, which are unable to synthesize vasopressin in their brains; and (2) the effects of intraventricular (IVT) injection of an oxytocin agonist on PRA.

Resting PRA was elevated in Brattleboro rats and the increase in PRA produced by the serotonin-releasing drug p-chloroamphetamine was greater than normal. The PRA responses to immobilization and to head-up tilt were also potentiated.

The effect of IVT administration of the oxytocin agonist [Thr^4, Gly^7]-Oxytocin on PRA was studied in conscious rats, and the effects of the same compound on arterial blood pressure and heart rate were studied in inactin anesthetized rats. 0.1 and 1 nmol had no effect on PRA 10 min after injection, but 2 and 5 nm produced significant increases. Mean PRA in controls injected with artificial spinal fluid was 10.6±1.4 ng AI/ml/3hr compared to 20.6±3.1 and 23.7±2.7 in rats receiving 2 and 5 nmol of the agonist. There were no significant changes in arterial blood pressure or heart rate.

Although preliminary, these findings suggest that oxytocin-secreting efferents to the brain stem or spinal cord may mediate increases in renin secretion. The vasopressin-secreting neurons may exert inhibitory effects. However, the results in Brattleboro rats could also be explained by hypertropy of the juxtaglomerular cells due to chronic stimulation of renin secretion because of the vasopressin deficiency. (Supported by NASA Grant NAGW 490, the Am. Heart Assoc., Smokeless Tobacco Res. Council, and USPHS Grant HL29714).

CENTRAL EFFECTS OF CORTICOTROPIN-RELEASING FACTOR (CRF) ON PENTOBARBITAL-INDUCED ANESTHESIA AND HYPOTHERMIA IN RAT 245

T.Imaki, T.Shibasaki, A.Masuda, H.Demura, K.Shizume
Institute of Clinical Endocrinology, Tokyo Women's Medical College, Tokyo 162, Japan

We examined the effect of CRF on pentobarbital (PbNa)-induced sleeping time and hypothermia in rats. Polyethylene tube was implanted into the right lateral ventricle of Wistar male rats weighing 180-200g 4 days before the experiment. Peptide solution or vehicle alone was administered through the ventricular cannula just before PbNa injection (50 mg/Kg). Vehicle administered rats were used as a control. The duration between loss of the righting reflex and recovery of this reflex was considered to be sleeping time. Rectal temperature was recorded 0, 20, 40 and 60 min. after PbNa injection. The temperature of the experimental room was about 23°C.

Intraventricular administration of CRF significantly shortened sleeping time induced by PbNa in a dose dependent manner (Control: 69.2±5.6 min., 0.2 nmol CRF: 52.4±4.1 min., 2 nmol CRF: 44.7±2.8 min., P<0.01), whereas peripheral administration of CRF had no effect on sleeping time (Control: 88.2±5.8 min., 2 nmol CRF: 92.7±5.7 min.). CRF at a dose of 0.2 nmol significantly reversed hypothermia induced by PbNa (Rectal temperature at 60 min.,; Control: 36.51±0.14°C, 0.2 nmol CRF: 37.14±0.18°C P<0.05). When administered peripherally, CRF did not affect rectal temperature. CRF antagonist, α-helical CRF 9-41, at the dose of 2 nmol reversed the antagonistic effects of 0.2 nmol of CRF on PbNa (Sleeping time; Vehicle alone: 79.0±4.8 min., 0.2 nmol CRF: 45.2±3.0 min., 0.2 nmol CRF + 2 nmol α-helical CRF : 63.2±3.0 min., Rectal temperature; Vehicle alone: 35.81±0.22°C, 0.2 nmol CRF: 36.95±0.20°C, 0.2 nmol CRF+ 2 nmol α-helical CRF: 36.38±0.32°C.).

These results suggest that CRF antagonizes the pharmacological effects of PbNa on anesthesia and hypothermia via the central nervous system and that CRF antagonist, α-helical CRF 9-41, attenuates the effect of CRF on PbNa.

POSSIBLE ROLE OF LEUMORPHIN, AN OPIOID PEPTIDE, IN CENTRAL REGULATION OF FLUID BALANCE IN RATS 246

H. Imura, N. Nakao, T. Yamada, H. Itoh, S. Shiono, M. Sakamoto, N. Morii, A. Sugawara, Y. Saito
Kyoto University Faculty of Medicine, Kyoto, Japan

Leumorphin is a 29 amino acid peptide derived from preproenkephalin B, having potent opiate-like activity. Since immunoreactive leumorphin exists in high concentrations in the rat hypothalamus, we studied the effect of intracerebroventricular (icv) injection of leumorphin on drinking behavior and vasopressin release in rats. Icv injection of leumorphin dose-dependently inhibited water intake induced by water deprivation. Drinking induced by icv injections of angiotensin II (AII) and carbachol was also dose-dependently inhibited by leumorphin. The effect of leumorphin was potent; 0.6 pmol of leumorphin inhibited AII-induced drinking and 6 pmol of leumorphin inhibited deprivation-induced drinking. Although leumorphin stimulated general locomotor activity, a larger dose (0.3 nmol) was required for significantly enhanced motor activity. It is unlikely, therefore, that antidipsogenic effect of leumorphin was due to the interference by other behavioral effects. The effect of leumorphin was partially counteracted by naloxone and naloxone alone partially inhibited drinking. To further explore the physiological significance of antidipsogenic effect of leumorphin, anti-leumorphin antiserum was injected icv. This tended to enhance drinking behavior induced by AII and water deprivation. Dynorphin 1 - 17, another opioid peptide derived from preproenkephalin B, was almost as active as leumorphin in inhibiting drinking. Icv injection of AII also caused vasopressin release in conscious, unrestrained rats and this effect was almost completely inhibited by icv injection of leumorphin.

These results suggest that leumorphin together with other preproenkephalin B-derived peptides plays a role in the central regulatory mechanisms of body fluid balance.

LINKAGE OF ADRENAL MEDULLARY OPIOID RECEPTORS TO GTP-BINDING PROTEINS, PERTUSSIS TOXIN SUBSTRATES 247

K. Kamikubo, H. Murase, M. Niwa*, K. Miura, M. Nozaki*, and K. Tsurumi*
Departments of Internal Medicine (III) and *Pharmacology Gifu University School of Medicine, Gifu 500, Japan.

GTP-binding regulatory proteins (G proteins) play crucial roles in signal transduction of membrane receptors. At least three G proteins (Gs, Gi and Go) have been identified, which mediate hormonal regulation of adenylate cyclase, phospholipase C, K channel, Ca channel etc.. Gi and Go are known to be ADP-ribosylated by pertussis toxin (PT). In this study, we have examined effects of guanine nucleotides and PT on the bovine adrenal medullary opioid receptor system in an attempt to clarify modes of actions of opioid peptides in this tissue.

In control membranes, Gpp(NH)p inhibited specific binding of (3H)D-Ala-D-Leu-enkephalin ((3H)DADLE) by increasing the dissociation constant. Gpp(NH)p enhanced (3H)diprenorphine binding to control membranes. In PT-treated membranes, (3H)DADLE binding was reduced to 80% of that in control membranes. Furthermore, Gpp(NH)p inhibition of (3H)DADLE binding was almost abolished following the PT treatment. Contrary, (3H)-diprenorphine binding to PT-treated membranes was enhanced to 120% compared to control membranes. These actions of PT on opioid binding were paralleled with (32P)ADP-ribosylation of membrane proteins.

DADLE and levorphanol inhibited adenylate cyclase activity in rat brain striatal membranes. However, they little inhibited adenylate cyclase activity in both control and PT-treated membranes of bovine adrenal medulla.

The present results indicate that adrenal medullary opioid receptors are linked to G proteins, substrates for PT. Rat brain striatal opioid receptors are coupled to inhibition of adenylate cyclase via Gi (Kamikubo et al. Japan. J. Pharmacol. 31, 175; Kamikubo et al. Japan. J. Pharmacol. 32, 893). In contrast, it is unlikely that G proteins linked to adrenal medullary opioid receptors are directly coupled to adenylate cyclase.

EFFECT OF CENTRAL LHRH MANIPULATION ON THE SKIN TEMPERATURE RESPONSE IN AN ANIMAL MODEL FOR THE HOT FLUSH 248

Michael J. Katovich, J.W. Simpkins and J. O'Meara
Department of Pharmacodynamics, University of Florida, Gainesville, FL 32610

There are numerous reports of a temporal relationship between LH secretion and a subsequent flushing response in menopausal women. We have developed an animal model for the hot flush which also demonstrates a surge in LH secretion preceeding the elevation in skin temperature in the rat. In the present study, we utilized central administration of an LHRH agonist and antagonist to evaluate the skin temperature response in our animal model. Ovariectomized female rats were fitted with unilateral cannula in the lateral ventricle (LV). One week later these animals were mildly restrained to allow for continuous measurement of tail skin temperatures (TST). Administration of 5, 10, or 20 µg of the LHRH agonist (des-Gly^{10},[im-Bzl-D-His^{6}]-LHRH Ethylamide) into the LV produced a similar elevation of TST of $4^{o}C$ in the morphine-dependent rats. However, elevations of $0.4 \pm 0.4^{o}C$, $1.2 \pm 0.6^{o}C$ and $4.0 \pm 1.0^{o}C$ were observed in the control animals at the respective doses. Central administration of naloxone was without effect in controls but produced a $5^{o}C$ rise of TST in the morphine-dependent rat while central administration of 10 µl of the saline vehicle produced no changes in TST in either group. Thus, it appears that the morphine-dependent rat is more sensitive to the LHRH agonist and the temperature response is similar to that observed following administration of a dose of naloxone which we have previously shown to produce an LH surge and elevation in TST. An LHRH antagonist ([D-$Phe^{2,6}$,Pro^{3}] - LHRH) at a concentration of 10 or 20 µg/10 µl in the LV blocked the rise in TST associated with systemic administration of naloxone (1 mg/kg, sc) in morphine-dependent rats. Collectively, these data indicate that activation of central LHRH receptors may initiate the temperature response observed during the hot flush and further support the hypothesis that activation of the LHRH neuron may be involved in the pathogenesis of the hot flush syndrome. (Supported by NIH grant HD 8133-03)

HYPOTHALAMIC MU OPIOID RECEPTORS DURING PREGNANCY AND AFTER PARTURITION. 249

P. Limonta, D. Dondi, R. Maggi, M. Motta, F. Piva
Department of Endocrinology, University of Milano, Italy.

It is known that brain β-endorphin (β-E) concentration increases in pregnant rats. It was then analyzed whether also the binding characteristics of hypothalamic mu receptors, to which preferentially β-E binds, undergo some modifications during pregnancy and after parturition. The number of binding sites (Bmax) and the affinity constant (Ka) for 3H-dihydromorphine (3H-DHM), a typical mu receptor ligand, were measured by a receptor binding assay in hypothalamic membrane preparations derived from rats killed at 7, 15, 22 days of pregnancy and 6-18 hours after parturition, and from lactating and non lactating dams killed 6-8 days post-partum. Females killed in the day of estrus served as controls. In all the groups considered also serum prolactin levels were measured by radioimmunoassay. The results show that the number of hypothalamic mu receptors increases during pregnancy, being significantly higher than in controls at days 15 and 22 of pregnancy, decreases immediately after parturition, and remains low in the postpartum period regardless of whether females are lactating or not. The Ka for 3H-DHM did not change in the hypothalami of the different groups of animals. Prolactin serum titers were significantly increased at day 22 of pregnancy and 6-8 days after parturition in lactating females. Conclusions: 1) the observed increase of hypothalamic mu receptors before parturition confirms that the opioid tone is enhanced during pregnancy. 2) No clear correlations appear to exist between the number of hypothalamic mu receptors and serum prolactin levels. 3) Possibly, during pregnancy and after parturition opioid system(s) are involved in mechanisms other than hormone release control (pain perception, maternal behavior?) (Supported by a grant from the C.N.R., no. 85.00715.56).

IN VIVO ACTH TREATMENT ALTERS IN VITRO RESPONSE OF TESTICULAR INTERSTITIAL CELLS TO HCG 250

D.R. Mann, M.M. Smith, C. Nelson, C.L. Free
Morehouse School of Medicine, Atlanta, GA 30310.

We reported previously that ACTH infusion for 3 days reduces basal testosterone (T) secretion and T response to GnRH in adult male rats. These effects occur independent of an effect on LH secretion. In this study, we determined the effect of ACTH on sensitivity of interstitial cells to HCG. Male rats were treated for 3 days, or 4 or 8 wk with 20 ug/day of ACTH using minipumps. ACTH treatment for 3 days reduced serum T values relative to control values. Serum corticosterone (B) was elevated 15-fold by ACTH. Interstitial cells from these rats were incubated for 2 or 4 h with or without 5 IU of HCG. Basal T production and T response to HCG was reduced 50% by prior ACTH treatment. At 4 h, basal and HCG-stimulated T production by interstitial cells from ACTH-treated rats did not differ from controls. Four wk of ACTH treatment increased adrenal weight, lowered testes and seminal vesicles weight, and reduced body weight gain. In these rats, serum B was elevated 50-fold, serum T was reduced by 50%. Basal and HCG-stimulated T secretion by interstitial cells from ACTH-treated rats was less than 40% of control values. At the end of 8 wk of ACTH treatment, rats showed a degree of escape from the effects of ACTH. During the last 2 wk of treatment, body weight gain was comparable to control rats. Moreover, adrenal weights were less, and seminal vesicles and testes size greater after 8 wk than after 4 wk of ACTH treatment. Serum B in rats at 8 wk of ACTH treatment was lower, and serum T comparable to control values. Interstitial cells from these rats exhibited normal basal and HCG-stimulated T secretion. These data show that ACTH treatment is associated with a reduction in the sensitivity of the testes to gonadotropin. However, when treatment is extended beyond 4 wk, the adrenals cease to respond to ACTH, causing a decline in adrenal activity, and the testes recover their normal sensitivity to gonadotropin. (DRR-08006).

EFFECTS OF CHOLECYSTOKININ ON RENAL FUNCTION IN SHEEP 251

J.G. McDougall, A.R. Coker, J.P. Coghlan, D.A. Denton, B.A. Scoggins
Howard Florey Institute of Experimental Physiology & Medicine, Parkville, Vic. 3052 Australia.

A relationship between delivery of sodium into the gastrointestinal tract and renal function has been postulated by a number of authors. Reported renal effects of a number of neuropeptides, including VIP and neurotensin, have been contradictory and may depend on the state of experimental animal and the species. In this paper the effects of cholecystokinin on renal function are examined.

Experiments were undertaken on conscious sodium replete sheep in which the renal artery and vein of a sole kidney were chronically cannulated. Cholecystokinin octapeptide (sulphated CCK_8) was infused for 2 h into the renal artery of 6 sheep at 4.5, 15, 45 and 150 µg/h on separate occasions. Sodium excretion increased in a dose related manner - from 157 ± 13 to 232 ± 21 µmol/min at 45 µg/h ($p<0.001$) and from 131 ± 16 to 335 ± 30 µmol/min ($p<0.001$) at 180 µg/h in the first hour of infusion. Urinary excretion of potassium, calcium and chloride all increased, but glomerular filtration rate and effective renal plasma flow were unchanged. CCK_8 was infused at the equivalent rate into the venous circulation and similar changes in renal function were observed. Sodium excretion increased from 171 ± 18 to 221 ± 23 µmol/min ($p<0.05$) at 45 µg/h and from 98 ± 12 to 224 ± 31 µmol/min ($p<0.001$) at 180 µg/hr. The data suggest that cholecystokinin stimulates natriuresis in conscious sheep via a second natriuretic mechanism or by release of a natriuretic hormone such as ANP.

The natriuretic response is specific to CCK_8 and was not observed following infusion of CCK_8 (unsulphated form), CCK_4, VIP, neurotensin, secretin or somatostatin.

POSSIBLE ROLE OF DYNORPHIN IN THE PATHOPHYSIOLOGY OF TRAUMATIC BRAIN INJURY. 251a

TK McIntosh and AI Faden. University of California, San Francisco.

Endogenous opioids have been implicated as secondary pathophysiologic factors in spinal cord injury and brain ischemia. However, there is no information available regarding the role of specific opioid peptides or of the mechanism of action of opiate antagonists in brain trauma. Cats (2.75-3.25 kg) were anesthetized with sodium pentobarbital (40 mg/kg), intubated, paralyzed with pancuronium (0.6 mg/kg) and artificially ventilated with 70% nitrous oxide and 30% oxygen; they were subsequently subjected to fluid-percussion (FP)-induced brain injury (3.2-3.6 atmospheres). Regional concentrations of leucine-enkephalin (ir-Enk), beta-endorphin (ir-Bep) and dynorphin A (ir-Dyn) were measured by radioimmunoassay at 2 h after injury (each n=10). Changes in regional cerebral blood flow (CBF) were measured in a second group using radioactive microspheres at 5 time points: 10 min prior to injury; and 15 min, 30 min, 1 h and 2 h after injury (n=8). A third group of animals was treated with the opiate antagonist WIN44,441-3 (0.2 mg/kg) or its stereoisomer (WIN44,441-2) (n=8/group).

Tissue concentration of ir-Dyn were significantly elevated in the caudate nucleus ($p < 0.05$), frontal cortex ($p < 0.01$), medulla ($p < 0.001$) and pons ($p < 0.01$) where injury, evidenced by histological examination, was most severe. The increase in ir-Dyn but not ir-Bep or ir-Enk was significantly correlated with a fall in CBF that occurred at 2 h post-injury in frontal cortex ($p < 0.01$), medulla ($p < 0.01$) and pons ($p < 0.01$). WIN44,441-3 caused a significant increase in CBF to midbrain ($p < 0.05$), brainstem ($p < 0.01$) and frontal cortex ($p < 0.05$). Administration of the inactive stereoisomer WIN44,441-2 was without effect on CBF. These results suggest that dynorphin, by contributing to the post-traumatic decline in cerebral blood, may play a role in the pathophysiology of secondary brain injury after trauma. These actions appear to be due to effects at opiate receptors, most likely the kappa-receptor.

Existence of peptidergic nerves and morphological changes of the smooth muscles in the congenital aganglionic intestine of rats 252

M. Oki, T. Domoto, T. Gonda, K. Inoue and S. Note
Shimane Medical University, Shimane, Japan

The distribution of cholinergic, adrenergic and peptidergic nerves in the large intestine was studied in the congenital aganglionosis rat(AGR), using the PAP method and antisera to VIP and substnace P; and by the acetylcholinesterase staining technique. Morphometric analysis of the muscle layers and smooth muscle cells was carried out with a digital planimeter.

The thickness of muscle layers of the aganglionic colon and rectum decreased significantly (1/2 and 1/1.3, respectively, of values in their control segments); cross sectional area of circular muscle cells was not significantly changed, so changes resulted from a decreased number of smooth muscle cells. Degenerative changes of the smooth muscles in the aganglionic segments were much reduced with advancing age in rats. A considerable number of peptidergic and acetylcholinesterase positive fibers were present in the aganglionic intestine but were not observed in the constricted ileum. We assumed that these extrinsic nerves in the AGR-intestine might relate to the differentiation and growth of the muscle cells throughout the organogenic process.

HETEROGENEITY OF OXYTOCIN RECEPTORS ON RAT AND SHEEP MYOMETRIAL CELLS 253

V. Pliška, J. Heiniger, H. Albertin-Kohlhauf
Institute of Animal Science, Swiss Federal Institute of Technology, ETH Zentrum, CH-8092 Zürich, Switzerland

High values of dissociation constants (K_d) for oxytocin (OTC) in rat myometrial plasma membranes as reported by Soloff & Swartz (J. Biol. Chem. *249*, 1376) and by Crankshaw et al. (Eur. J. Biochem. *86*, 341) markedly contrast with low pA_2 values for inhibitors structurally similar to OTC. We have therefore investigated the OTC binding to rat and sheep myometrium using short-time monolayer cultures of myometrial cells (0 to 12 days, 37°C, medium F10-Seromed). Cells were prepared from uteri of freshly slaughtered ewes (age: >6 months) or decapitated young rats (age: 4 to 7 weeks) by a trypsin/collagenase/dispase treatment. Prior to enzyme treatment, endometrium and perimetrium layers were mechanically removed, and the myometrium was minced. Quickly sedimenting cells (largely fibroblasts) were discarded after 1 h incubation. Experiments carried out with tritiated OTC (6 to 26 Ci/mmol) in a conc. range 3×10^{-10} to 4.5×10^{-4}M and suspensions of vital cells at low Mg conc. (3mM Ca) indicate populations of binding sites with K_d approx. 5×10^{-9}, 5×10^{-7} and $>10^{-5}$ mol/l (22°C). Binding on all three sites was displaceable by "cold" OTC; dissociation rate constants computed from the displacement experiments were 10^{-4} and 2×10^{-3} s^{-1} (probably first two sites). Binding sites with $K_d \approx 5\times10^{-7}$ seem to be identical with OTC receptors for uterotonic response *in vitro*: 1) pA_2 values for OTC analogues acting as inhibitors are in the range 6 to 8; 2) computation of K_d for OTC from side chain contributions to pA_2 obtained by the Free-Wilson analysis (Pliška, Experientia *34*, 1190) yield a K_d value close to 10^{-7} mol/l; and finally, 3) a similar value can be obtained from dose-response analysis carried out on rat uterus after stepwise partial irreversible inhibition of the OTC receptors (Pliška & Marbach, Eur. J. Pharmacol. *49*, 213; Pliška, J. Receptor Res. *4*, 371).

Supported by Swiss National Science Foundation, Grant 3.478-83, and by FFVFF Foundation, Zürich.

THE ACTION OF THE LATERAL HYPOTHALAMIC AREA ON NEURONS IN THE REGION OF THE SUBFORNICAL ORGAN WITH EFFERENT PROJECTIONS TO THE HYPOTHALAMIC PARAVENTRICULAR NUCLEUS IN THE RAT 254

H. Saito, J. Tanaka, H. Kaba, K. Seto
Kochi Medical School, Nankoku, Kochi, Japan

The neurons in the subfornical organ (SFO) have efferent projections to the hypothalamic paraventricular nucleus (PVN), and activation of these SFO neurons alters the excitability of neurohypophyseal neurons in the PVN. Recent tracing studies have identified angiotensin II (AII)-immunoreactive pathways from the lateral hypothalamic area (LHA) to the SFO, suggesting the possibility that the LHA may modulate the excitability of neurohypophyseal neurons in the PVN through an influence on AII sensitive SFO neurons projecting to the PVN. Thus, we examined the effects of microiontophoretic application of AII and electrical stimulation of the LHA on the activity of neurons in the region of the SFO with efferent projections to the PVN and the effects of microiontophoretic application of the antagonist on responses to AII or LHA stimulation.

Twenty neurons in the region of the SFO were antidromically identified by electrical stimulation of the PVN in male rats under urethane anesthesia. The activity of all identified units in the region of the SFO was excited by microiontophoretically (MIPh) applied AII and the effect of AII was blocked by MIPh-applied saralasin (Sar), an AII antagonist, suggesting that neurons in the region of the SFO with efferent projections to the PVN have AII receptors.

Electrical stimulation of the LHA excited the activity of 11 identified units in the region of the SFO, but did not affect the remaining units. The excitatory response of all identified units to LHA stimulation was blocked by MIPh-applied Sar.

These results suggest that the LHA has an excitatory influence on the activity of neurons in the region of the SFO with efferent projections to the PVN and that the influence may be mediated by AII receptors.

EFFECTS OF LONG-ACTING SOMATOSTATIN ANALOGUE IN A CASE OF MULTIPLE ENDOCRINE NEOPLASIA WITH α SUBUNIT-SECRETING PITUITARY ADENOMA, ZOLLINGER-ELLISON AND HYPERPARATHYROIDISM 254a

G. Sassolas, J.C. Souquet, J.A. Chayvialle, C. Partensky and B. Loras
Centre Médecine Nucléaire, Hop Cardiologique, Lyon, France.

The long-acting somatostatin analogue, SMS 201-995, has been reported to exert beneficial effects in some cases of endocrine tumors of the digestive tract and in acromegaly. Its therapeutic value in patients with multiple endocrine neoplasia (MEN) remains to be delineated. In a 51 year-old woman, a pituitary adenoma, immunocytochemically defined as an alpha-subunit secreting adenoma was partially removed in 1983; plasma alpha-subunit levels remained elevated thereafter (11 ng/ml; N<1 ng/ml) and CT scan disclosed a suprasellar remnant tumor. In march 1985, a grade V melanoma of the left arm was removed. Three months later, an hemorragic duodenal ulcer led to the detection of an endocrine tumor of the pancreatic tail, confirmed by ultrasound-guided cytoponction. Fasting plasma gastrin was elevated (800pg/ml) and further increased under 3CU/kg/hr secretin. SMS 201-995 (100µg subcutaneously twice daily) normalized plasma gastrin and basal acid secretion within three days, and was since pursued resulting in complete ulcer healing with steady, normal gastrin levels. Hypercalcemia with elevated parathormone levels (6.5UI/l; N<4.5UI/l) developed under SMS 201-995 treatment during the last four months and required surgical removal of 4 hyperplastic parathyroid glands. Plasma α subunit concentrations progressively decreased to normal values (0.8ng/ml). Head CT scan performed after 11 months of SMS treatment was normalized. This case i) represents a rare MEN type I with a α subunit secreting pituitary adenoma, pancreatic gastrinoma and parathyroid hyperplasia in a patient with a melanoma, ii) examplifies the dramatic effect of SMS 201-995 on at least some gastrin-secreting tumors, and iii) suggests that this agent may inhibit pituitary adenoma secretions other than GH.

NUTRITIONAL MODULATION OF THE EXERCISE-INDUCED INCREASE OF HYPOTHALAMIC NOREPINEPHRINE TURNOVER 255

U. Schweiger, J. Leifeld, M. Seidl, K.M. Pirke
Max-Planck-Institut für Psychiatrie, D-8000 München 40, F.R.G.

Peripheral and central norepinephrine (NE) turnover is reduced in different forms of starvation in rat and man under baseline conditions. As starvation frequently is associated with hyperactivity we compared the effects of exercise on NE turnover - as assessed by its major metabolite 3-methoxy-4-hydroxy-phenylethylene-glycol (MOPEG) - in the medio-basal-hypothalamus (MBH) under different nutritional situations.

4 groups of 13 animals were studied. Two groups were fed ad libitum. Two groups were semistarved with a high-protein low-carbohydrate diet to induce a weightloss of about 20% of initial weight. After 3 weeks one ad lib. fed group and one semistarved group was submitted to 1 hour of wheel-running exercise (10 m/min). Total MOPEG in MBH was assayed using a HPLC method.

MOPEG concentration in the MBH under resting conditions was 10.6 pMol (± 1.1 SEM) in the ad lib. fed group and 8.7 pMol (± 0.5) in the semistarved group. Exercise increased MOPEG under both nutritional conditions, but significantly (p 0.01) less in semistarved rats (19.4 pMol ± 1.8) as compared to ad lib. fed rats (30.1 pMol ± 1.7).

Data indicate that functional reactivity of central noradrenergic systems may be impaired to a greater extent by starvation than is reflected by the alterations of baseline activity.

GNRH PROHORMONE IMMUNOREACTIVTY IN THE PRIMATE FOREBRAIN AND HYPOTHALAMUS 256

T.Song, K. Nikolics, P.H. Seeburg, P.C. Goldsmith
Reproductive Endocrinology Center, Dept. of Ob/Gyn and Repro. Sci., Univ. of Calif., San Francisco, CA 94143

The structure of the prohormone for human and rat gonadotropin releasing hormone (proGnRH) includes the GnRH decapeptide followed by a 56 amino acid GnRH-associated peptide (GAP). GAP has been localized in neurons and median eminence terminals in the rat (Philips et al., Nature 316:542, 1985). In this study, we compared immunostaining for GnRH and GAP in 2 female and 3 male fetal rhesus macaques aged 109-156 days gestation. Serial frontal Vibratome sections (40 microns) were immunostained with antisera against GnRH (LR1, R. Benoit), against GAP 1-11 (24A), or against GAP 26-40 (KN-1) using the PAP technique. Solid phase absorption with GnRH or GAP confirmed the specificity of these antisera.

Most GAP immunoreactive (GAP+) neurons were bipolar in shape (like GnRH+ neurons), but a few multipolar and unipolar examples were seen depending upon the plane of section. Interneuronal contacts were rare. Cell counts showed a slightly greater number of GnRH+ than GAP+ neurons (527 vs. 472) in paired sections from 12 equispaced levels between the septum and mammillary bodies (4.4 mm). GAP+ cell bodies were concentrated in the septo-preoptic area (44.3%; n=3), the supraoptic-lateral hypothalamic region (23.1%; n=3), and medial basal hypothalamus (16.4%; n=3). GAP+ fibers were present throughout the forebrain and hypothalamus, and formed well-defined pathways such as the periventricular and ventral hypothalamic tract. They were also abundant in the infundibulum and median eminence, forming an elaborate network in the palisade zone. However, GAP+ fibers and terminals immunostained somewhat less densely than GnRH+ fibers in comparable regions.

These results indicate that proGnRH (GAP) is present in the same population of neurons as GnRH in the primate brain. They also suggest that post-translational products of proGnRH are present in GnRH perikarya, axons and axon terminals, and that GnRH and GAP may be cosecreted into hypophysial portal blood in the rhesus macaque.

Supported by NIH Grant HD 10907.

MORPOHOMETRIC AND TOPOGRAPHICAL ORGANIZATION OF CAPILLIARIES WITHIN THE RAT SUBFORNICAL ORGAN. 257

N.M. Sposito, P.M. Gross, J.D. Fenstermacher. Dept. Neurol. Surg., SUNY Stony Brook, NY 11794

Previous studies of cell types and capillaries in the rat subfornical organ (SFO) indicate a topographical organization suggestive of differences in function within it. Anatomically, the SFO is divided into: 1) central and lateral zones in the coronal plane, and 2) 3 regions in the sagittal plane -- rostral, central and caudal. Using light microscopic morphometry, we evaluated capillary densities, surface areas (SA), volume fractions, and diameters within the SFO in brains from albino, Long-Evans and homozygous Brattleboro rats perfusion-fixed with aldehydes. Capillary density was greatest in the central zone of the central region and lowest in the rostral region. In albino rats, the central zone had 616 capillary profiles/mm2 whereas the lateral zone had 257. The SA of central zone capillaries was 22.0 ± 6.7mm2/mm3 (mean ± SD) compared to 12.1 ± 6.9 mm2/mm3 in the lateral zone. The volume fraction of central zone capillaries was 2.51 ± 0.79% compared to 1.14 ± 0.43% in the lateral zone. The diameter of capillaries was larger in the lateral zone -- 5.1 ± 0.4 um vs. 4.6 ± 0.3 um in the central zone. There were wide pericapillary labyrinths in the central zone of the central and caudal regions especially where capillaries were in close proximity to the ventricular surface. Larger blood vessels lacking pericapillary spaces were predominant in the lateral zone and rostral region. The capillary bed of the rat SFO displays a topographical organization that may correlate with the predominant neural cell function and type for that corresponding part of the SFO. The lateral zone and rostral regions have relatively low capillary density and contain the main efferent fiber projections from the SFO. Capillaries in the central zone and region are great in number and are located within the area of angiotensin II afferent terminals to the SFO.

PHENCYCLIDINE AND OPIATE BINDING SITES IN HYPOTHALAMUS AND PITUITARY CELLS 258

S.S. Stojilkovic, M.L. Dufau, K.J. Catt
Endo. & Reprod. Res. Branch, NICHD, Bethesda, Maryland

Specific binding sites for [^{3}H]phencyclidine (PCP, 1-(1-phenylcyclohexyl)piperidine) were characterized in membranes from rat hypothalamus (Ht), anterior pituitary (AP) and neurointermediate lobe (NIL), and in primary cultures of anterior pituitary cells (AC), enriched gonadotrophs (G) and lactotrophs (L).

Bound [^{3}H]PCP was displaceable by 10 nM to 10 μM unlabeled PCP, and specific binding in the presence of 100 μM PCP constituted 50, 65 and 90% of total binding at 22°C for Ht, NIL and AC, respectively. Scatchard analysis revealed a single class of relatively high affinity [^{3}H]PCP-binding sites (Kd=190, 98, and 110 nM for Ht, NIL, and G, respectively) with estimated maximal binding capacity of 1.32 pmol/mg Ht, 153 fmol/mg NIL, and 0.98 pmol/10^6 G cells. [^{3}H]PCP bound with similar affinity to AC and L but not to AP membranes. Other drugs, including naloxone, etorphine and (-)ethylketocyclazocine, did not inhibit [^{3}H]PCP binding even at concentrations of 100 μM or more. [^{3}H]etorphine bound with high (nM) affinity to Ht and NIL membranes, and with relatively lower affinity in AC (etorphine>cyclazocine>naloxone>naltrexone>morphine sulfate). PCP did not inhibit [^{3}H]etorphine binding to Ht, NIL and AC. The etorphine binding sites in AC are probably related to the inhibitory actions of etorphine and morphine sulfate on LH release in vitro. In contrast, PCP stimulated LH release in cultured AC, and markedly enhanced the secretory response to GnRH.

The presence of etorphine and PCP sites in hypothalamus and anterior pituitary cells, and the influence of opiates and PCP on basal and GnRH-induced LH release, reflect the existence of additional regulatory systems for the local control of pituitary function. The direct inhibitory effects of etorphine and morphine are probably mediated by κ receptors, whereas the stimulatory PCP sites may correspond to σ receptors, providing two distinct opiate-like receptor subtypes for modulation of gonadotropin secretion.

THE EFFECT OF HIGH POTASSIUM ON ATRIAL NATRIURETIC FACTOR RELEASE FROM RERIFUSED RAT HYPOTHALAMUS 259

I. Tanaka, Y. Oki, M. Sakamoto, T. Inagami*, H. Imura**, K. Nakao**, T. Yoshimi
Hamamatsu University School of Medicine,Hamamatsu,Kyoto University School of Medicine**Kyoto, Japan, Vanderbilt University School of Medicine* Nashville, Tennessee

The release of immunoreactive atrial natriuretic factor(IR-ANF) from the perifused rat hypothalamus was examined *in vitro* using a radioimmunoassay(RIA) for ANF.

The antiserum was produced in a rabbit immunized with α-human ANP conjugated with BSA using glutaraldehyde. This antiserum recognized α-rat ANP, the cross-reactivity of which was 100%. The separation of antibody bound and free labelled α-rat ANP was effected by adding PEG. The final dilution of the antiserum was 1:5,000 and the minimum detectable quantity of α-rat ANP was 10 pg/tube. The hypothalamic blocks were obtained from male Wistar rats and cut saggitally through the center of the median eminence. Four hypothalamic halves were placed in a incubation chamber adapted to the perifusion apparatus. The flow rate of the standard medium consisting of KRB buffer containing 10mM glucose, 1mM PMSF, 50μg/ml bacitracin and 0.2% BSA saturated with a 95%O_2-5%CO_2 gas mixture was 0.2ml/min and every 5-min fraction was collected. The collected samples were lyophilized and reconstituted with the assay buffer and subjected to RIA for ANF or gel chromatography.

The high potassium medium(K^+=50mM) caused a significant increase in the release of IR-ANF, which returned to the basal level when the medium was changed to the standard medium. This effect of high potassium concentration was abolished when Ca^{++} was removed from the medium. Gel chromatographic study on a Bio-Gel P-10 column revealed that the major component of IR-ANF released from the hypothalamus eluted near the elution position of synthetic ANF IV.

These findings suggest a possible role of ANF as a neurotransmitter or a neuromodulator in the central nervous system.

SUBFORNICAL ORGAN AND HYPOTHALAMIC PARAVENTRICULAR NUCLEUS CONNECTIONS WITH MEDIAN PREOPTIC NUCLEUS NEURONS IN RATS 260

J. Tanaka, H. Kaba, H. Saito, K. Seto
Kochi Medical School, Nankoku, Kochi, Japan

Recent anatomical tracing studies have revealed that the subfornical organ (SFO) neurons have angiotensin II (AII)-immunoreactive efferents to the median preoptic nucleus (MnPO) that in turn projects to the hypothalamic paraventricular nucleus (PVN), suggesting the importance of these pathways for the control of body fluid balance. The objectives of current study were thus to characterize the action of these pathways on the activity of vasopressin (VP)-secreting neurons in the PVN.

In urethane-anesthetized male rats, electrical stimulation in the region of the SFO produced excitation or inhibition of the activity of MnPO neurons that were antidromically identified by electrical stimulation of the PVN. The activity of identified MnPO neurons excited by SFO region stimulation was also excited by microiontophoretically (MIPh) applied AII, while the remaining neurons were not affected. The excitatory responses induced by not only SFO region stimulation but also MIPh-applied AII were blocked by MIPh-applied saralasin (Sar), an AII antagonist, whereas the inhibitory responses induced by SFO region stimulation were not affected. These results suggest that the SFO efferents have both excitatory and inhibitory influence on the activity of MnPO neurons projecting to the PVN, and that the excitatory influence may be mediated by AII receptors.

Electrical stimulation in the MnPO produced excitation or inhibition of the activity of putative VP-secreting neurons in the PVN. On the other hand, microinjected AII into the MnPO produced either an excitation or no effect in the activity of putative VP-secreting neurons in the PVN.

These data speculate that AII sensitive MnPO neurons projecting to the PVN may act to enhance the activity of putative VP-secreting neurons in the PVN in response to the excitatory inputs from the SFO.

ACCUMULATION OF SEROTONIN AND COEXISTENCE WITH TYROSINE HYDROXYLASE IN HYPOTHALAMIC NEURONS OF ACUTELY STALK-SECTIONED BABOONS 261

K.K. Thind, J.E. Boggan, T. Song, P.C. Goldsmith
Reproductive Endocrinology Center, Dept. of Ob/Gyn and Repro. Sci., University of Calif., San Francisco, CA 94143

The distribution of serotonin (5HT) and tyrosine hydroxylase (TH) was examined in the hypothalamus of juvenile baboons, 24 hours after infundibular stalk section (SS) via the infratemporal approach. Simultaneous immunostaining for 5HT (PAP) and TH (colloidal gold) was performed on Vibratome sections from 3 operated and 1 control female. Light microscopy revealed bilateral profusion of fine 5HT immunopositive (5HT+) fibers, presumably axons, in the suprachiasmatic nucleus and ventromedial hypothalamus (VMH). In addition, focal accumulations of swollen and heavily stained 5HT+ fibers occurred on the side of the surgical approach. Enlarged fibers were densest in the medial preoptic area, lateral and VMH, and the median eminence. The absence of such staining in contralateral areas or in control sections suggested the response was due to trauma.

TH immunoreactivity (TH+) in VMH cell bodies and axons was only slightly increased over that in controls. Areas of 5HT+ and TH+ overlap (e.g. the medial VMH and periventricular zone) were examined by electron microscopy. 5HT+ profiles were mostly unmyelinated axons (up to 10 microns in diameter) and irregular varicosities. A few myelinated 5HT+ axons were also observed. TH+ perikarya, dendrites, axons and terminals contained 15 nm gold particles. Colocalization of 5HT and TH was present in a number of varicosities in SS but not control animals. Both single and double-labeled profiles occurred in individual thin sections, thus ruling out antibody cross-reactivity.

These results indicate that (1) hypothalamic 5HT fibers project to the median eminence in primates, (2) 5HT+ fibers become more visible after SS due to accumulation of transmitter without neurotoxins or monoamine oxidase inhibitors, (3) focal 5HT+ immunoreactivity in the hypothalamus can increase dramatically after distant and mild surgical trauma, and (4) coexistence of 5HT and TH in single neurons can occur after acute SS and/or trauma in experimental animals. These findings have important neuroendocrine implications, and suggest acute functional plasticity in expression of 5HT and TH synthesis in mature primate brain.

Supported by NIH Grant HD 10907 (PCG).

INFLUENCE OF PROSTAGLANDINS ON PITUITARY PORTAL BLOOD FLOW (PPBF) 262

W.Z. Traczyk, U. Szkudlarek

Department of Physiology, School of Medicine, Lodz, Poland

The concentration of hypothalamic hormones in the pituitary portal blood is regarded as the principal factor by which hypothalamus controls anterior pituitary secretion. On the contrary, the regulation of the PPBF has been scarcely investigated.

For the estimation of PPBF in urethane/chloralose anaesthetized male rats the transpharyngeal approach and exposure of the pituitary stalk according to Worthington (1966) was applied. Several methods of measuring the PPBF were checked including continuous measurement of portal vessel calibre using the stereomicroscope, television camera and video monitor. Because of pituitary stalk respiratory movements a more accurate method was established of determination of hemoglobin amount in 10-min samples of continuously washed and collected blood from the cut pituitary portal vessels. The PPBF was estimated in ten consecutive 10-min periods. The extreme differences between means of PPBF for control periods were between 2 and 22%.

During 5th or 6th period a slow injection of 0.2 ml solution through the external carotid artery into the internal carotid artery was performed. Injection of 20 µmol of TRH or 56 nmol of $PGF_{1\alpha}$ had no influence on the PPBF. After injection of 56 nmol of PGE_1 the PPBF significantly increased to the same value as during 10-min hypoxia with hypercapnia induced by the increase of the respiratory dead space by 3 ml.

Our data indicate that PGE_1 is the essential factor increasing significantly the PPBF.

RENIN-RELEASING FACTOR IN RAT AND BOVINE HYPOTHALAMUS L.D. Van de Kar and J.H. Urban. Loyola Univ. of Chgo., Sch. Med. Dept. Pharmacol. Maywood, IL 60153 263

Previous studies from our lab have demonstrated that stimulation of brain serotonergic receptors causes a renin-releasing factor (RRF) to appear in the blood. The RRF was found to be a heat stable peptide with a molecular weight between 5,000 and 10,000 daltons. Since lesions in the hypothalamus prevent the effect of the serotonin releaser p-chloroamphetamine (PCA) on renin secretion, we decided to investigate whether the hypothalamus contains renin-releasing substances. Rat hypothalamic, pituitary and cerebellar tissue was homogenized in boiling water and then placed in a boiling water-bath for an additional 10 min. After centrifugation, the extracts were lyophilized to dryness, resuspended in saline and added to kidney slices to test for renin-releasing activity. The hypothalamic extract contained the highest renin-releasing activity, followed by the cerebellar extract. The pituitary extract contained no renin-releasing activity at all. In a second experiment, a bovine hypothalamus (12.3 g) was homogenized with boiling water (123 ml) and an aliquot (4.5 ml) was treated as described above. The remaining solution (± 120 ml) was fractionated by ultrafiltration into fractions of molecular weight ranges of 1,000-5,000; 5,000-10,000; and 10,000-20,000 daltons. Testing these fractions in our renin-release bioassay (using kidney slices) revealed that the M.W. = 1,000-5,000 and the M.W. = 5,000-10,000 fractions contained renin-releasing substances, whereas the M.W. = 10,000-20,000 fraction had very little renin-releasing activity. Digestion of these fractions with a wide spectrum protease (pronase) for 4 hours completely eliminated their renin-releasing activity, suggesting that these renin-releasing substances are peptides. These studies suggest that the plasma-borne renin-releasing factor may originate in the hypothalamus.

IN VIVO RELEASE RATES OF ADRENAL NEUROPEPTIDES IN THE RAT MEASURED BY A NOVEL DIALYSIS METHOD 264

R. Vaupel, H. Jarry, E.-M. Düker, W. Wuttke
Div. Clin. Exp. Endocr.,Dept. ObGyn.,Univ. Göttingen,FRG

Colocalization and corelease of adrenal catecholamines and neuropeptides has been reported previously (1). These results prompted us to study whether a stressful stimulus which is known to cause release of adrenal catecholamines, would also induce a simultaneous secretion of neuropeptides within the adrenal gland. We employed a recently described in vivo dialysis method (2) to assess the release of several neuropeptides within the adrenal. Plasma prolactin levels were measured to confirm the stressful conditions.

The adrenal gland of intact males was implanted with the dialysis system and the jugular vein was catheterized. One day after surgery, the adrenal dialysis system was connected to the perfusion pump and Ringer's solution was used for dialysis (1ml/h); dialysate fractions were collected at 15 min intervals and blood was withdrawn at the end of each fraction period after a 2 h equilibration period.

The basal release rates of Met-Enkephalin (Met-Enk), Substance P (SP) and CCK were constant during the pre-shock period. Application of electric foot shock stress resulted in a marked increase of adrenal Met-Enk and SP release. Plasma prolactin levels rose during the time of exposure to foot shock. After termination of the stressful stimulus, prolactin levels returned to basal values within 15 - 30 min. Intra-adrenal Met-Enk and SP release remained elevated for at least 1 h after the cessation of the stress stimulus. In contrast, adrenal CCK release was not altered by application of foot-shock stress.

The results demonstrate that peptides such as SP and Met-Enk are released in high concentrations within the adrenal and secretion is increased under stressful conditions. Possibly they may exert paracrine effects. Obviously, a subtype of chromaffin cells producing catecholamines and CCK is not addressed by electric foot shock stress.

(1) Stine, S.M., Yang, H.C., Costa, E. 1980 Neuropharmacol 19:683; (2) Jarry, H., Düker, E.-M., Wuttke, W. 1985 Neurosc Let 60:273

USE OF EVOKED POTENTIALS (EEG) FOR EVALUATION OF NEUROPEPTIDE FUNCTIONS IN MAN 265

Voigt, K., Bickel, U., Born, J., Fehm, H. L.
Institute of Clinical Pharmacology, Free University of Berlin, Hindenburgdamm 30, 1000 Berlin 45

While devoid of the endocrine activity of adrenocorticotropin, the sequence ACTH 4-10 has retained the behavioral activity of ACTH 1-39. It modulates attentional behavior in animals and humans and has been shown to influence components of acoustic-evoked potentials in humans that are related to stimulus processing.

Four healthy male volunteers took part in the EEG study. They had to detect signal stimuli (tone pips) in a train of standardpips in one ear while ignoring standard and signal stimuli in the contra lateral ear (Hillyard paradigm). Differences in the amplitude of late components in the recorded evoked potentials between attended and unattended channel represent a measure of selective attention. 45 min. prior to testing the subjects received one of four doses of synthetic ACTH 4-10 as i.v. bolus injection (o, 0.1, 1, 10 mg).

In another group of six male volunteers the plasma kinetics were measured by a specific radioimmunoassay after i.v. injection of 125 µg/kg body weight ACTH 4-10. Detection limits of the assay in plasma samples extracted on polystyrene cartridges are 30-50 pg/ml.

ACTH 4-10 decreased the amplitude difference between attended and unattended channel compared to the zero-dose (control). The effect of 0.1 mg did not reach significance, while 1 mg and 10 mg were significantly effective. Following bolus injection plasma levels of ACTH 4-10 rapidly decrease. The kinetics can be described by a two compartment model with a half life of distribution of 0.3 to 0.5 min. and a half life of 3.6 to 9 min. in the elimination phase.

The central effects of peripherally administered ACTH 4-10 as represented by modulation of evoked potentials are elicited in a dose dependent manner. These effects are detectable at times when levels of this rapidly eliminated peptide have already decreased to the femtogram per ml range in peripheral blood. So far it remains unknown whether the primary site of action for ACTH 4-10 lies within the central nervous system.

METABOLISM OF DEHYDROEPIANDROSTERONE BY DISCRETE BRAIN REGIONS AND HYPOPHYSIS OF THE RAT. 266

J. Weidenfeld, H. Schiller, I. Chowers
Laboratory of Experimental Endocrinology, Dept. of Neurology, Hadassah University Hospital and Dept. of Internal Medicine, Bikur Cholim Hospital-Hebrew University Medical School, Jerusalem, Israel

Dehydroepiandrosterone (DHA) is an important precursor of hormonally active steroids in peripheral tissues. Its ability to be metabolized in brain tissue has not been yet determined. We studied the metabolism of DHA in various brain areas and in adenohypophysis of the rat.

Slices of brain tissue from discrete brain areas and hypophysis were incubated with 1,2 ^{3}H-DHA. The incubation products were separated by chromatography in various systems. Products were identified by formation of derivatives and by reverse isotopic dilution. Aromatization of DHA was determined by the incorporation of ^3H_2O into the incubation medium.

In the adenohypophysis the following metabolites were isolated: DHA-sulphate, androstenedione and 5α-androstane-3α, 17β-diol (3,5, diol).

In hypothalamic tissue from male or female rats, no conversion of DHA to DHA-sulphate could be detected. Conversion to androstenedione was observed only in hypothalami of male rats. No conversion to estrogens could be demonstrated. In hippocampus, amygdala, or septum of male rats no conversion of DHA to DHA-sulphate was detected; these areas were active in converting DHA to androstenedione or 3,5, diol.

The formation of these metabolites was enhanced in septum as compared with other brain areas examined. No aromatization of DHA could be detected in hippocampus or amygdala; significant aromatization of DHA was observed in the septum. In parietal cortex no metabolism of DHA occurred.

The findings show that specific brain areas and the adenohypophysis are able to convert DHA to several metabolites with biological activity. The physiological significance of these conversions remain to be elucidated.

COMPARISON OF IMMEDIATE AND DELAYED REPLACEMENT OF CORTICOSTERONE AFTER ADRENALECTOMY ON ACTH. 267

S. F. Akana, C. S. Cascio, L. Jacobson, N. Levin, J. Shinsako and M. F. Dallman. UCSF, San Francisco, California 94143 USA.

We have previously reported that pellets of a 25% mixture of corticosterone:cholesterol implanted subcutaneously at the time of adrenalectomy normalizes plasma and pituitary ACTH levels, thymus weight and body weight compared to sham-operated rats 5 days after surgery (AJP 249:R527, 1985). In these experiments we determined the early effects of adrenalectomy and pellet implantation (2-72h) on pituitary and plasma ACTH content compared to sham-adrenalectomy or adrenalectomy. Compared to sham, plasma ACTH in adrenalectomized rats was elevated at all times post-surgery ($p<0.05$) and pituitary content was reduced at 2 and 12h ($p<0.05$). Corticosterone replacement resulted in normal plasma and pituitary ACTH levels at all times after adrenalectomy, compared to sham-adrenalectomy. By contrast to the maintenance of normal ACTH observed when corticosterone was supplied at surgery, implantation of corticosterone 5 d after adrenalectomy resulted in a marked increase in pituitary ACTH content 1 and 3 days later ($p<0.05$). Plasma ACTH levels were decreased to the normal range at all times after implantation whereas plasma corticosterone levels were maintained between 6-10 µg/dl over this same period of time. We conclude from these studies that 1. replacement of corticosterone at adrenalectomy prevents the usual perturbation of the adrenocortical system following adrenalectomy; and 2. the major rapid effect of corticosterone is on ACTH secretion rather than synthesis. When corticosterone is supplied to the activated corticosterone-free system, corticotropes adjust only slowly to the abrupt decrease in drive to the pituitary.

(Supported, in part, by AM28172 and HL29714.)

ACETYLCHOLINE AND SEROTONIN REGULATION OF HYPOTHALAMIC CRH RELEASE IN VITRO. 268

A.E.Calogero, R.Bernardini, L.Tamarkin, T.Tomai, A.Luger, P.W.Gold, D.L. Loriaux and G.P.Chrousos.
DEB, NICHD, NIH and CPB and BPB, NIMH, Bethesda, MD

Indirect studies assessing bioassayable CRH or plasma ACTH secretion suggest that acetylcholine (ACh) and serotonin (5HT) may influence the basal, circadian and stress-responsive components of hypothalamic CRH secretion.

To more directly explore the possible role of these neurotransmitters on CRH secretion we measured their effects on the release of immunoreactive CRH (iCRH) from rat hypothalami in short-term culture. The sensitivity of the CRH RIA (3.7±0.2 pg/tube) enabled us to use one hypothalamus per well.

Dose-response studies (10^{-11}-10^{-5} M) were performed immediately after dissection or after a 24h preincubation period. Following each treatment, neuronal depolarization with 60mM KCl led to a 5-fold increase of iCRH release. In the experiments performed immediately after explantation, ACh and 5HT failed to cause significant iCRH secretion at all concentrations used. Twenty four hours after explantation, ACh and 5HT were able to stimulate iCRH release at the 10^{-9} - 10^{-5}M concentration range (Table).

PERCENT INCREASE (MEAN+SE) OF iCRH RELEASE

	10^{-11}M	10^{-9}M	10^{-7}M	10^{-5}M
ACh	30±20	340±150*	174±49*	166±79*
5HT	230±114*	304±60*	221±82*	288±160*

*$p<0.05$

Addition of 10^{-8}M ACh or 10^{-7}M 5HT in the media during the 24h preincubation inhibited the release of iCRH in response to an equimolar pulse of the respective but not the other neurotransmitter. This could reflect desensitization of the hypothalamic CRH neuron to the action of the respective neurotransmitter.

We conclude that 1) our system is suitable for studying the regulation of CRH secretion in vitro; 2) both ACh and 5HT stimulate hypothalamic iCRH release in vitro at physiologic concentrations; and, 3) ACh and 5HT act on the CRH-secreting neuron independently of each other.

THE ROLE OF GABA IN THE HYPOTHALAMO-PITUITARY ADRENAL (HPA) AXIS IN THE RAT. 270

E.A.Campbell, *P.R.Scraggs, *A.R.H. Altaher, B. Gillham and *M.T.Jones.
Departments of Biochemistry and *Gynaecology, United Medical and Dental Schools(St. Thomas's Campus), London.

The involvement of GABA as an inhibitory neurotransmitter in the control of CRF release from the hypothalamus has been established for many years. The present study set out to determine the effect on the HPA axis in the rat of experimentally raising GABA levels in vivo by treatment with the GABA transaminase inhibitors sodium valproate(1mg/ml in the drinking water for 3months) or γvinyl GABA(single i.p. injection of 250mg/kg or 1g/kg 18hours prior to killing).

Hypothalamic CRF levels were unaltered except following the higher dose of γ vinyl GABA when it was reduced by nearly 50%. Pituitary responsiveness both in vivo (plasma ACTH response to ether and laparotomy stress) and in vitro (ACTH released in response to CRF) was suppressed following all treatment regimes. In contrast in vitro responsiveness of the adrenal to 17nM synacthen was enhanced following sodium valproate or 250mg/kg γ vinyl GABA.

GABA is present in the adrenal and levels are increased following γvinyl GABA treatment. We therefore determined the effects of this drug and also sodium valproate on the corticosterone(B) release from dispersed adrenal cells incubated in vitro. Sodium valproate had no consistent significant effect on basal or stimulated B release either in the presence or absence of GABA. However γ vinyl GABA (40-50µM) added to the incubation medium consistently increased basal B release and either had no effect or inhibited stimulated release. This is a similar pattern to the plasma B changes observed following 1g/kg γ vinyl GABA where basal B was increased but the plasma B response to stress was decreased.

Thus the increased adrenal responsiveness observed in vitro may be a dose related phenomenon and also may be dependent on longer term changes in the adrenal cortex rather than an acute effect on the adrenal.

The authors thank Sanofi UK and Merrill Dow for gifts of sodium valproate and γ vinyl GABA respectively.

THE EFFECTS OF DEXAMETHASONE ON CENTRAL AND PERIPHERAL ACTH SYSTEMS IN RATS 271

M. Carnes, C.M. Barksdale, N.H. Kalin, M.S. Brownfield, S.J. Lent
Wm. S. Middleton Veterans Hospital and University of Wisconsin, Madison, Wisconsin

To investigate the simultaneous effects of dexamethasone on peripheral and central ACTH systems, rats were treated with dexamethasone or saline for four days. Pituitary, plasma, hypothalamus and cerebrospinal fluid (CSF) were then collected and analyzed for ACTH immunoreactivity. Additionally, hypothalamic tissue extracts were analyzed for corticotropin releasing hormone (CRH).

Peripherally, dexamethasone significantly lowered pituitary and plasma levels of ACTH. Centrally, hypothalamic ACTH content significantly increased while CSF ACTH significantly decreased with dexamethasone treatment. Hypothalamic CRF showed a small but not statistically significant decrease.

These results 1) suggest that prolonged exposure to dexamethasone affects central as well as peripheral ACTH activity, 2) corroborate our previous findings in rhesus monkeys of decreased CSF ACTH in response to dexamethasone treatment, 3) suggest that dexamethasone may inhibit the release of ACTH from hypothalamic neurons into CSF, and 4) provide evidence that the effect of dexamethasone on pituitary ACTH is more immediate than its effect on hypothalamic CRH.

SEROTONIN-OPIOID INTERACTIONS ARE NOT MEDIATED THROUGH $5HT_2$ RECEPTOR SUBTYPE 272

F.Facchinetti,°E.Martignoni,°°S.Marini,AR.Genazzani
Dept.of Obstetrics and Ginecology,University of Modena, °Dept.of Neurology,University of Pavia,°°Janssen Italia, Roma-Italy

The most part of serotonin (5HT) ligans such as methisergide, cyproheptadine,etc. binds to both $5HT_1$ and $5HT_2$ subtypes. Recently, a new compound, Ritanserin (R 55667, Janssen,I) which binds specifically only to $5HT_2$ receptors and has not activity against $5HT_1$ mediated effects have been available. In order to better define the influence of 5HT upon Proopionmelanocortin (POMC) related peptides release, this study deals with the effects of Ritanserin pretreatment on 5hydroxytryptophane (SOHTP)-induced B-Endorphin (B-EP), B-Lipotropin (B-LPH) and Cortisol secretion.

Seven healthy young male volunteers were submitted to 2 stimulation tests with 5-OHTP (Sigma Tau, I), before and after 4 days of treatment with Ritanserin (20 mg/die for the 1st and 2nd day and 10 mg/die for the 3rd and 4th day). After overnight rest, 200 mg of 5-OHTP were given p.o. and blood samples were taken twice before(-30 and 0) and every 60 minutes for the 4 hours following the drug administration. Plasma cortisol, B-EP and B-LPH concentrations were measured in each sample by RIA, after silicic acid extraction and Sephadex G 75 column chromatography. Ritanserin treatment does not modifie the basal levels of the three hormones. The integrated area of response (subtracted of basal value) to 5-OHTP was similar in basal conditions (Cortisol 7.6± 2.1 ug min/ml; B-EP 1.1± 0;1 pmol min/ml; B-LPH 1.9±0.4pmol min/mol) and after Ritanserin (5.1±1.4,0.9±0.3 and 1.5±0.6,respectively).

These data confirm that 5-HT exerts a stimulatory action on POMC-related peptides in humans. The lack of Ritanserin inhibition of 5-OHTP induced POMC-related peptides secretion suggests that the positive effect of 5HT upon endorphines is mediated through hypothalamic adenylate cyclase-dependent receptors. The role of $5\text{-}HT_2$ subclasse of receptors in physiological and pathological conditions remain to be explored, but they do not seem involved in mediating the central serotonin-opioids interaction.

EFFECT OF CHRONIC HYPERPROLACTINEMIA ON CATECHOLAMINE CONTENT AND RELEASE FROM ADRENAL TISSUE 273

J.J. Fernández Ruiz; M. Cebeira; C. Agrasal; J.A.F. Tresguerres*; J.A. Ramos; A.I. Esquifino
Department of Biochemistry and Human Physiology*. F.Medicine. U.Complutensis. Madrid. Spain.

In order to study the effect of chronic hyperprolactinemia on catecholamine (CA) synthesis and release from the adreno-medullary tissue, female rats bearing an additional anterior pituitary gland under the right kidney capsule since day 30 of life and their sham operated controls, were sacrified 45 days after the grafting and their plasma prolactin (PRL) levels measured using a specific RIA method. Dopamine (DA), norepinephrine (NE) and epinephrine (E) levels in plasma and their contents in adreno-medullary tissue were determined by a radioenzymatic assay.

Grafted rats showed a significant increase in plasma PRL levels as compared to controls (21.6 ± 3.1 ug/l vs 6.1 ± 0.3 ug/l), without modification of plasma DA levels (0.6 ± 0.2 ug/l vs 0.8 ± 0.3 ug/l). However a significant increase in plasma NE and E levels were detected (NE: 4.2 ± 1.1 ug/l vs 1.7 ± 0.5 ug/l; E: 2.9 ± 0.5 ug/l vs 1.6 ± 0.2 ug/l). DA content in the adreno-medullary tissue of grafted rats was increased (29.1 ± 6.8 ng/mg protein) whereas both NE and E were decreased (NE: 33.2 ± 6.8 ng/mg protein; E: 65.9 ± 11.8 ng/mg protein) as compared to controls (DA: 12.0 ± 3.6 ng/mg protein; NE: 79.3 ± 22.1 ng/mg protein; E: 188.9 ± 32.1 ng/mg protein).

The results obtained suggest that the grafting induced chronic hyperprolactinemia was able to increase the synthesis and release of CA from the adreno-medullary tissue.

PRL-kit were generously provided by the NIH. This work has been possible through a FISS Foundation Grant (Madrid, Spain).

EFFECT OF PASSIVE IMMUNIZATION AGAINST CORTICOTROPIN RELEASING-FACTOR (CRF) ON THE POST-ADRENALECTOMY CHANGES IN CRF BINDING SITES IN THE RAT ANTERIOR PITUITARY GLAND. 274

M. Grino, V. Guillaume, E. Castanas, B. Conte-Devolx, and C. Oliver.
Laboratoire de Neuroendocrinologie Expérimentale, INSERM U 297, Faculté de Médecine Nord, Bd P. Dramard, 13326 Marseille Cédex 15, FRANCE.

Specific binding sites for CRF have been identified recently in the anterior pituitary gland. The number of these sites decreases rapidly after adrenalectomy (Wynn et al. Endocrinology 116, 1653-1659, 1985). These changes may be related either to a desensitization of the CRF receptors through an increased CRF release in hypophysial portal blood or to a direct effect of the suppression of circulating glucocorticoids at the level of the anterior pituitary.

In order to examine this mechanism, we have measured the concentrations of CRF binding sites in the anterior pituitary gland of intact and adrenalectomized rats after immunoneutralization of endogenous CRF with a specific antiserum anti-rat CRF (CRF-AS). The binding characteristics of (^{125}I) Tyr-ovine CRF have been determined on anterior pituitary membranes obtained from 24h-adrenalectomized or sham operated rats, injected with CRF-AS or normal rabbit serum (NRS) (0.5ml at the time of surgery and 0.5ml 4h before the experiment). Nine rats have been used in each group 3 pituitaries being pooled for each binding study.

In NRS injected rats, the number of CRF binding sites (fmol/mg protein) was significantly lower after adrenalectomy (12.5± 0.9) than after sham surgery (20.7±2.6). In CRF-AS injected rats, a similar decrease in CRF binding sites was observed in adrenalectomized rats (12.2 ± 1.7 vs 20.5±2.2 in sham-operated rats). CRF-AS injection induced a 50% reduction in plasma ACTH levels in both groups. The affinity of CRF for its binding sites was not significantly altered in all the groups studied.

These results indicate that CRF receptors desensitization is not involved in the post-adrenalectomy decrease of CRF binding sites. They suggest that glucocorticoids act directly at the level of the pituitary gland to modulate the number of these sites.

Grants from INSERM CRE 83 40 07

EFFECTS OF OVINE CRF, VASOPRESSIN AND METYRAPONE UPON PLASMA LEVELS OF ACTH AND CORTISOL IN STRESS-SENSITIVE AND STRESS-RESISTANT PIGS 275

J. Hari, V. Pliška
Institute of Animal Science, Swiss Federal Institute of Technology, ETH Zentrum, 8092 Zürich, Switzerland

The responsiveness of domestic pigs to various stressors is generally high and seems to increase with the intensity of breeding. In order to clarify the genetic component associated with this sensitivity, we investigated functional parameters of the hypothalamo-hypophyseal-adrenal-axis (HHA) in two specific breeding lines of Swiss Landrace pigs. These lines originated from a common ancestral population and were developed into positive ("lean") and negative ("fatty") lines, as classified according to production traits. A subpopulation showing a strong reaction to halothane,a commonly used stressor in pig, occurs only within the positive line. We measured the ACTH and cortisol levels in pigs of each breeding line after i.v. administration of i) oCRF (1 µg/kg body weight), ii) lysine vasopressin (LVP; 0.4 µg/kg), iii) a combined injection of oCRF and LVP (1 µg + 0.4 µg/kg), iv) metyrapone (30 mg/kg) and v) an oCRF-injection (1 µg/kg) 4 h after the metyrapone administration. Blood samples were withdrawn from the jugular vein through a surgically inserted permanent catheter. Release of ACTH following CRF and metyrapone administration was significantly greater in the negative line. ACTH responses were only slightly scattered within groups of identical lines and ages; however, these responses seemed to be independent of stress sensitivity, and in particular, of the reaction to halothane. The responses in the two lines did not differ when LVP alone, or in combination, was used for stimulation. Moreover, there was a possible effect of age. The increase of cortisol levels was approximately equal in all experiments. Therefore,the release of ACTH and of cortisol (measured as the peak level or as total amount of the hormones released after stimulation) was not correlated for individual experimental groups. A genetic influence on the HHA clearly exists within the two lines, but could not yet be fully interpreted in terms of stress sensitivity. Genetic variability may exist, e.g. in the peptide hormones involved.

EFFECT OF SYNTHETIC ATRIAL NATRIURETIC PEPTIDE ON ACTH AND CORTICOSTERONE SECRETION IN RATS 276

K. Hashimoto, S. Suemaru, T. Hattori, M. Sugawara, H. Inoue, T. Takao, J. Kageyama, Z. Ota
Third Department of Internal Medicine, Okayama University Medical School, Okayama 700, Japan

The effect of synthetic atrial natriuretic peptide (ANP) was examined on the in vivo and in vitro release of ACTH and corticosterone. In in vivo experiments, ANP (0.5-10 µg/kg) was injected into the jugular vein catheters in unanesthetized freely moving rats. Then, hemorrhage stress (withdrawal of 2-ml blood) and handling stress (handling the rats for 15 sec) were given immediately after and 5 min after ANP injection, respectively. Corticotropin-releasing factor (CRF, 4 µg/kg), arginine vasopressin (AVP, 2 µg/kg) and angiotensin II (A II, 4 µg/kg) were injected into the jugular catheters at 5 or 10 min after ANP injection. Blood samples were drawn via the jugular catheters 3-4 times before and after these manipulations. In in vitro experiments, the effects of ANP on ACTH and corticosterone secretion were examined using monolayer cultured anterior pituitary cells and isolated adrenal glands.

In in vivo experiments, hemorrhage, handling stress, CRF, AVP and A II evoked a significant plasma ACTH and corticosterone elevation. ANP inhibited the hemorrhage-induced ACTH elevation, whereas it did not affect the handling stress-, CRF-, AVP- and A II-induced ACTH elevations in unanesthetized freely moving rats. ANP did not affect the basal and CRF-induced ACTH release in pituitary cell cultures. A high dose of ANP (10^{-6} M) reduced basal corticosterone secretion from the adrenal gland, while the corticosterone response to ACTH was not affected.

These results suggest that ANP inhibited the hemorrhage-induced ACTH release but that it did not affect the ACTH secretagogues-induced ACTH release in vivo and in vitro. The mechanism of ANP inhibition on the hemorrhage-induced ACTH secretion remains to be clarified.

EFFECTS OF BACLOFEN ON HYPOTHALAMO-PITUITARY-ADRENOCORTICAL (HPA) FUNCTION IN RATS 277

A. Häusler
Res. Dept., Pharm. Div.,
CIBA-GEIGY Ltd., 4002 Basel, SWITZERLAND

An inhibitory role of GABA in the control of HPA function in rats is suggested by a number of in vitro studies with GABAergic agents. The final goal of the present study was to test in vivo whether baclofen, a GABA-B agonist, given systemically to male rats at a dose of 5 mg/kg (s.c.) also has an inhibitory effect on HPA function. As a basis for the in vivo study, the effect of baclofen on ACTH and corticosterone secretion was studied in vitro.

In vitro, ACTH secretion was studied in a perifusion system with dispersed anterior pituitary cells obtained from adrenalectomized rats given baclofen 18 h prior to decapitation. ACTH release, induced by corticotropin releasing factor (CRF, 5-50 ng/ml) was reduced (40-60% of controls). Corticosterone release, stimulated by ACTH (10-1000 ng/ml) from incubated adrenal fragments obtained from baclofen-pretreated rats was increased (170-200% of controls). Baclofen added in vitro had no effect on ACTH secretion in the absence of CRF or on corticosterone release in the presence or absence of ACTH.

In vivo, HPA activity was studied by monitoring urinary corticosterone excretion. Baclofen given either at 0800 h or at 1600 h (time of low and increasing HPA activity, resp.) significantly increased HPA activity (>1000% and 270% of controls, resp.). This net stimulatory effect of baclofen on HPA activity could be due to the increase in adrenocortical responsiveness to ACTH shown in vitro which overrides the inhibitory effect of baclofen at the hypothalamo-pituitary level.

It is concluded that the modulatory role of GABA in HPA control may not be confined to the hypothalamo-pituitary unit alone, but may also be extended to the adrenal gland.

THE EFFECT OF CORTISOL ON MEMBRANE POTENTIAL OF THE HIPPOCAMPUS CELLS IN VITRO 278

S.Y. Hua, Y. Z. Chen
Second Military Medical College,Shanghai, China

It is generally believed that glucocorticoids function by exerting their effects on cytosol and nuclear receptors. But recently some evidences have indicated that the hormone does influences the electrical activities of the nerve cells.

Glucocorticoid has a variety of influences on central nervous system. It also has a feedback action on ACTH secretion. The effective loci may be pituitary, hypothalamus, or prehypothalamic structures of which the hippocampus is the most suggestive one.

Using slices of rat hippocampus, we attempted to investigate the machanisms by which the hormone works. In 8 intracellularly recorded cells, six of them responded to the drug with hyperpolarization, one of the six showed a decreasing spontaneous discharges. The other two did not respond to the drug.

Our result for the first time shows that cortisol has a hyperpolarizational effect on the hippocampal cells. It is suggested that this effect may be involved in the feedback action of cortisol. The significance of the present result in relation to other central nervous activities was discussed.

A NOCTURNAL RISE IN CORTICOSTERONE MAY BE REQUIRED FOR NORMAL ACTH RESPONSES TO STRESS IN RATS. 279

L. Jacobson, S.F. Akana, M.F. Dallman
Department of Physiology, UC San Francisco, CA 94143

The role of circadian and stress-induced changes in glucocorticoids in the ACTH response to stress is not well understood. We have previously found that adrenalectomized rats provided with constant corticosterone (B) levels via a subcutaneous corticosterone-cholesterol pellet have normal resting morning ACTH, but exhibit enhanced stress-induced ACTH release relative to sham-operated (SHAM) rats. (Akana, Endocrine Soc. Abst. 1986) We now report that stress-induced hypersecretion of ACTH in the adrenalectomized, corticosterone-pelleted (PELLET) rat does not continue indefinitely; after 2' restraint stress, PELLET rat ACTH levels return to those of SHAMS in 1-4 h. Hypersecretion of ACTH was also elicited in PELLET rats by laparotomy under pentobarbital anesthesia, indicating that this response is not specific to psychogenic stimuli. However, SHAM and PELLET ACTH responses to 0.1 & 0.5 ug rCRF were not different. To distinguish between the requirement for stress-induced or circadian increases in B in normalizing the ACTH response to stress, adrenalectomized rats were given 25 ug/ml B in the drinking water (WATER). WATER rats exhibited a rise in plasma B commencing with the nightly activity period; morning B levels were similar to those in SHAMS (<1ug/dl). Like PELLET rats, WATER rats had normal thymus weight and morning ACTH levels relative to SHAMS, but lacked adrenals to modify B in response to stress. However, WATER rats did not differ from SHAMS in their ACTH response to ip injection, a stress previously found to cause hypersecretion of ACTH in PELLET rats. We conclude that the stress-induced hypersecretion of ACTH in PELLET rats, at least within the first hour after stress, does not involve increased pituitary sensitivity to CRF, appears to be a consequence of the loss of the circadian rise in B, and may reflect a general mechanism for feedback regulation of ACTH responses to stress.

Supported in part by AM28172 and HL29714

COORDINATE ENDOCRINE ROLES FOR ADRENAL MEDULLA AND CORTEX IN STRESS 280

D. Jefferys and J.W. Funder
Medical Research Centre, Prince Henry's Hospital, Melbourne, Australia 3004.

Naive rats placed in 15 cm of water at 25°C in a plexiglass cylinder 15 cm in diameter spend progressively more time immobile over a 15 minute initial exposure (1). Intact, adrenalectomized (adrx), hypophysectomized (hypox) or adrx-hypox rats show indistinguishable levels of progressive immobility over the initial test period. Retested 24 hours later, rats without adrenals are immobile for only approximately 30% of five minute retest period, compared with 60-70% for intact and hypox rats. The effect of adrx is reversed by dexamethasone, corticosterone, ketazocine or dynorphin 1-17 at the time of test (but not retest), but not by catecholamines, morphine, D-Ala^2-Leu^5-enkephalin or deoxycorticosterone (2,3). Naloxone, but not its quaternary analogue, equivalently blocks the incorporation of information into memory in intact rats and adrx rats treated with glucocorticoids or opioids (4). In contrast, the kappa-selective opiate antagonist MR2266 was without effect in intact or glucocorticoid replaced rats, but blocked the effect of ketazocine in adrx rats. These findings prompted the hypothesis that the incorporation of information into memory is mediated either by glucocorticoids or a kappa-selective opioid pathway, both of which act through a common, non-kappa opioid relay within the blood-brain barrier.

To test this hypothesis we have used RU38486 to block glucocorticoid action, and the long-acting nicotinic antagonist mecamylamine to block adrenal medullary opioid release. Administered alone, neither agent affects memory; administered together, they block memory to the levels seen in adrx rats, or in hypox rats given MR2266 or mecamylamine. We interpret these data as clearly defining the necessary role of the adrenal in the incorporation of learned experience into a behavioral repertoire after mild to moderate stress.

1. Porsolt RD et al (1977) Nature 266:730-732.
2. Jefferys D et al (1983) Eur J Pharmacol 92:99-103.
3. Jefferys D et al (1985) Eur J Pharmacol 107:331-335
4. Jefferys D et al (1984) Eur J Pharmacol 103:205-210

THE ROLE OF THE ADRENAL MEDULLA IN MODULATING THE STRESS-INDUCED RELEASE OF PITUITARY HORMONES. 281

O. Khorram and S.M. McCann
Department of Physiology, Univ of TX Hlth Sci Center, Dallas, Texas 75235

Catecholamines can have direct effects on the pituitary gland to affect hormone release and β_2 adrenoreceptors are present in the anterior pituitary and neurointermediate lobe. To determine if adrenal medullary secretions can alter stress-induced release of pituitary hormones, adrenal medullectomized (MEDX) male rats (Zivic Miller Labs) were used 1 week after operation. One day prior to experiment a cannula was implanted in the jugular vein for withdrawal of blood samples. A baseline blood sample was withdrawn. The animals were then immobilized for a period of 1 hour and blood samples were withdrawn at 5, 15, 30 and 60 minutes. Plasma levels of prolactin (PRL), growth hormone (GH) and α-MSH were measured by RIA. In the sham-operated and MEDX groups GH levels were significantly and similarly lowered within 5 min and remained low throughout. Plasma PRL levels significantly increased within 5 min in both groups. In the sham-operated animals PRL levels increased up to 15 min returning to baseline values thereafter, whereas in the MEDX there was a constant increase in PRL levels. The increase in PRL levels in the MEDX group was significantly higher than in the sham-operated group at 5, 15, 30 and 60 min. Plasma α-MSH levels also increased in both groups within 5 min but were not different from each other at any time point. Measurement of β_2 receptors in the anterior pituitary using ^{125}I-iodocyanopindolol 1 week after medullectomy revealed a significant increase in the number of receptors. The increased number of β-receptors which have been shown to have a stimulatory effect on PRL secretion may account for the greater increment in plasma PRL in the MEDX group. These studies indicate that peripheral catecholamines can significantly alter the stress-induced release of PRL but not GH or α-MSH.

(Supported by NIH grant HD 09988).

STRESS-INDUCED RELEASE OF β-ENDORPHIN, ACTH AND CATECHOLAMINES: MEDIATION VIA THE HISTAMINERGIC SYSTEM 282

U. Knigge, S. Matzen, F.W. Bach, P. Bang, J. Warberg
Inst. of Medical Physiology C, University of Copenhagen, and Dept. of Clinical Chemistry, Gentofte Hospital, Denmark

We investigated whether histamine (HA), which serves as a central neurotransmitter might be involved in restraint-stress induced release of β-endorphin (β-END), ACTH, and catecholamines (CA) in male rats.

7 days prior to experimentation a permanent cannula was implanted intracerebroventricularly (icv). On the day of the experiment restraint-stress was applied to one group of rats which were fixed on their bag for 5 min and then decapitated. Another group of rats received an icv infusion of 30 µg HA 15 min before decapitation. In other experiments HA antagonists were infused icv 15 min prior to induction of restraint-stress or administration of HA. Control rats were infused icv with saline and left undisturbed for 1 hour before decapitation. Trunk blood was collected and plasma analysed for hormones.

β-END: The β-END level was increased 2.5 fold by HA. This effect was inhibited 70% by the H_2-antagonist cimetidine (CIM; 100 µg icv) and 48% by the H_1-antagonist mepyramine (MEP; 100 µg icv). The antagonists had no effect on basal β-END secretion. The β-END response to restraint-stress was abolished by CIM whereas MEP inhibited the response only 50%.

ACTH: HA increased the ACTH level 2.5 fold. Neither CIM nor MEP had any effect on this release. Restraint-stress stimulated the release of ACTH 4.5 fold. This effect was not inhibited by HA antagonists.

CA: The plasma levels of dopamine (DA), norepinephrine (NE), and epinephrine (E) were increased almost 2 fold by HA. CIM prevented this response while MEP had no effect. Restraint-stress caused a 2 fold increase in all three CA. The response of DA and NE was abolished by both CIM and MEP. The E response was unaffected by CIM and partly (50%) inhibited by MEP.

The results indicate that HA participates in the mediation of restraint-stress induced release of β-END and peripheral CA whereas other neurotransmitters seem to be involved in stress-induced release of ACTH.

DEXAMETHASONE FEEDBACK TO CRF AND AVP AT THE PARAVENTRICULAR NUCLEUS 283

K.Kovács, J.Z.Kiss, G.B.Makara
Institute of Experimental Medicine, Hungarian Academy of Sciences, Budapest, Hungary

The site of inhibitory action of glucocorticoids on the hypothalamic corticotropin releasing factor (CRF) and arginine vasopressin (AVP) was studied using a combination of glucocorticoid implantation and immunocytochemistry. Adrenalectomy increased the number and the staining intensity of the neurons containing CRF-like immunoreactivity in the anterior and medial parvocellular subdivisions of the paraventricular nucleus (PVN) and induced the appearance of AVP-like immunoreactivity in the same cell population. These effects of adrenalectomy were inhibited only by those dexamethasone implants, which were placed close to the PVN. Unilateral implantation of dexamethasone into the PVN inhibited the adrenalectomy induced changes in CRF and AVP immunostaining only on the implanted side. Dexamethasone implants placed into the hyppocampus decreased the effect of adrenalectomy in the PVN while similar implants into the amygdala and cerebral cortex were uneffective. These results suggest that the primary site of glucocorticoid feedback inhibition on the hypothalamic secretagogues of adrenocorticotropin is the paraventricular nucleus.

ENDORPHIN MODULATION OF THERMAL ADAPTATION TO EMOTIONAL STRESS 284

K. Kubo, S. Tsuzuki, and T. Sasaki
Dept. Bioregulation, Inst. Med. Gen., Kumamoto Univ. Med. Sch., Kumamoto 862, Japan

The effects of IIIrd ventricular injection of β-endorphin (ED) on rectal temperature (Tr) and oxygen consumption ($\dot{V}O_2$) under emotional stress (immobilizing with wire mesh for 3 hours) were studied in the rats in a warm-environment. The stress induced a fall in Tr with a decrease in $\dot{V}O_2$. Repeating the stress once a day for 10 days, the hypothermic responses diminished day by day, and a recovery to the pre-stress level during the stress occurred in $\dot{V}O_2$ by day 9.

ED induced hyperthermic responses in a non-stress state, but if injected at 1 hr of first stress it enhanced the progress of hypothermic responses induced by stress stimuli. On day 10 of repeated stresses, however, ED at 1 hr of stress induced hyperthermic responses, indicating that thermal adaptation developed by day 10. Naloxone did not suppress the rapid progress of hypothermia during initial 1 hr of stress, but eliminated the ED enhancement of hypothermia and maintained Tr level of 1 hr of stress. Endogenous ED may be involved in the modulation of metabolic thermoregulation during stress but not in the mediation of the stress stimuli.

Furthermore, effects on thermal adaptation of either priming of ED or naloxone at 1 hr of every stress during the repeated stresses were studied. The diminishment of hypothermic responses in initial 1 hr of stress normally progressed by repeating the stresses did not occur even on day 10 in the rats primed with ED, but it accelerated in the rats primed with naloxone. Thus endogenous ED appeared to inhibit the development of thermal adaptation to the stress.

Present data suggest that ED in the brain may act to suppress responsiveness of thermoregulatory mechanisms to thermal input under both stress and non-stress states, and to inhibit the development of adaptational changes in the brain in response to the stress stimuli.

CORTICOTROPES ARE INSENSITIVE TO STEROID FEEDBACK SIGNAL IN VIVO. 285

N. Levin*, M. Blum, C. Cascio*, J.L. Roberts and M.F. Dallman* *UC San Francisco, CA 94143 USA and Columbia Univ College of Phys & Surg, New York, NY 10032 USA.

We have examined the effect of a range of constant corticosterone (B) levels in adrenalectomized rats to determine the major site of feedback on ACTH. Adult male Sprague-Dawley rats received either medial basal hypothalamic (MBH) lesions or sham lesions; 2d later all rats were adrenalectomized and provided with fused B: cholesterol pellets placed s.c. At this time, MBH lesioned rats received mini-pumps preloaded to deliver either 5ug/d rCRF or 1ug/d inactive $rCRF_{3-41}$. Rats were decapitated 5d later and blood, anterior pituitaries and brains were collected. Data are presented as $\bar{X}$±SEM and were analyzed by nonparametric ANOVA. Plasma B levels were 0.8±0.1, 2.5±0.2, 7.1±0.5 and 18.3±2.4 ug/dl in the 0, 20, 40 and 80% B pellet groups, respectively.

SHAM-MBH (8/gp)	Plasma ACTH (pg/ml)	Pit ACTH (ng/ug prot)	Pit POMC mRNA (POMC/poly A+)
0% B pellet	363±67	.59±.05	1.79±.36
20 "	119±18	.58±.06	1.95±.28
40 "	35±8	.41±.06	1.05±.25
80 "	23±4	.35±.09	.98±.13
MBH-CRF (5/gp)			
0% B pellet	85±12	.36±.04	.84±.10
20 "	80±26	.43±.08	.80±.14
40 "	48±11	.31±.04	1.01±.24
80 "	56±15	.37±.04	.71±.15
MBH+CRF (5/gp)			
0% B pellet	176±55	.45±.18	1.30±.22
20 "	294±108	.53±.11	1.25±.29
40 "	323±109	.44±.11	1.22±.14
80 "	64±22	.48±.13	.74±.23

In Sham-MBH rats, B reduced plasma and pituitary ACTH and POMC mRNA levels in a dose related manner. In lesioned rats lacking hypothalamic drive (MBH-CRF) B did not suppress any of these variables. In lesioned rats receiving exogenous CRF (MBH+CRF) plasma ACTH levels were reduced only at the highest B dose, while neither pituitary ACTH or POMC mRNA exhibited significant sensitivity to B. We conclude that the anterior pituitary is relatively insensitive to B and that the primary effect of adrenalectomy is removal of B from brain feedback sites.

EFFECTS OF ETHANOL ON NALTREXONE INDUCED STIMULATION OF ANTERIOR PITUITARY, ADRENAL AND GONADAL HORMONES IN WOMEN 286

J.H. Mendelson, N.K. Mello
Harvard Medical School-McLean Hospital, Belmont, MA

Alcohol abuse by women and chronic ethanol self-administration by female rhesus monkey causes severe derangements in menstrual cycle and reproductive hormone function. However, acute administration of ethanol to women and female rhesus monkey does not change plasma levels of pituitary gonadotropin or gonadal steroid hormones. The purpose of this study was to determine if acute alcohol administration affected Naltrexone perturbated pituitary, adrenal and gonadal hormonal responses in women. We recently reported that oral administration of Naltrexone, a long-acting opioid antagonist, may be used as a provocative test for anterior pituitary hormone function in women (Mendelson et al., Pharmacol Biochem Behav 24:309-313, 1985). Eighteen healthy, normally cycling, women provided informed consent for participation in these studies. Nine were studied during the early follicular phase and nine during the mid-luteal phase of the menstrual cycle. Blood samples were collected for LH, estradiol, prolactin, ACTH and cortisol analyses prior to and following administration of Naltrexone plus alcohol or alcohol placebo. Naltrexone produced a significant increment ($P < .01$) in plasma LH, prolactin, ACTH and cortisol levels during both the follicular and luteal phases of the menstrual cycle. Alcohol administration produced a significant augmentation of the prolactin response and enhanced the LH response following Naltrexone. Naltrexone and alcohol placebo did not induce any significant changes in plasma estradiol or progesterone levels. Alcohol (but not alcohol placebo) significantly stimulated ($P < .001$) an increase in plasma estradiol levels following Naltrexone administration. We postulate that Naltrexone perturbation of prolactin and pituitary gonadotropins is enhanced by concurrent acute alcohol intake as a consequence of ethanol induced stimulation of plasma estradiol levels.

PVN LESIONS COMPLETELY ABOLISH STRESS-INDUCED INCREASES IN PITUITARY CYCLIC AMP IN VIVO 287

J.L. Meyerhoff, G.J. Kant and E.H. Mougey
Neuroendo. Branch, Dept. Medical Neurosciences, Walter Reed Army Institute of Research, Washington, D.C. 20307-5100

We have previously shown that stress elevates pituitary cyclic AMP in vivo. These increases were associated with increased plasma levels of pituitary hormones derived from proopiomelanocortin (POMC) and released by corticotropin releasing factor (CRF). CRF is one of several substances reported to increase pituitary cyclic AMP in vitro. The paraventricular nucleus (PVN) of the hypothalamus has been identified as a major center involved in the regulation of ACTH secretion from the anterior pituitary gland, and recently CRF-containing neurons in the PVN have been shown to project to the median eminence of the hypothalamus. To determine the role of the PVN in the stress-induced increase of pituitary cyclic AMP in vivo, we lesioned the PVN bilaterally in male Sprague-Dawley rats.

Radiofrequency lesions of the PVN were performed under Chloropent anesthesia, using coordinates derived from the atlas of Paxinos and Watson. Sham-operated rats were anesthetized and subjected to electrode penetration without lesioning. Lesioned and sham-operated rats were subjected to intermittent, variable-interval footshock at 1.6 mA intensity (5 sec shock duration, approximately 30 shocks during a 15 min session). The stressed rats were killed by decapitation immediately after exposure to footshock. Unshocked groups of lesioned and sham-operated rats were decapitated immediately upon removal from their home cages.

Footshock increased pituitary cyclic AMP over twofold in the sham-operated rats. Lesions of the PVN completely abolished the stress-induced increase in cyclic AMP, without affecting resting levels in unstressed rats. In sham-operated rats, footshock increased plasma levels of ACTH, beta-endorphin, and beta-lipotrophic hormone sixfold, fourfold and ninefold, respectively. Each of these increases was markedly attenuated by PVN lesions. The present experiment demonstrates that an intact PVN is required for footshock to produce increases in pituitary cyclic AMP in vivo. These results provide strong support for the role of pituitary cyclic AMP as a component of the CRF-mediated neuroendocrine response to stress.

INFLUENCE OF RESTRAINT STRESS ON THE NOCTURNAL PROLACTIN SURGE OF PSEUDOPREGNANT ANIMALS 288

M. Morehead and R.R. Gala
Dept. of Physiology, Wayne State Univ., Detroit, MI 48201

Pseudopregnancy (PSP) was induced in female Sprague-Dawley rats by electromechanical stimulation of the cervix on the day of metestrus in animals exhibiting 2-3 normal 4 or 5 day cycles. Six to 9 days after cervical stimulation blood samples (0.4 ml) were obtained from a chronic atrial catheter implanted 7 days earlier in adrenalectomized (ADX) and sham operated animals. The nocturnal (N) prolactin (PRL) surge peaked at 0400h in both ADX and sham control animals. In the ADX animals the surge began 2 hrs earlier, however the peak level and extinction of the surge were similar to that of sham controls.

Restraint stress for 3 hrs (tieing the hind legs together with plastic coated bell wire) resulted in a rapid and marked decrease in the PRL surge in both the intact and ADX animals. One hr after initiation of stress the N PRL surge had decreased to 9% of the initial 0400 hr value compared to only 46% of the initial 1800 hr value for the afternoon surge. Control animals sampled during the N surge at the same time as stressed animals had a PRL decrease to 56% of the initial 0400h PRL value 1 hr later. The PRL value of control animals sampled during the proestrus afternoon surge simultaneously with the stressed animals was 72% of initial value 1 hr after the initiation of sampling.

The initiation of sampling 2 hrs prior to the N surge did not prevent the decrease in plasma PRL in non-stressed animals. Sampling control and stressed animals on separate nights prevented the decrease in the controls.

It is concluded that: (1) 3 hrs of restraint stress decreases the N PRL surge in PSP rats and ADX does not alter the response; (2) the N PRL surge appears to be more sensitive to stress than the proestrus afternoon surge; and (3) sampling stressed and non-stressed rats simultaneously suppress the N surge of non-stressed rats. (Supported by WSUSM BRSG Grant #NS52-S07 RR05384-24).

POMC-DERIVED HORMONE RESPONSES TO MAXIMAL TREADMILL EXERCISE 289

M. Oleshansky, J. Zoltick, R. Herman, E. Mougey and J. Meyerhoff
Dept Medical Neurosciences, Walter Reed Army Institute of Research, Washington, D.C. 20307-5100

Neuroendocrine responses to stress reflect the severity of a stressor and an individual's capacity to cope with that stressor. Running at 60-80% of the maximal oxygen consumption has been reported to increase plasma levels of β-endorphin (β-EP). One study noted that the increase in plasma β-EP levels in trained long distance runners after a strenuous run appeared to be inversely correlated with years of training. To further characterize the role of fitness in neuroendocrine responses to exercise, we administered a maximal exercise treadmill test (ETT) to subjects ranging from highly fit to unfit. We found that the pattern of recovery of proopiomelanocortin (POMC)-derived peptides after a maximal ETT is inversely correlated with fitness.

Twenty healthy male subjects, age 39.8±2.5 years (mean ± S.E.M.), exercised on a treadmill until exhausted at a constant rate of 3.3 mile/hr with a 5% increase in grade every three min. Mean maximal ETT time was 15.2±0.7 min (range 8.9-19 min). Plasma was collected: (A) thirty min after resting supine; (B) fifteen min after standing, just prior to exercise; (C) upon exercising to a heart rate of 140 beats/min; (D) immediately following maximal exercise; and (E) fifteen min after exercise. β-EP, β-LPH and ACTH were assayed by RIA.

(pg/ml)	A	B	C	D	E
β-LPH	59±5	64±6	76±6	238±27	222±32
β-EP	3.4±0.4	4.3±0.6	7.2±1.0	36.0±5.0	30.0±5.7
ACTH	16±3	22±4	30±6	66±9	70±16

The plasma levels of β-EP, β-LPH and ACTH increased dramatically in nearly all subjects during a maximal ETT. These changes were independent of the duration of maximal exercise (an index of fitness), suggesting that fitness did not influence the magnitude of the neuroendocrine responses in this exercise protocol. On the other hand, the changes in the plasma levels of these peptide hormones over fifteen minutes after maximal exercise were inversely correlated with the duration of maximal exercise. This finding suggests that the more fit an individual, the faster his POMC-derived hormones recover from a brief, vigorous physical stressor.

CHOLINERGIC AND SEROTONERGIC STIMULATION OF HYPOTHALAMIC CRF RELEASE IN VITRO 290

M.J. Owens, M.A. Smith and C.B. Nemeroff, Departments of Pharmacology and Psychiatry, Duke University Medical Center, Durham, N.C., USA

Considerable controversy exists concerning the role of various neurotransmitters on the activity of the hypothalamic-pituitary-adrenal (HPA) axis. Norepinephrine, acetylcholine and serotonin have been reported to stimulate HPA activity by some investigators, whereas others have reported these neurotransmitters to inhibit HPA activity. These early studies were conducted using a bioassay in which a perfusate thought to contain CRF was used to release ACTH from pituitary cell cultures. Bioassays such as these lack specificity because ACTH can be released by a variety of substances (e.g., vasopressin, oxytocin, epinephrine). In the present study, we have determined the effects of several neurotransmitters on CRF release using a specific and sensitive radioimmunoassay (RIA).

Male Sprague-Dawley rats were decapitated and a hypothalamic block was dissected using rostral-caudal boundaries of the optic chiasm and mammillary bodies, respectively, and dorsally to a point just above the third ventricle. Two such blocks were immediately placed in a test tube containing 0.6ml of a modified Kreb's-Henseleit buffer which was gassed with 95% O_2/5% CO_2 and the pH adjusted to 7.4 at 37°C. At ten minute intervals the buffer was removed and stored at -70°C until assayed for CRF. Our RIA uses ^{125}I-rCRF as a tracer and has a sensitivity of 0.625pg CRF/tube. The buffer was replaced by either fresh buffer in the case of basal release, or buffer containing the neurotransmitter under investigation. Basal release was measured for five consecutive ten minute intervals, and then the test substance was added during the 50-60 minute interval and once again restimulated during the 80-90 minute interval.

By the 40-50 minute epoch, basal release had stabilized to 6.8pg CRF/500µl incubation buffer. High potassium concentrations [40mM KCl] stimulated CRF release 1100% above basal levels. Serotonin [10µM] and carbachol [10µM] stimulated CRF release 550% and 300% above basal levels, respectively. In contrast to these results using whole hypothalamic blocks, carbachol and serotonin did not stimulate significant CRF release from minced hypothalami, though high potassium concentrations stimulated CRF release 900% above basal levels in this preparation.

These studies are concordant with the hypothesis that serotonergic and cholinergic neurons stimulate CRF release, resulting in HPA axis activation. Absence of neurotransmitter effects in minced hypothalami suggest that the projections of CRF neurons from the paraventricular nucleus (PVN) to the median eminence must be intact to respond to serotonin and acetylcholine. These neurotransmitters most likely act on PVN CRF containing perikarya and/or dendrites.

DOPAMINERGIC MODULATION OF THE SEPTO-HIPPOCAMPAL CHOLINERGIC SYSTEM UNDER STRESS. 291

J.M. Rabey, V.H. Gilad, G.M. Gilad.
The Center for Neurosciences and Behavioral Research, The Weizmann Institute of Science, Rehovot, Israel.

The effects of pharmacological interference with dopaminergic neurotransmission, using the agonist apomorphine or the antagonist sulpiride, on high affinity choline uptake and newly synthesized acetylcholine release by hyppocampal synaptosomal preparations, were examined in rats subjected to immobilization stress.

Increased dopamine uptake by septal synaptosomal preparations was taken as evidence for increased mesoseptal dopaminergic activity in response to stress. Apomorphine treatment failed to alter choline uptake or acetylcholine release in unhandled rats, but prevented the increase of these cholinergic parameters in response to acute stress. In contrast, after treatment with sulpiride both choline uptake and acetylcholine release were increased, as they did after acute stress. However, acute stress of sulpiride treated rats produced similar changes as either treatment alone. We conclude that the mesoseptal sopaminergic system plays an important role in modulating the activity of the septo-hippocampal cholinergic system under stress.

Plasma cortisol and beta endorphin after dexamethasone in Parkinson Disease 292

J.M. Rabey, M.Zohar, Z.Oberman and E. Graff
Department of Neurology, and Department of Chemical Pathology, Tel Aviv Medical Center, Sackler School of Medicine, Tel Aviv University, Israel.

We have measured plasma level of cortisol(RIA, Diagnostic Product Corporation) and beta endorphin(RIA Immuno-Nuclear Corporation),before and after dexametha-sone, 1 mg. in twenty seven idiopathic non depressed, parkinsonian patients.

Fifteen patients showed a normal cortisol depression while twelve patients showed cortisol "resistance". Basal pre-dexamethasone cortisol levels were significantly different(p 0,005)between thw two groups (13,5mg/100 ml+3,75 and 19,3+4,99 respectively).

Beta endorphin was examined in 15 patients. Seven patients showed high levels of beta endorphin after dexamethasone, while eight patients showed a normal depression. Predexamethasone beta-endorphin levels did not show a significant difference among the two groups (10,33pg/1+6,84 and 9,15 pg/1+ 6,23 respectively).

The results presented did not show a correlation between cortisol and beta endorphin supression after dexamethasone.

Interesting, we observed that anxiety behavior was always associated with a non-supression of both cortisol and beta endorphin. Ye, while some patients with anxiety were also cortisol supressive, all of them showed beta endorphin non supression. The results indicate that beta endorphin plasma levels after dexamethasone supression test could be a useful biological tool for the evaluation of anxiety, at least in parkinsonian patients.

EFFECT OF ETHANOL ON CRF RELEASE *IN VITRO* 293

E. Redei, B. Branch, A.N. Taylor
Dept. of Anatomy, UCLA and West LA/Brentwood VA, Los Angeles, CA 90024

In order to determine the site and mechanism of action of ethanol on the hypothalamic-pituitary-adrenal axis we studied the CRF response of superfused rat hypothalamus to ethanol (20, 40, 80, 200 mg/dl). For each *in vitro* superfusion experiment, three age-matched female Sprague-Dawley rats were sacrificed by decapitation, blocks of hypothalami removed within 2 min and presuperfused for 45 min. When a stable baseline level of CRF release was attained various doses of ethanol were applied as a bolus in a counterbalanced design. Two-minute fractions were collected continuously and analyzed for CRF content by RIA.

Basal CRF release as well as CRF response to ethanol showed multiphasic patterns, therefore data was subjected to Pulsar algorithm to determine pulsatile characteristics of CRF release. Ethanol did not produce significant changes in overall mean CRF levels at any dose. However, at doses of 20 and 40 mg/dl ethanol attenuated pulse amplitude of CRF significantly compared to mean pulse amplitude of basal release (67.1 ±6.0 (SE) and 75.6±21.3 vs 131.1± 17.9 pg/ml CRF, in five independent experiments, p 0.01 and p 0.05, respectively).

The highest dose (200 mg/dl) also decreased peak amplitude significantly (67.2±9.2 pg/ml CRF, p 0.05), while the 80 mg/dl dose produced no change (91.0±19.3 vs 131.1±1.7.9 pg/ml CRF, NS). There were no significant changes in pulse duration or interpulse interval in response to ethanol at any dose.

Major conclusions from these results are: (1) Frequent sampling is necessary to reveal the temporal characteristics of the hypothalamic CRF response to ethanol. (2) Acute exposure to low doses of ethanol *in vitro* inhibits the temporal release of CRF but induces release of ACTH directly at the pituitary, as we reported previously, suggesting that ethanol at low doses has its primary site of stimulatory action on the corticotrophs.

ALDOSTERONE SELECTIVITY OF TYPE I CORTICOID RECEPTORS IN RAT ANTERIOR PITUITARY 294

K. Sheppard and J.W. Funder
Medical Research Centre, Prince Henry's Hospital, Melbourne, Australia 3004.

We have previously shown renal Type I (mineralocorticoid) and hippocampal "corticosterone (B) preferring" receptors to have identical intrinsic steroid specificity in vitro (Krozowski & Funder, P.N.A.S. 80:6056, 1983). In the present study we have examined Type I receptors in colon, parotid, and pituitary, and have evaluated the role of tissue sequestration of corticosterone by in vivo and in vitro studies on 10-day old rats, which have with negligible circulating and tissue transcortin levels. Adrenalectomized adult Sprague-Dawley rats were injected s.c. with ^{3}H-aldosterone (^{3}HA) or ^{3}H-corticosterone (^{3}HB), with X100 RU28362 to exclude tracer from Type II glucocorticoid receptors. Rats were sacrificed after 10-180 min and specific receptor binding determined. ^{3}HB bound negligibly in all tissues except hippocampus; in contrast, ^{3}HA bound well and was well retained in kidney, colon, parotid and pituitary. Ten-day old rats injected with either ^{3}HA or ^{3}HB and X100 RU28362 showed an identical pattern of high ^{3}HA binding and low ^{3}HB binding, in all tissues except hippocampus. In vitro cytosol studies showed that B > A as a competitor for tracer binding to Type I sites in all the above tissues. We interpret these data as evidence (a) for an in vivo, post-receptor binding specificity conferring mechanism, distinct from extravascular transcortin, in kidney, colon, parotid and pituitary, enabling the selective retention of aldosterone rather than corticosterone and (b) that Type I receptors both in classical mineralocorticoid targets (kidney, colon, parotid) and in pituitary may thus represent physiologic aldosterone receptors.

Supported by the National Health & Medical Research Council of Australia.

STRESS-INDUCED ALTERATIONS IN NEUROTENSIN-LIKE IMMUNOREACTIVITY (NTLI) IN RAT BRAIN AND ADRENALS. 295

M.A. Smith, A.Y. Deutch, P.B. Chappell, G. Bissette, L. O'Connor, R.H. Roth, and C.B. Nemeroff. Dept. of Psychiatry, Duke Univ. Med. Ctr., Durham, N.C. and Yale Univ., New Haven, Ct.

Neurotensin (NT) is a peptide distributed in the brain and GI tract which induces a variety of behavioral and physiological effects including protection against stress-induced gastric ulcers. In the present study we investigated the ability of various stressors to alter NTLI in the brains and adrenals of adult male rats.

First we examined the effect of 3 hrs of immobilization at 4°C on brain NTLI. After decapitation, the brains were dissected into 10 regions, and NTLI was extracted in 1 N HCL, lyophilized and quantitated by radioimmunoassay. Measurable NTLI (pg/mg protein ± SEM) was found in all 10 brain regions. However only the midbrain showed an increase in NTLI (1070 ± 21) in the stressed group compared to a non-stressed control group (867 ± 32), ($p<0.001$). A trend for a decrease in NTLI occurred in the caudate nucleus.

Next we exposed rats to 20 mins of mild foot-shock stress and measured NTLI by RIA and 3,4-dihydroxyphenylacetic acid (DOPAC) by HPLC. DOPAC was elevated in the ventral tegmental area (VTA) and prefrontal cortex indicating that stress induced increases in dopamine turnover in these areas. The only significant increase in NTLI in the group receiving foot-shock compared to a non-stressed control group occurred in the VTA, (539 ± 31) vs (427 ± 42), ($p<0.05$). A trend towards decreased NTLI was again seen in the caudate nucleus.

Finally we measured NTLI in rat adrenals after acute stress (3 hrs of cold-restraint) and chronic stress (2 weeks of a series of stressors including cold swim, ether etc.). Adrenal NTLI was 3.4 ± 0.5 pg/mg wet weight in controls. NTLI increased to 4.7 ± 0.7 after acute stress and to 8.4 ± 0.6 following chronic stress.

These results indicate that two different stressors cause similar increases of NTLI in the midbrain of rats. Moreover acute and chronic stress increased NTLI concentrations in the adrenals. The role of NT during stress is unknown, but it may be important in the regulation of dopamine neurons in the VTA and elsewhere.

BRAIN CORTICOTROPIN-RELEASING FACTOR (CRF) AND PITUITARY-ADRENAL RESPONSIVENESS IN CHRONICALLY STRESSED RATS 296

S. Suemaru, K. Hashimoto, T. Takao, T. Hattori, M. Sugawara, H. Inoue, J. Kageyama, Z. Ota
Third Department of Internal Medicine, Okayama University Medical School, Okayama, Japan

The brain CRF concentration and pituitary-adrenocortical responsiveness were examined in chronically stressed rats. Male Wistar rats were exposed to the ether-cold-restraint stress for 30 min daily for 2 to 3 weeks and decapitated 20 hrs after the last stress session. One group of chronically stressed rats was exposed to a novel stress, 15 min exposure to the same stress, and then decapitated. The median eminence (ME), the rest of the hypothalamus (rHY), the cerebral cortex, the neurointermediate lobe (NIL) and anterior lobe of the pituitary (AP) were dissected out and truncal blood was obtained. CRF concentrations in ME, rHY, the cerebral cortex and NIL were measured using rat CRF-RIA, and ACTH content in AP and plasma ACTH and corticosterone (B) concentrations were measured by RIAs. The synthetic rat CRF or AVP was injected intravenously to the jugular vein catheters of chronically stressed rats in freely moving conditions, and blood samples were drawn before and 5, 15 and 30 min after injection for plasma ACTH and B measurements.

CRF in ME and ACTH in AP were increased, whereas the resting plasma ACTH and B levels were unchanged in chronically stressed rats compared with control rats. The chronic stress did not affect CRF concentrations in NIL and cerebral cortex. The novel acute stress increased the hypothalamic CRF concentration and the ratio of plasma B to ACTH in chronically stressed rats compared with the non-chronically stressed rats. The plasma ACTH response to exogenous CRF was relatively blunted, whereas that to AVP was relatively exaggerated in chronically stressed rats.

These results suggested that the hypothalamic CRF secretion was facilitated in chronic stress, which might cause a down-regulation of CRF receptors resulting in the blunted ACTH response to a subsequent stress or an exogenous CRF, whereas an increased releasable pool of ACTH resulted in the exaggerated ACTH response to AVP, and that the sensitivity of adrenal cortex to ACTH was increased in chronically stressed rats.

DIFFERENCES IN (3H)CORTICOSTERONE AND (3H)DEXAMETHASONE BINDING CHARACTERISTICS TO HYPOTHALAMUS, HIPPOCAMPUS AND ANTERIOR PITUITARY GLAND. 297

W. Sutanto and B.D. Allen. Human Physiology, Royal Holloway and Bedford New College, Egham Hill, Egham, Surrey TW20 0EX, ENGLAND.

Glucocorticoids have profound influence on the functioning of the central nervous system (CNS). The effects include the feedback action on the secretion of CRF from the hypothalamus (HYP) and of ACTH from the anterior pituitary gland (AP). The hippocampus (HIPP) exerts inhibitory influence on the hypothalamo-pituitary-adrenocortical (HPA)-axis and some of this influence represents mediation of feedback inhibition by glucocorticoids. In each case, the steroids exert their actions by interacting with specific cytosolic receptors prior to the translocation to the nucleus where they influence the genome.

Corticosterone (B) and dexamethasone (Dex) bind to the cytosolic macromolecules and they are believed to occupy different binding sites in the CNS. The present study shows that both steroids bind to cytosols from HYP, HIPP and AP with similar high affinity but their binding characteristics to these tissues are affected differently by various steroids.

Binding competition studies were carried out as described in Allen, et al, (1986). The results show that RU 28362 (a glucocorticoid) and RU 38486 (an antiglucocorticoid) at equimolar concentration or less are competitors with (3H)Dex and (3H)B in HIPP but only with (3H)Dex in HYP or AP. 11-epicortisol and 17α-hydroxyprogesterone at 10^{-7} M are better competitors for (3H)Dex than for (3H)B in the 3 tissues.

In the light of evidence in the past 10 years that not all B receptors can be occupied by Dex, the present results provide further proof of heterogeneity of glucococorticoid binding sites in the CNS.

Reference : Allen, B.D., et al. J. Physiol. (1986) In the Press.

We would like to thank Dr R. Deraedt (Roussel-Uclaf Pharmaceutical Company, France) for the generous gift of RU 28362 and RU 38486.

CENTRAL ADRENERGIC AND NORADRENERGIC STIMULATORY CONTROL OF THE CRH-ACTH AXIS IN THE RAT. 298

A. Szafarczyk, G. Alonso, F. Malaval, R. Gibaud, I. Assenmacher
Neuroendocrinology Lab. - UA 1197 CNRS - Dept of Physiology, Univ. Montpellier II - F 34060 Montpellier, France.

The concept that brain catecholamines (CA) exert a stimulatory control on ACTH was inferred from the recent demonstration that a catecholaminergic denervation of the hypothalamus by micro-injection of 6-OHDA into the ventral noradrenergic bundle (VNAB), leading to a 80 - 90 % fall in hypothalamic concentrations of adrenaline (Ad) and noradrenaline (NA) -but not dopamine-, dramatically reduced the diurnal stimulated and stress-induced ACTH release (A. Szafarczyk et al., Amer. J. Physiol., 249, E219, 1985).

Immunocytochemical studies additionally revealed that the decrease of CRH immunoreactivity, normally induced by colchicine, in axons of the external median eminence was significantly inhibited in the VNAB lesioned rats, which points to an obliteration of CRH release. In an attempt to characterize further the nature of the stimulatory CA control on the CRH-ACTH axis, we measured the effect on plasma ACTH of i.c.v. injections of CA agonists and antagonists, and of the latter in correlation with ether-stress. Results indicated that (1) stress-like ACTH surges followed both i.c.v. Ad or NA in a dose response relationship , and with a higher effectiveness for Ad vs NA on an equimolar basis ; (2) NA-triggered ACTH release was inhibited exclusively by a pretreatment with an α_1 blocker (prazosin), while the response to Ad was equally decreased with an α_1 or a β blocker (propranolol) ; (3) a pretreatment with α_1 or β or both blockers, at least halved the stress-induced ACTH surge. Taken together the data favor the theory that the CA, and especially the Ad innervation of the CRH neurons, provided a stimulatory component to the stress-induced ACTH release.

RELEASE OF CORTICOTROPIN-RELEASING FACTOR FROM RAT HYPOTHALAMUS IN VITRO

299

T. Takao, K. Hashimoto, S. Suemaru, T. Hattori, J. Kageyama, Z. Ota
Third Department of Internal Medicine, Okayama University Medical School, Okayama 700, Japan

Corticotropin-releasing factor (CRF) release from rat hypothalamus was examined in vitro using an incubation method and a perifusion method. One or two hypothalami were incubated in a polyethylene tube with 1 ml of Krebs-Ringer bicarbonate buffer (KRBG) containing glucose (0.2%), bovine serum albumin (0.25%), bacitracin (100 μg/ml) and ascorbic acid (1 mM). All tubes were placed in a water bath (37°C) and gently shaken in a 95% O_2-5% CO_2 atmosphere. A series of two incubations were performed at 45 min intervals after 30 min preincubation, and test substances were added to the medium in the second incubation. In the perifusion method, 6-8 hypothalami were placed in a small column in a 37°C water bath, and perifused with KRBG at 200 μl/min. Test substances were dissolved in KRBG and were added into the perifusion medium through bypass tube. CRF concentration in the incubation medium and the perifusion medium were measured by a specific CRF radioimmunoassay, of which sensitivity was 2 pg/tube.

The high K^+ concentration (56 mM) evoked a 6-8 fold increase in the CRF release from the hypothalamus during 45 min incubation. However, serotonin, norepinephrine, angiotensin II, atrial natriuretic peptide did not evoked statistically significant change of CRF release in this incubation system. In the perifusion system, high K^+ concentration also evoked a marked CRF release. Serotonin and acetylcholine stimulated CRF release, while norepinephrine did not show significant change of CRF release. Angiotensin II stimulated CRF release from perifused hypothalami.

These results suggest that the perifusion method is more sensitive than the incubation method to examine the effect of amines and peptides on CRF release and that serotonin, acetylcholine and angiotensin II stimulated CRF release from the hypothalamus.

EFFECT OF STRESS ON NEUROPEPTIDES AND THEIR RECEPTORS OF RAT CNS

300

H. Takayama, H. Kuroda, N. Ogawa, Z. Ota
Third Department of Internal Medicine and Institute for Neurobiology, Okayama University Medical School, Okayama Japan

It is well known that a variety of stressors induced a significant alteration in the metabolism and/or function of various neurotransmitters in the CNS as well as peripheral nervous system. For example, it has demonstrated that various environmental stresses exhibit a significant decrease in cerebral noradrenaline, dopamine and opioid peptides contents. On the other hand, little is known about the other neuropeptide systems under stressful situations. Therefore, we attempted to examine whether or not an environmental stress affects both the concentration and the receptor binding of neuropeptides using an immobilization stress (IM-stress).

Male Sprague-Dawley rats were stressed by immobilization for 0.5 to 3 hours. The concentration and the receptor binding of substance P (SP), methionine-enkephalin (ME) and thyrotropin releasing hormone(TRH) were determined in the eight brain regions and the spinal cord by radioimmunoassay and radiolabeled receptor assay, respectively.

The concentration of SP was decreased in the septum, striatum and hippocampus, and the SP receptor binding was decreased in the septum, amygdala+piriform cortex and hypothalamus. The concentration of ME was not changed, but the ME receptor binding was decreased in the septum. The concentration of TRH was decreased in the frontal cortex, septum, amygdala+piriform cortex and pons+medulla oblongata, but increased in the spinal cord. The TRH receptor binding was decreased in the septum, amygdala+piriform cortex and hypothalamus.

These results show that IM-stress affects neuropeptide receptor as well as neuropeptide concentration and the septum is a very important region under IM-stress. Moreover, the effect of stress on neuropeptide-mediated neural system can become clearer after measurement of the receptor levels.

ACTH RESPONSE TO CHRONIC INTRAVENTRICULAR ADMINISTRATION OF ANTI-CORTICOSTERONE IN THE RAT

301

J.E. Van Zuylen, A.N. Taylor, S. Gholami, E. Redei
Dept. of Anatomy, UCLA, Los Angeles, CA 90024

The purpose of this study was to examine how the removal of glucocorticoid negative feedback from suprapituitary sites influences ACTH secretion. Cerebral cannula were stereotaxically implanted into the lateral ventricle of female Sprague-Dawley rats weighing 342±5 (SE) g. Osmotic minipumps filled with corticosterone antiserum or normal rabbit serum (NRS) (mean fill volume of 244.4±1.6 mg with flow rates of 0.46 ul/hr) were inserted subcutaneously into the interscapular region and joined to the cerebral cannula for infusion.

Blood samples were taken by cardiac puncture one week after the start of infusion. Animals were decapitated at the end of the second week, trunk blood collected and ACTH and corticosterone (CS) measured by RIA. Hypothalami were removed, extracted and assayed for CRF content by RIA. Adrenal and thymus weights were measured.

At one week, plasma ACTH and CS levels were significantly elevated in rats infused with anti-corticosterone compared to NRS controls (885.5±317 vs 24.3±10.8 pg/ml ACTH, p=0.01, n=6; and 240.6±49.7 vs 129.3±30.1 ng/ml CS, $p<0.05$). However, after two weeks, plasma levels of ACTH and CS, CRF content of hypothalami and adrenal weights were not significantly different in the two groups; while thymus weights were significantly lower (149.9±9.1 vs 233.8±9.0 mg, $p<0.01$) in rats infused with anti-CS compared to controls.

In summary, binding of free CS by anti-CS produced an increase in ACTH levels similar to adrenalectomy suggesting that the primary site for negative feedback action of glucocorticoids is suprapituitary. The lack of effect after two weeks of chronic infusion might represent insufficient amounts of anti-CS to bind free CS in the brain, possibly due to the previously elevated ACTH and CS levels seen at one week.

QUANTITATIVE ANALYSIS OF ADRENOCORTICAL SECRETION IN RESPONSE TO ACTIVATION OF PERIPHERAL NERVE FIBER GROUPS OF DIFFERENT DIAMETERS

302

Z.Z. Wang, Y.Z. Chen
Second Military Medical College,Shanghai,China

Electrical stimulation of the somatic afferents may be considered as a pure neurogenic stimulus, and the purpose of the study was to determine to what extent the different peripheral somatosensory neural afferents participate in the activation of the adrenocortical responses. The influence of graded electrical stimulation of the sciatic nerve on corticosterone secretion was investigated in nembutal-anaesthetized rats. Serum corticosterone level was not changed during a short or long period of sciatic nerve stimulation with the current intensity capable of exciting A-alpha fiber. A significant elevation of serum corticosterone was elicited by activation of A-delta or/and C fiber group, the response to activation of A-delta and C fibers was more obvious than that to A-delta fiber only. Following the cessation of the stimulation, serum corticosterone level rapidly increased, reach its maximum at about 5-10 minutes and the high level last up to 90 min. Correlations between the patterns of corticosterone secretion and the current intensity, duration and frequency of stimulation were quantitatively analysed. These results indicate that activation of high threshold small myelinated or unmyelinated afferent was essential for the adrenocortical secretion responses. The physiological significance of the effects of somatic afferent stimulation and its possible role in the neurogenic stress are discussed.

303

PLASMA CORTICOTROPIN-RELEASING FACTOR, CORTISOL, AND CORTISOL-BINDING GLOBULIN DURING THIRD TRIMESTER PREGNANCY

C. D. A. Wolfe, E. A. Linton[2], P. R. Scraggs, E. A. Campbell[1] and M. T. Jones
Department of Gynaecology and [1]Biochemistry, St. Thomas's Hospital Medical School and [2]Protein Hormone Unit, St. Bartholomew's Centre for Clinical Research, London.

Biologically active corticotropin-releasing factor (CRF) has been extracted from human term placenta and elevated plasma levels of this peptide have been reported in the third trimester of pregnancy.

Using a direct sensitive, specific two-site immunoradiometric assay (IRMA) for CRF, we have demonstrated in a group of 80 normal pregnant subjects, levels rising from 50 ± 15 pg/ml at 28 weeks to 1462 ± 182 pg/ml at 40 weeks and 1680 ± 101 pg/ml in labour. Post-partum levels return to normal within 15 hours. CRF levels show no diurnal variation and are unaffected by changes in posture or during myometrial contractions. Sequential measurements of total cortisol by RIA in the same patients shows a rise to term reaching levels of 1000-2000 nmoles/l in labour. In contrast to CRF, however, cortisol does show a diurnal variation and post-partum levels remain elevated for several days.

In five subjects, we also measured cortisol-binding globulin (CBG) in the same samples. In one subject with CRF levels at the top of the normal range, CBG and cortisol were also high, whereas in two subjects with low CRF values, CBG was also low and cortisol was at the lower end of the normal range.

CRF values were unchanged following treatment for premature labour with high dose dexamethasone, except in one subject in whom CRF was undetectable 12 hours after treatment but returned to normal subsequently.

Thus there appears to be some correlation between CRF, cortisol and CBG levels during third trimester pregnancy, but placental CRF is not under the same control mechanisms as hypothalamic CRF in that it shows no diurnal variation and, in general, is non-suppressible with high-dose dexamethasone even although there are specific glucocorticoid receptors in the placenta.

304

INHIBITION OF PLASMA RENIN ACTIVITY BY CORTISOL.

C.E. Wood and J. Silbiger, Department of Physiology, University of Florida College of Medicine, Gainesville, FL 32610

Previous studies from this laboratory have demonstrated that in preterm fetal sheep, increases in plasma cortisol (F) concentration equal in amplitude to fetal F stress responses, suppress plasma renin activity (PRA). The purpose of this study was to investigate the possibility that this negative interaction exists in adult sheep. Five conscious ewes with chronically prepared carotid arterial loops were infused intravenously with F (6 µg/kg/min) or vehicle (5% ethanol in 0.9% saline) for 5 hours. Each ewe participated in both F- and vehicle- infusion experiments. One hour after the end of F or vehicle infusion, renin secretion was stimulated by hypotension produced by infusion of sodium nitroprusside (20 µg/kg/min, i.v.). Data were analyzed by one- and two-way ANOVA; hormones were measured by RIA. F infusion increased plasma F from 26 ± 3 to 46 ± 8 ng/ml; during vehicle infusion plasma F decreased from 15 ± 4 to 9 ± 4 ng/ml. F infusion decreased hematocrit from 29 ± 2 to 26 ± 1%, while vehicle infusion did not significantly change hematocrit from 30 ± 2%. The decrease in hematocrit during F infusion may have been caused by influx of fluid into the vascular space. Basal PRA in vehicle- and F-infused groups were 0.4 ± 0 and 0.2 ± 0.1 ng AI/ml/hr and did not change. It is possible that suppression of basal PRA was not demonstrated because levels were low initially. Nitroprusside decreased mean arterial pressure equally in both groups. In vehicle-infused ewes PRA increased from 0.4 ± 0 to 4.6 ± 0.4, while in F-infused ewes PRA increased from 0.2 ± 1 to 3.3 ± 0.4 ng AI/ml/hr, a significantly smaller response. We conclude that physiological increases in ovine plasma F inhibit PRA responses to nitroprusside-induced hypotension. This suppression of PRA by F may result from an increase in vascular volume and may therefore be reflex in nature. (Supported by NIH grant HD17705 and by a grant from The Florida Affiliate of The American Heart Association).

305

HYPOTHALAMIC LHRH CONTENT IN NEONATALLY ESTROGENIZED-STERILE FEMALE RATS IS HIGHER THAN THAT IN INTACT CYCLING RATS

M. AIHARA(1), S. HAYASHI(2), K. WAKABAYASHI(3), and H. KOBAYASHI(1) (1)Dept. Biol.,Toho Univ.,Funabashi, Chiba 274, (2)Dept.Anat./Embryol.,Tokyo Metropol.Inst. Neurosci., Fuchu, Tokyo 183, (3)Inst. Endocr., Gunma Univ., Maebashi, Gunma 371, Japan.

Administration of 10 µg estradiol benzoate(EB) for 5 consecutive days into the newborn female rats of the Sprague-Dawley strain induced extreme reduction in gonadotropic activity in adulthood. Administration of EB and progesterone into these sterile female rats caused an increase in the blood LH levels, but it was only about 1/10 of that in the control female rats which had received no neonatal EB injections. The LHRH content in the diencephalon of these rats was assessed at around 50, 100 and 240 days of age, and compared with that of control rats. Immediately after decapitation, a diencephalon block (ca W6xD4xL10 mm) was trimmed out and mounted on a cryostat stage. Serial frontal sections of 400 µm thickness were made. The LHRH content in the acid extract of these samples was measured by radioimmunoassay.

Two clear peaks in the rostro-caudal LHRH distribution were detected which were divided at the suprachiasmatic nucleus (SCN) region. No clear difference in the distribution pattern of the LHRH was detected among the groups. Total amount of the LHRH in the hypothalamus was calculated separately for the rostral and medio-basal halves which were divided at the SCN region and the total was also compared in the sterile and control rats at varying ages. The LHRH content was higher in the rostral parts in the sterile rats at 50 and 240 days of age and in the mediobasal parts at 50 days compared with that in the control rats. At 100 days of age, no significant difference in the LHRH content in either half was detected between the sterile and the control rats. These results indicate that the gonadotropic activity in the neonatally estrogenized rats does not directly reflect the hypothalamic LHRH content. Thus, it is likely that neonatal administration of EB affected hypothalamic mechanisms relating to the LHRH releasing systems.

306

IS THERE A DEFECTIVE CENTRAL COORDINATION OF OVARIAN ACTIVITY IN AGING RATS ?

M. Cioni, L. Greco, H. Zachi Pour, U. Scapagnini, B. Marchetti
Dept. of Pharmacology,Catania University, 95125 Italy

Loss of fertility during midlife occurs in female of many mammalian species. The development of reproductive acyclicity represents, perhaps, one of the most dramatic examples of neuroendocrine changes with age. In the present study we have investigated whether loss of cycles in female rats is accompanied by changes of hypothalamic and gonadal LHRH activity as well as ovarian noradrenergic tone. Middle-aged (8-11 months) rats displayed lower hypophyseal LHRH receptor (R) activity in the morning of proestrus, compared to young animals, while in constant estrous (CE) rats pituitary LHRH-R numbers were similar to values measured in young estrus control. Stimulation of the medial preoptic area produced a significant increase of LHRH-R within the pituitary of both young and old rats, suggesting that the pituitary LHRH-R per se is not intrinsically impaired with age, but the neural signals impinging on the "LHRH pulse generator" are altered. Ovarian LHRH-R are high in old rats and levels are reduced by intraovarian injection of a potent LHRH-antagonist, while β - adrenergic R are markedly lost in old CE rats. Ovarian denervation performed at estrus, markedly decreased estradiol and progesterone plasma levels in intact rats on the afternoon of proestrus, while in middle-aged rats the response was significantly reduced. Results demonstrate a disruption in central and peripheral mechanisms regulating hypothalamic and gonadal LHRH activity, associated with a decreased efficiency of peripheral adrenergic neural tone in aging rats. It is speculated that a defective neural signal impinging in the gonadal milieu might participate in the establishment of gonadal failure observed with aging.

DELAYED SEXUAL MATURATION DURING PREPUBERTAL CHRONIC CANNABINOID TREATMENT: ASSOCIATED REDUCTION IN SERUM PROLACTIN 307

E. Field, L. Tyrey, Duke University, Durham, N.C. 27710

Δ-9-tetrahydrocannabinol (THC) delays the onset of vaginal cyclicity and ovulation in pubertal rats when chronically administered from 27 days of age until the onset of sexual maturity. The mechanism by which THC delays pubertal development is unclear. The present study was conducted to determine whether THC treatment initiated at different prepubertal ages would be equally effective in delaying sexual maturation and if prepubertal alterations in pituitary hormone secretion were associated with the pubertal delay.

Pair-fed female rats were treated twice daily with THC (10 mg/kg, ip) or vehicle beginning at 24, 27, or 30 days of age. Pairs of anestrous animals from each treatment group were decapitated 2 hr after the second daily injection at 24, 27, or 30 days of age to determine serum LH and PRL levels. Other animal pairs were treated up to the first day of full vaginal cornification.

Chronic THC treatment delayed the first estrus by 4.4 days in the group treated beginning at 27 days of age ($p<0.05$), but no differences in the age at sexual maturation were found between THC- and vehicle-treated animals when treatment was begun at 24 or 30 days of age. Animals that experienced pubertal delay exhibited a transient suppression of serum PRL at 27 days of age ($p<0.05$), an effect not observed in animals treated from 24 days of age. Prepubertal THC treatment also was associated with a reduced incidence of high LH values thought to represent pulsatile LH secretion.

The current study confirms our previous report that prepubertal exposure to THC beginning at 27 days of age delays the onset of sexual maturity in the female rat and further defines the time during which THC exposure results in pubertal delay. The failure of THC treatment initiated at 24 days of age to delay the age at first estrus likely reflects tolerance development to THC action. Although the evidence is only correlative, it is possible that THC-induced inhibition of PRL secretion could contribute to delayed follicular maturation and vaginal cyclicity. (Supported by DA 02006.)

DECREASED IMMUNOREACTIVE GNRH AND PROGNRH HYPOTHALAMIC NEURONS IN JUVENILE PRIMATES 308

P.C. Goldsmith, K.K. Thind, T. Song, S.E. Monroe
Reproductive Endocrinology Center, Dept. of Ob/Gyn and Repro. Sci., Univ. of Calif., San Francisco, CA 94143

Puberty in primates (at 3-4 yr.) is preceded by a period of high gonadotropin secretion and responsiveness to GnRH in neonates, followed by decreased secretion and responsiveness in juveniles (6-36 mo.) (Monroe et al., Biol. Repro. 29:422, 1983). Since these changes suggest altered hypothalamic GnRH secretion, we examined whether the GnRH neuronal system reflects these events. Frontal Vibratome sections from various ages and both sexes of *Macaca mulatta* and *fascicularis*, and *Papio cynocephalus* and *anubis* were immunostained with antisera against GnRH (LR1, R. Benoit) or its prohormone (proGnRH) (24A, P. Seeburg) using the PAP technique. The location, distribution, number, and staining intensity of immunoreactive (+) neurons from comparable levels were surveyed using light microscopy. Late fetal (110-160 d.) and neonatal (2-5 d. post-partum) animals had the most numerous proGnRH+ and GnRH+ neurons, correlating with high LH and FSH levels reported at this time. Numbers of GnRH+ cell bodies averaged ~40/section in the septo-preoptic area (S-POA) and ~15/section in the medial basal hypothalamus (MBH). Juvenile (2-2.5 yr.) primates had less immunoreactive and fewer GnRH+ neurons/section than neonates, particularly in the S-POA (~75% fewer) and MBH (~50% fewer). Adult macaques and baboons (4-8 yr.) contained more GnRH+ neurons/section than juveniles, ~50% more in the S-POA and ~30% more in the MBH, but less than fetal and neonatal animals. These results suggest that reproductive quiescence in prepubertal primates may be due to decreased GnRH neuronal activity. Taken together with previous data, they also suggest that GnRH synthesis and secretion are high in late fetal and neonatal animals, and low in juveniles. Since immunostaining for proGnRH and GnRH persists throughout development, they also support the concept that synthesis rather than post-translational processing is suppressed during the prepubertal period.

Supported by NIH Grants HD10907 (PCG) and HD11979.

DIFFERENTIAL EFFECTS OF NEONATAL AND ADULT ANDROGEN EXPOSURE ON THE GROWTH HORMONE (GH) SECRETORY PATTERN IN THE MALE RAT 309

J-O Jansson, L.A. Frohman
Div. of Endocrinology and Metabolism, Univiversity of Cincinnati College of Medicine, Cincinnati, OH 45267

The secretory pattern of GH in the rat is sex differentiated with males exhibiting lower baseline levels and higher and less frequent pulses. We have studied the interaction of androgen exposure during neonatal and adult life on the pattern of GH secretion.

Neonatal male rats were gonadectomized (NGX) or sham operated on day 1-2 of life and injected immediately after surgery with testosterone propionate (250 µg SC) or vehicle. At 90-130 days of age, rats were bled every 20 min between 9-17 h from an indwelling iv catheter. Some NGX rats were then given depot testosterone (15 mg/kg IM) and sampled again after 5-10 days. Plasma GH (RIA) pulsatile secretory patterns were analyzed by the PULSAR program. GH pulses were markedly lower in NGX (77±8 ng/ml) than in sham operated (264±35 ng/ml) rats, while the baseline GH levels were increased by NGX. In NGX rats given neonatal testosterone, high GH pulses were restored (191±29 ng/ml) and baseline levels were increased. In comparison to intact male rats, the pulses were shorter (55±8 vs 110±4 min, $p<0.01$) and more frequent (3.9±0.7 vs 2.5±0.1 pulses/8 h, $p<0.05$), and baseline GH levels were markedly higher ($p<0.01$). In contrast, NGX rats treated with testosterone during both neonatal and adult life displayed a GH pattern indistinguishable from that in normal males with high (243±24 ng/ml) and long-lasting (103±8 min) pulses every 3 h (2.7±0.2 pulses/8 h) and a low baseline. Masculine GH patterns were also seen in NGX rats given testosterone only during adult life.

The results indicate that neonatal androgen exposure results in an overall stimulation of GH secretion including higher pulses. However, only adult androgen exposure can produce a GH secretory pattern consisting of high pulses every 3 h separated by a low baseline, that is characteristic of normal male rats.

DEVELOPING NEUROENDOCRINE SYSTEMS AS TARGETS FOR DRUGS AND PEPTIDE HORMONES 310

W. Lichtensteiger, M. Schlumpf and U. Ribary
Inst. of Pharmacology, University of Zürich, Zürich, Switzerland

The temporal coincidence between critical phases in the organization of neuroendocrine systems and the ontogeny of forebrain transmitter systems raises the possibility of multiple interactions. We are investigating two aspects, i.e., the possibility of indirect drug actions on fetal brain through changes in neuroendocrine systems, and the possible role of peptide hormones in brain ontogeny.

1. Drug actions were studied on the gonadal axis of the rat fetus. We found that nicotine administered to pregnant rats from GD 12, suppressed the GD 18 testosterone peak and caused a loss of sexual dimorphism in the preference for saccharin-containing drinking water in adulthood (Lichtensteiger and Schlumpf, Pharm. Biochem. Behav. 23, 439, 1985). The same treatment also resulted in persistent alterations in forebrain catecholamine metabolites. The nicotine-induced metabolite pattern changed from prenatal through postnatal to adult life, with sex differences during postnatal development. In adulthood, prenatally nicotine-exposed males exhibited reduced levels of MOPEG, DOPAC, and HVA, whereas their female littermates showed only a reduction of HVA.

2. Little is known on the role of peptide hormones in brain ontogeny. We analyzed interactions between the developing brain and alpha-MSH. The acute feedback reaction of rat tubero-hypophyseal DA neurons to i.p. alpha-MSH develops towards the end of the first postnatal week. When alpha-MSH antiserum was injected i.v. on post natal days 5 + 6, i.e., on two days characterized by a prominent peak of plasma MSH, we observed a complete disappearance of the feedback response to alpha-MSH in adult rats; the reaction to i.p. prolactin was, however, preserved. This observation points to a specific effect of alpha-MSH on the developing DA neurons. There appears to exist a critical period, since antiserum injection in the second week of life was ineffective.

ELECTRICAL STIMULATION OF THE HYPOTHALAMUS INDUCES DIFFERENTIAL LH RELEASE AT TWO DEVELOPMENTAL STAGES IN IMMATURE FEMALE GUINEA PIGS 311

M.D. Loose, E. Terasawa
Wis. Regional Primate Research Ctr., Univ. of Wisconsin, Madison, WI 53715-1299

Previously, we observed in prepubertal female guinea pigs (18 days of age) that there were either no LH pulses or significantly fewer LH pulses with small pulse amplitude as compared to LH pulses in pubertal females (46 days of age). To investigate whether the immature LH pattern before puberty reflects the inability of LHRH neurons to respond to a signal for release or reflects the lack of the neural stimulus for LHRH release, we applied electrical stimulation (ES) to the arcuate nucleus and adjacent areas in prepubertal and pubertal female guinea pigs. Female guinea pigs ovariectomized 2 weeks earlier and implanted with an electrode 2 days earlier were stimulated at 18 (n=13) or 46 (n=10) days of age. ES (15 Hz, 0.5 msec, 200 μA or 500 μA) was applied for two minutes. Blood samples were collected from the unanesthetized animals through a jugular catheter every 10 min for 3.5 h with additional samplings at 2.5 and 5 min post-stimulation. After the last ES, 7.5 ng LHRH/100g B.W. was injected i.v. LH was estimated using RIA. Results are: 1) During the prestimulation period, mean LH levels and the LH pulse frequency were significantly lower in the day-18 group than the day-46 group ($p<0.01$). 2) The 500 μA ES resulted in significant LH release in both age groups ($p<0.005$). Similarly, the 200 μA stimulation induced LH release in both groups but with smaller amplitude than the 500 μA stimulation. 3) However, the magnitude of the LH increase after the 500 μA ES in the day-18 group (373±99 ng/ml) was significantly ($p<0.01$) smaller than that in the day-46 group (908±109 ng/ml). 4) LHRH injection induced a slightly smaller LH release (503±119 ng/ml) in the day-18 group than that (704±78 ng/ml) in the day-46 group. These results indicate that LHRH neurons in prepubertal females are capable of releasing LHRH if depolarized. Therefore, the neural circuit activating pulsatile LHRH release may not be fully established before the onset of puberty. (Supported by NIH grants RR00167 and HD11355.)

AGING AND BRAIN K OPIOID RECEPTORS 312

R. Maggi, D. Dondi, F. Piva
Department of Endocrinology, University of Milano, Italy.

It has been recently observed in this laboratory that the number of mu opioid receptors decreases significantly in the whole brain and in the hypothalamus of aged male rats. Also K receptors are present in high concentrations in the brain. Consequently, it was deemed of interest to analyze whether also this subclass of brain opioid receptors is affected by aging. This study was performed by measuring with a binding receptor assay the maximal binding capacity (Bmax, index of the number of receptors) and the affinity constant (Ka) for 3H-Bremazocine (3H-BRZ) in membrane preparations derived from the hypothalamus, amygdala, mesencephalon, hippocampus, thalamus, frontal poles, anterior and posterior cortex, isolated from the brains of 2 and 19 month old male rats. In order to obtain the binding of 3H-BRZ only to K receptor, the ligand was added to membrane preparations from each animal after protection of mu and delta receptors with 3H-dihydromorphine and 3H-D-ala-2-D-leu-enkephalin, respectively. The results obtained show that the Bmax for 3H-BRZ is significantly higher in the amygdala and thalamus of old rats than in the same areas of young animals; no changes of the Bmax for 3H-BRZ were observed in aged rats in the other regions selected. The Ka for 3H-BRZ did not change in any of the structures under study. Conclusions: 1) aging, in addition to mu receptors, affects also the number of K receptors in selected regions of the rat brain; 2) the increase of the number of K receptors in the amygdala might have some bearing on the decrease of serum gonadotropins observed in senescent male rats, since the amygdala is involved in the nervous circuits influencing the hypothalamo-pituitary axis.

(Supported by C.N.R. grant no. 85.00715.56)

SELECTIVE INCREASE OF TYPE I CORTICOSTEROID RECEPTORS IN HIPPOCAMPUS OF SENESCENT RATS AFTER CHRONIC TREATMENT WITH A BEHAVIORALLY POTENT $ACTH_{4-9}$ ANALOG 313

J.M.H.M. Reul, J.A.D.M. Tonnaer, E.R. de Kloet
Rudolf Magnus Institute for Pharmacology, Utrecht, and Organon Scientific Development Group, Oss, The Netherlands

In rat brain, two receptor systems can be distinguished for corticosterone (CORT). First, the type I CORT receptor (CR), which is exclusively localized in neurons of the septal-hippocampal complex and recognizes CORT as sole agonist. Secondly, the type II glucocorticoid receptor (GR), which shows highest affinity for synthetic glucocorticoids (dexamethasone) and is widely distributed in rat brain.

CR is under any condition for more than 90% occupied with endogenous CORT, while GR becomes occupied concurrent with rising CORT levels after stress or during circadian variation. Moreover, GR and not CR is subject to autoregulation by its principal endogenous ligand. In contrast, CR displays circadian variation and is regulated by neurotrophic factors. It is thought that CR mediates tonic influences of CORT, while GR is involved in the feedback action of CORT on stress-activated brain processes.

Cytosol binding assays and in vitro autoradiography have revealed that senescence affects CR and GR capacity in rat brain. The number of CR sites in the senescent rat hippocampus (28-30 months old) was 52% decreased in comparison with the young control (3 months old). GR number in the old rat hippocampus was decreased to a lesser extent: 28%. In hypothalamus and amygdala, age-induced decrease of GR was 15-16%. Chronic treatment of senescent rats with a behaviorally potent $ACTH_{4-9}$ analog (ORG 2766) selectively increased the number of hippocampal CR towards the level found in young animals. In young rats, ORG 2766 treatment was ineffective on CR and also the GR capacity in young and old rats was not affected by ORG 2766 treatment. No effect of age or ORG 2766 was found on the relative binding affinity of CR and GR.

It is concluded, that the number of hippocampal CR sites is a sensitive index for brain aging and treatment of neurotrophic peptides as is shown in the present study with ORG 2766.

Supported by FUNGO grant 13-49-030.

AGE-RELATED CHANGES IN MOLECULAR FORMS OF POMC-DERIVED PEPTIDES IN THE BRAIN OF RATS 314

C.W. Wilkinson and D.M. Dorsa
Geriatric Research, Education and Clinical Center, American Lake and Seattle VA Medical Centers, and University of Washington, Seattle, Washington

Age-associated changes in molecular forms of peptides of the pro-opiomelanocortin (POMC) family were investigated in specific regions of the rat brain by using a combination of reverse phase high pressure liquid chromatography and radioimmunoassays. Brains were removed from ten 8-month-old and ten 24-month-old male Fischer 344 rats, dissected and frozen. Individual tissue fragments were boiled in 1 M acetic acid, sonicated, and centrifuged. Supernatants were applied to ODS-silica cartridges and eluted with 80% acetonitrile (ACN) containing 0.1% trifluoroacetic acid (TFA). Peptides were separated on a 5 μm, 330 Å pore, C_{18} reverse phase column with a gradient of ACN against water, both containing approximately 0.1% TFA. Eluate fractions were collected and assayed for β- and γ-endorphin-like immunoreactivity (βE-LI, γE-LI).

Hypothalami from adult (8-month-old) rats contained predominantly βE 1-31 with smaller amounts of βE 1-27 and 1-26. Only 5% of the βE-LI co-eluted with α-N-acetylated forms of βE. In hypothalamic extracts from old rats more than 30% of the βE-LI co-eluted with acetylated forms of βE, and over 35% of the βE-LI co-eluted with acetylated or unacetylated βE 1-26. Individual elution profiles were much more variable among old rats. Acetylated γE was much more prevalent among old (35%) than among adult rats (3%).

In midbrain extracts, no significant age-related differences in proportions of forms of βE- or γE-related peptides were found. In both groups more than 65% of the βE-LI co-eluted with βE 1-31 and more than two-thirds of the remainder co-eluted with unacetylated forms of βE 1-27 and 1-26. Approximately 60% of midbrain γE-LI co-eluted with γE and approximately 15% with acetylated γE.

Changes in molecular forms of POMC-derived peptides in rat brain occur with aging, and these changes are anatomically specific.

AGE- AND STRAIN-RELATED DIFFERENCES IN VASOPRESSIN AND OXYTOCIN RELEASE. 315

V. Zbuzek*, A.R. Fuchs+, V.K. Zbuzek*, W.Wu*
*UMDNJ, New Jersey Medical School, Newark, New Jersey 07103 and +Cornell University Medical Center, New York, New York 10021.

We have studied the influence of age and strain on the release of vasopressin (VP) and oxytocin (OT) from isolated, individually superfused neurohypophyses (NH) of male Fisher 344 (F344) and Sprague-Dawley (SD) rats, 2-3 and 26-30 months of age. VP and OT release measured by RIAs was analyzed as follows: initial traumatic, basal, evoked by electrical and 56 mM K+ stimulation, and total.

The age-related differences in VP release were greater and did not parallel those of OT release. Expressed per mg NH, basal VP release was significantly lower in aged rats of both strains whereas basal OT release did not change. When expressed per whole NH, basal VP release decreased significantly in SD rats only, whereas basal OT release significantly increased in aged rats of both strains.

Expressed per mg NH, traumatic release of both VP and OT and their release following electrical and 56 mM K^+ stimulation were lower in aged than in young rats of both strains. When expressed per whole NH, the age-related decline in OT release was not significant, whereas VP release declined significantly. The age-related difference in VP release was more prominent in SD compared to F344 rats.

The results indicate that: 1) The impairment of basal and stimulated VP release appears to be unique for this neuropeptide rather than a part of general neuroendocrine disturbances associated with the aging process. 2) Age-related differences in VP release are more prominent in SD than in F344 rats.

Supported in part by USPHS Grant AG02778.

MODULATION OF CIRCADIAN AND PULSATILE THYROTROPIN-RELEASE BY THYROID HORMONES, GLUCOCORTICOIDS AND SOMATOSTATIN 316

G.Brabant, A.Esslinger, R.D.Hesch and A.von zur Mühlen
Dept.Clin.Endocrinol, Med. Hochschule D-3 Hannover F.R.G.

The recent developement of sensitive assay methods for thyrotropin(TSH) made it possible to reevaluate the suppressive influence of thyroid hormones, glucocorticoids and somatostatin (SST) on TSH secretion in greater detail not only under conditions of hypothyroidism but also in euthyroid subjects.

Methods: 5 healthy male volunteers(age 23 to 29 years) were studied by sampling blood every 10 min over 24 h. Studies were performed under basal conditions, an 8 h infusion of 50µg T_3, 250µg T_4, 500µg SST starting at 7pm or a bolus of 4mg dexamethason(dex) at 7 and 10 pm. At the end of each experiment a TRH-test was performed. In separate experiments the pituitary reserve was tested under dex 1 and 9 h after the last dex-bolus. TSH was measured by a sensitive radiometric assay(maximal CVintraassay:7.3%). Pulse analysis: visuell and by PULSAR-program.

Results: In addition to the expected circadian pattern TSH exhibited a pulsatile secretion pattern(5 +/-0.6 pulses/24 h). Infusion of T_3, T_4 lead to a prolonged suppression of basal TSH after about 4 h. In contrast, SST immediately suppressed TSH levels, but thyroid hormones as well as SST seemed not to affect the TSH pulsatility. The application of dex, however, immediately lowered TSH secretion and completely suppressed TSH pulses. TSH in the TRH-tests was not impaired in all test situations under dex, but under T_3, T_4 and SST.

Discussion: As shown previously TSH is not only secreted in a circadian pattern, but also with pulses of low amplitude(Brabant et al 1986). This pulsatile TSH secretion being preserved under SST-infusion makes it unlikely that it is driven by episodic SST-changes as discussed for growth hormone. However, our results on the complete disappearance of TSH-pulses under dex together with a normal response to exogenous TRH suggests a hypothalamic action of dex and a hypothalamic origin of TSH pulses. In contrast, the suppression of TSH by thyroid hormones indicates that they most likely exert their negative feedback on the level of the pituitary as again pulsatility is preserved.

POSSIBLE PROLACTIN MEDIATED EFFECT OF MELATONIN ON REPRODUCTIVE AXIS IN FEMALE RATS. 317

A.I. Esquifino*; M.A. Villanúa and J.A.F. Tresguerres.
Dpts. of Biochem. and Physiol. Faculty of Medicine. Complutense University. 28040 Madrid. SPAIN

In order to study if melatonin (M) exerts its inhibitory effects on the reproductive axis through prolactin (PRL) modifications, female rats of the Wistar strain, kept under a 12:12 light/dark period and bearing a pituitary graft under the kidney capsule, from day 30 of life and their age-matched sham operated (SO) controls have been used in this study.On day 90 of life, they were submitted to daily i.p. saline (S) or M administration (1mg/kg/day) during 10 days. Injections were given 5 h. prior to the start of the darkness period. Changes in basal PRL, LH and FSH levels under this conditions were examined on days 1, 2,3,5 and 7, using specific RIA methods. Additionally both M and S injected groups received 50 µg of Estradiol Benzoate (EB) s.c. on day 7. Blood samples were drawn basally and after 24,31,48,55 and 72 h, for the measurements of the above mentioned hormones. An increase in plasma PRL levels was detected in M treated SO rats as compared to S injected controls. On the contrary a marked decrease of previously high PRL levels was seen in pituitary grafted M treated groups. M administration did not alter LH levels in SO rats as compared to S control rats, but a recovery in plasma LH levels, reaching SO control values was found in M treated grafted rats. Plasma FSH levels showed an increase in M injected SO animals, whereas the increase shown in S treated grafted group is reduced with the M treatment. PRL was not able to respond to the EB administration in grafted rats, whereas a pulsatile response was shown in S injected SO group, with higher values found in the afternoon. M treatment restaured PRL pulsatility in grafted animals. S treated SO rats exhibited a plasma LH pick 31 h. after EB administration but this was reduced in the grafted group. M administration was not able to modify the plasma LH response to EB in controls but induced a marked increase in grafted rats. However M did not modify FSH response patterns to EB in any group. All these data suggest a PRL mediated modulatory role of M on LH but not on FSH secretion mechanisms in pituitary grafted rats.

This work has been possible through Grant nº 83/108 from the Spanish-USA Joint Comitte.

CHRONIC ADMINISTRATION OF METHAMPHETAMINE DISORGANIZES THE CIRCADIAN LOCOMOTOR RHYTHM IN THE RAT 318

T. Hiroshige, K. Honma, S. Honma, Y. Katsuno, T. Nagasaka, Y.Noe
Hokkaido University School of Medicine, Department of Physiology, Sapporo, 060 Japan

Amphetamine, a powerful CNS stimulant with a sympathomimetic action, was reported to show a peculiar effect on the circadian system. In order to obtain further informations on the nature of the drug action on circadian system, we examined effects of chronic administration of methamphetamine, a methyl derivative of amphetamine, dissolved in drinking water. When Wistar rats (both sexes) were given 0.005 or 0.01% methamphetamine solution over a period of more than 3 months, a marked change in the locomotor activity pattern ensued: in the first 2 months or so, they showed an augmented locomotor activity, thereafter activity onset started to phase-delay, followed by a similar change in activity offset. This gradual phase shift stopped when the activity offset reached a certain time of day and a rapid phase advance followed, resulting in restoration of the initial phase position. The gradual phase delay and rapid phase advance occurred periodically, which gave an impression of relative coordination. In some rats, the rhythm split into two activity components, one free-running with a period of approximately 29 hours and the other entraining to LD cycle. After methamphetamine withdrawal, the changes disappeared rapidly with some transients. Thus the changes were reversible. When plasma corticosterone level was monitored, the changes essentially similar to those of locomotor activity were observed. The drug-induced changes were persistent even in constant dark (DD) with the free-running period which was not affected by the drug administration. These results indicate that neither change of sensitivity to light nor lengthening of the intrinsic period is involved in the methamphetamine-induced changes of rat circadian rhythm. Possible mechanisms are discussed in relation to a two-oscillator model of the circadian system.

RELATIONSHIP BETWWEN SLEEP, MELATONIN AND GROWTH HORMONE IN NORMAL YOUNG MEN 318a

B. Roussel, P. Garry, B. Claustrat, R. Cohen, R. Amalberti and G. Sassolas
Centre Médecine Nucléaire, Hop. Cardiologique, Lyon, France.

Correspondance analysis was applied to elucidate the still controversial relationships between sleep-wake cycle and secretions of growth hormone and melatonin in normal man.

Six normal young men (21-28 years old) were involved in a study comprising from 20.00 h - 08.00 h continuous recording of sleep stages and blood sampling at 20 min intervals for determination of melatonin and growth hormone. Twelve nights were analyzed.

The patterns of hormone night secretion were classical : 2-3 secretory episodes for GH and pulsatile secretion for melatonin.

The 20 min of vigilance preceeding the blood sampling was classified in wake, stages 1, 2, 3, 4 and paradoxical sleep according to a taxonomic analysis based on sleep stages repartition.

Thus, for each 20-min period corresponded both a vigilance stage and a plasma concentration of GH and melatonin.

These date were analyzed by the correspondance method.

Vigilance appeared with a tripod aspect : summit being stage II and feet being PS, Δ sleep and wakefulness.

As regards the relationship between sleep and GH, the highest values of GH were temporally related with Δ sleep (3 + 4) and the lowest with wakefulness. Morever a relationship was observed between PS and medium values of GH.

In contrast no relationship was found between melatonin and sleep nor between melatonin and GH.

This approach using a multifactorial statistical methodology confirms the close temporal relationship between Δ sleep and maximal GH plasma concentration.

DAILY PATTERN OF SOMATOSTATIN CONCENTRATION IN HUMAN CEREBROSPINAL FLUID: CONNECTION WITH DISEASE ACTIVITY IN MULTIPLE SCLEROSIS. 319

K.V.Sørensen[1],T.Alslev[1],S.E.Christensen[2],N.B.Jensen[1] H.Ørskov[3].
Departments of Neurology, Aarhus, Odense, Viborg[1]-Second Clinic of Internal Medicine, Aarhus[2]-Institute of Exp. Clinical research, University of Aarhus, Denmark.

Somatostatin and albumin in cerebrospinal fluid and plasma growth hormone were measured in samples obtained hourly during a 24 h period using RIA. 18 patients participated in the study. 5 patients with multiple sclerosis in stable phase, 7 patients in relapse of the disease and 6 controls.

Cerebrospinal fluid somatostatin immunoreactivity averaged 166± 5,3 (SEM) pg/ml in the control subjects at noon when the study started and rose around midnight to a broad peak of 208 ± 3,8 pg/ml, decreased again to basal levels at about 5 a.m.,and exhibited another small peak 3 hours later. Almost identical values and variations were found in patients with multiple sclerosis during stable phase. Whereas patients in relapse exhibited constantly low values (99 ±9,2 pg/ml) throughout the 24 h period. Cerebrospinal fluid albumin was similar in the 3 groups and without oscillations. The diurnal patterns of plasma growth hormone were also similar in the 3 groups and unrelated to the observed variations in cerebrospinal fluid somatostatin, indicating that hypothalamic release was insignificant in the overall production and in these variations of cerebrospinal fluid somatostatin. The observation that the central nervous system releases somatostatin at lower levels during relapses in multiple sclerosis and that these do not oscillate normally, as they do in stable phases, may suggest that the constant low level represents passive spillover from somatostatin containing cells within the central nervous system while the oscillating levels above them are representative of active yet unknown neurophysiological functions which become reversibly extinct in relapses of multiple sclerosis. These changes may be secondary to the disease process, but it seems evident that the magnitude and the variform nature of cerebrospinal fluid somatostatin are dependable indicators of the disease activity.

INFLUENCE OF MELATONIN ON THE TESTICULAR REGRESSION INDUCED BY TESTOSTERONE PELLETS IN MALE RATS KEPT IN LONG OR SHORT PHOTOPERIOD. 320

M.K. Vaughan, S. Oaknin, B. Cozzi, K. Li, R.J. Reiter
Cellular & Structural Biology, Univ. Texas Health Science Center, San Antonio, Texas

The neuroendocrine-gonadal axis of the rat can be made responsive to the negative feedback effects of testosterone if the animals are subjected to short photoperiod (SP) (Wallen & Turek, Nature 289, 402, 1981). The effects of SP may be mediated by the pineal hormone melatonin (MEL); injections of MEL in rats kept in long photoperiod (LP) and bearing a silastic testosterone pellet (TP) might mimic the effects observed in SP-exposed, TP-treated rats. Since MEL pellets inhibit the action of MEL injections in the Syrian hamster, we tested the effect of MEL pellets in preventing the actions of MEL injections or SP in TP-treated rats kept in LP or SP.

Adult male rats (180-200 g) were kept in either 2:22 LD (lights on 1000-1200 h; 3 groups) or 14:10 LD (lights on 0600-2000 h; 5 groups). Three groups in 14:10 LD received a daily sc injection of 25 μg MEL between 1600-1800 h. MEL pellets (1 mg MEL/24 mg softened beeswax) were implanted biweekly in a group of MEL injected, TP-implanted rats kept in LP and in a group of TP-implanted, SP-exposed rats. Silastic TP implants (15 mm) were also made biweekly. Rats were killed at the end of 12 weeks of treatment and the testes weighed.

MEL injections in LP-exposed rats had no effect on testicular weight; similarly, exposure of rats to SP had no effects on gonadal weight. However, TP-implanted rats in both LP ($p < 0.001$) or SP ($p < 0.001$) showed a significant reduction in testicular weight; this was more pronounced in the SP-exposted rats ($p < 0.025$). MEL injections in TP-treated rats in LP exacerbated the inhibitory effects of TP alone ($p < 0.025$). MEL pellets were not found to statistically reverse the effects of MEL injections or SP but, in both instances, there was a marked trend at returning testicular weights to the level seen in TP-treated LP or SP-exposed rats.

In conclusion, TP reduced testicular weights in both LP and SP-exposed rats with the effect being more pronounced in SP-exposed animals. The observation that MEL injections exacerbate the effects of TP in LP animals and reduces the testicular weight to the same level seen in SP-TP-treated animals indicates that the effects observed with SP may be due to the pineal indole melatonin (Supported by NSF grant #8410592).

ESTRADIOL REGULATES MELATONIN ACTIVITY IN THE FEMALE RAT BRAIN 321

N. Zisapel and M. Laudon
Dept. of Biochemistry, Tel-Aviv University, Tel-Aviv 69978, Israel.

We have previously observed that the inhibitory effect of melatonin on stimulated dopamine release from brain hypothalami in vitro was abolished in long-term (2-4 weeks) ovariectomized (OVX) female rats and could be reinstated in the OVX rats by implantation of 17β-estradiol capsules. We therefore investigated the effects of short term treatment with estradiol in-vivo and in vitro, on the ability of melatonin to inhibit stimulated dopamine release from the hypothalami of OVX rats and on the density of melatonin binding sites in the female rat brain.

Reinstatement of the responsiveness to melatonin was observed in hypothalami of OVX rats shortly (2h) after a single subcutaneous injection of 17β-estradiol (200 ng). Incubation of hypothalami of OVX rats with estradiol in-vitro for 50-90 min resulted in a partial (i.e. up to 50%) time- and steroid-concentration dependent reinstatement of the ability of melatonin to inhibit the induced dopamine release. Such incubations with estradiol had no effect on the responsiveness of hypothalami of normal rats at Estrus to melatonin.

The specific binding of ^{125}I-iodomelatonin, a melatonin receptor probe, to synaptosomes prepared from whole brains and from hypothalami of the female rats was investigated. The densities of the binding sites in the preparations from whole brains and hypothalami of the OVX rats were lower by 70% and 30% respectively, than those in normal rats at Estrus. Reinstatement of most of the binding sites was observed in the brains and hypothalami of OVX rats shortly (2h) after a single injection of 17β-estradiol.

The results clearly show that 17β-estradiol directly modulates the responses of the dopaminergic neurosecretory system in the hypothalamus to melatonin. This phenomenon may primarily be associated with the estradiol-regulated changes in the density of melatonin receptors in the brain.

INTERLEUKIN-1 MODULATES SECRETION BY RAT PITUITARY CELLS IN MONOLAYER CULTURE 322

J.E. Beach, E.W. Bernton, J.W. Holaday, R.C. Smallridge, H.G. Fein
Divs. of Medicine and Neuropsychiatry, Walter Reed Army Institute of Research, Washington, D.C. 20307-5100

Interleukin-1 (IL-1) is a secretory product of stimulated macrophages with a variety of trophic functions. It induces proliferation of T-lymphocytes and augments secretion of fibrinogen, haptoglobin and vascular prostaglandins. It is also produced in the CNS by microglia and can induce slow-wave sleep and fever. Anterior pituitary hormones such as ACTH, endorphins, TSH, and PRL have direct effects on immune cell function. Therefore, the question arises whether IL-1 might directly affect pituitary cell secretion.

After enzymatic dispersion, rat pituitary cells were cultured in 24-well plates (300,000 cells/well) for 3 days in medium with 10% fetal bovine serum. Cells were then incubated for 4 h with serum-free medium, and then for 4 h with media containing mouse recombinant IL-1 (0.1 pM-10 nM). GH, LH, ACTH, and PRL were measured by RIA. Hormone levels during the second 4 h were divided by those during the first 4 h; these values were expressed as percentages of control well secretion ratios. The normal function of the cells was confirmed as ACTH was stimulated 995% by 100 nM CRF and LH 1424% by 100 nM LHRH.

IL-1 had concentration-related effects on the secretion of all hormones studied. Peak effects were observed at 0.1 pM, with lesser responses seen at greater concentrations, suggesting a maximal stimulation at physiologic levels. At 0.1 pM, IL-1 increased secretion of ACTH to 412% of control wells ($p<0.001$), LH to 374% ($p<0.001$), and GH to 213% ($p<0.01$). In contrast, PRL secretion was moderately inhibited (64% of controls, $p<0.01$).

Thus, IL-1 has potent, direct, and relatively generalized hypophysiotrophic effects, perhaps mediated through a common effector mechanism for regulation of pituitary hormone secretion. These effects may either enhance or regulate the metabolic and immunologic actions by which IL-1 mobilizes host defenses in response to infection or antigenic challenge.

NEUROENDOCRINE REGULATION OF RAT SPLEEN LYMPHOCYTES 323

R.Bernardini, G.Paciotti, R. Skwerer & L.Tamarkin, CPB/NIMH, Bethesda, MD 20892

Current evidence indicates a bidirectional communication between the neuroendocrine and immune systems. We investigated this hypothesis by examining the response of splenic lymphocytes to mitogenic stimulation following acute *in vivo* and *in vitro* neuroendocrine challenges. Rats were injected with TRH (100 ug/kg) or isoproterenol (ISO 2 mg/kg at time 0 and 2 h later). Control animals received saline. TRH-treated animals were sacrificed at 30 and 60 min after injection. ISO-treated animals were sacrificed 4 h after the first injection. Lymphocytes were harvested by disruption of the spleen and separated by Ficoll Paque gradient. Cells were plated at 10^6/well, stimulated for 72 h with Concanavalin A (0.62, 1.2, 2.5, 5, 10 ug/ml), then pulsed with 3H-thymidine and harvested. Results are presented as percent differences of peak lymphocyte growth of treated animals compared to controls.

		TRH		SAL	ISO	SAL
Time	0	30	60	30	4h	4h
Percent	100	27.9	67.1	93.7	20	100

In vitro lymphocyte stimulation with ISO (10^{-6}, 10^{-7} and 10^{-8}M) did not alter cell growth in response to Con A; peak levels were 108, 94, and 99% of controls respectively. *In vitro* experiments of TRH, TSH and prolactin are in progress. However dexamethasone (10^{-6}M) greatly reduced Con A stimulated growth to 1.6% of controls, suggesting the *in vivo* effect of ISO may result from a secondary corticosteroid release. To determine how circulating hormones may alter lymphocyte activity, two intracellular second messenger modulators were incubated with rat spleen cells *in vitro*. In the absence of mitogen both forskolin (10^{-6}M) and phorbol 12, 13-dibutyrate (10^{-6}M) diminish basal cell growth by 26% and 83% respectively. In the presence of Con A maximum lymphocyte growth was inhibited by 39% and 62% respectively. These data suggest that changes in hormonal levels can impact on the ability of lymphocytes to respond to an antigenic challenge. The mechanism by which hormones alter lymphocyte activity may involve both the phosphatidylinositol and the cAMP second messenger systems.

THYMOSIN REGULATES HORMONE SECRETION OF MOUSE CORTICOTROPHIC TUMOR CELLS 324

J.M. Farah, N.R. Hall, A.L. Goldstein, J.F. Bishop and T.L. O'Donohue Experimental Therapeutics, N.I.N.C.D.S. N.I.H., Bethesda, MD 20892 & Department of Biochemistry, The George Washington University, Washington, DC 20037

The thymus gland is increasingly associated with the regulation of the hypothalamic-pituitary-adrenocortical axis partly because the bovine thymic preparation, thymosin fraction 5 (TSN-5), has been found to stimulate the secretion of ACTH both *in vivo* and *in vitro* (Healy et al, 1983, Science 222:1353; McGillis et al, 1985, Fed Proc 44:3438). The purpose of the present study was to determine if TSN-5 similarly affects secretion of another proopiomelanocortin (POMC) peptide, β-endorphin, from AtT-20 corticotrophic tumor cells. Immunoreactive β-endorphin (iβ-E) was measured by a radioimmunoassay which detects all β-E peptides including their precursors, β-lipotropin and POMC. TSN-5 (600 μg/ml) significantly increased iβ-E release within 7 min (1.81±0.11 vs 0.96±0.08 ng/ml, mean ±SEM; N=6) and linearly increased release for 4 hrs to a maximum of 270% of control values. Release of iβ-E was increased in a dose-related manner by 10 to 600 μg/ml TSN-5, however, doses greater than 1000 μg/ml were increasingly less effective. Stimulation of iβ-E secretion by TSN-5 was inhibited by either glucocorticoid pretreatment or by calcium channel antagonists. Synergism of TSN-5 with maximally-effective stimulatory concentrations of either CRF or forskolin indicates that TSN-5 may influence corticotrophic cell secretion through a mechanism independent of cyclic AMP second messenger. The present results demonstrate that TSN-5 directly modifies hormone secretion by corticotrophic cell types and support the use of AtT-20 cells as an *in vitro* system for screening TSN-5 for its corticotrophic constituents and for investigating the cellular mechanisms by which thymic hormones regulate the synthesis and secretion of POMC-derived peptides in the anterior pituitary gland. Furthermore, these findings support the concept that products of the immune system may directly modulate the activity of neuroendocrine circuits.

NEURO-ENDOCRINE AND IMMUNOLOGICAL EFFECTS OF PHOSPHATIDYLSERINE 325

E. Galbiati, G. Calderini, E. Boarato, L. Mietto and A. Bruni
Fidia Neurobiological Research Laboratories, 35031 Abano Terme, Italy

Acute and chronic i.p. treatment with purified brain-cortex phosphatidylserine (BC-PS) induces a dose-dependent decrease of plasma prolactin (PRL) in male rats. This action is paralleled by a decrease of ^{32}P-incorporation into pituitary phosphatidyl-inositol as well as by a diminished protein-kinase C activity in the pituitary membrane. Since BC-PS has also been shown to stimulate hypothalamic dopamine and nor-adrenaline turnover, the effect on PRL secretion may reflect its action at this level.

Serine phospholipids are able to interact with immunocompetent cells. In particular, the acute i.v. injection to mice induces mast-cell-histamine release. Moreover, phosphatidylserine can specifically bind to macrophage and neutrophils. PS-activated macrophages are enabled to interact with mast-cells and to induce histamine release.

In view of the increasing evidence of a bidirectional link between neuro-endocrine and immune system it is likely that the interaction of serine-phospholipids with the immunocompetent cells may sequentially mediate the changes in the hypothalamic cathecolamines turnover and the variations in hormonal secretion.

THE THYMUS AS A NEUROENDOCRINE ORGAN 326

V.Geenen, J.J.Legros, M.P.Defresne, J.Boniver
University of Sart Tilman, B-23, B-4000 Liège, Belgium.

We have recently reported that the human thymus contains high amounts of oxytocin (OT) and associated carrier neurophysin (Np) (V.Geenen et al, Science, in press). OT has been characterized by specific RIA, biological assay and HPLC. Thymic OT concentration declined with increasing age of the patients and was particularly high in a myasthenic young man. The coexistence of OT and Np in equimolar amounts in the human thymus strongly suggested a local synthesis of OT.

Immunohistochemical studies revealed the presence of Np-containing stromal cells in subcapsular cortex (SCC) and medulla (M) of the human thymus. This distribution was very similar to that of epithelial cells identified by the monoclonal antibody A2B5 which usually recognizes a ganglioside expressed on membranes of neurones, neural crest-derived and neuropeptide-secreting cells (B.Haynes et al, J.Clin.Invest., 71, 9, 1983).

In mouse thymus, we observed a double staining of thymic epithelial cells in SCC and M with A2B5 and anti-Np, OT or vasopressin (AVP) antisera. Moreover, the lympho-epithelial complexes so-called "Thymic Nurse Cells" - whose origin is still unclear and which are supposed to play a major role in intrathymic T-lymphocyte differentiation - were also labeled with A2B5 and anti-Np, OT or AVP antisera.

From these data, we conclude :

1° The neuropeptides AVP and OT are synthesized in thymic epithelium in a similar way as in the hypothalamo-neurohypophyseal system.

2° The thymic neuroendocrine cells share the same distribution with A2B5+ cells, mainly in SCC and M.

3° As strongly suggested by immunocytochemical studies, the Thymic Nurse Cells could be derivatives from the embryonic neural crest. With regard to the previous observation of interleukin 2-like properties for AVP and OT (H.Johnson et al, J.Immunol., 129, 983, 1982), the neuroendocrine secretory activity of these cells may represent an important factor in the control of T-lymphocyte differentiation.

(V.Geenen is "Aspirant of the Belgian FNRS".)

HUMAN INTERLEUKIN 1 β STIMULATES ACTH RELEASE FROM RAT ANTERIOR PITUITARY CELLS IN A CAMP AND PROSTAGLANDIN E_2 INDEPENDANT-MANNER 327

Ph. Kehrer[1], R.C. Gaillard[1], J-M. Dayer[2], A.F. Muller[1].
Clinique Médicale[1] et Division d'Immunologie[2] et d'Allergie. Dept. of Medecine, University Hospital CH-1211 Geneva 4 / Switerland.

There is a body of evidence that endocrine and immune systems do influence each other. Interleukin 1 is a peptide released by macrophage undergoing an immune response. It has been shown to induce ACTH release from AtT-20 pituitary tumor cells. In this work, using human recombinant interleukin 1 β (IL1β) expressed at Biogen SA Geneva, we analyzed the ability of this peptide to induce ACTH relase from normal rat anterior pituitary cells in culture and we investigated the transduction mechanism involved in this secretion.

As bioassay we used the monolayer culture of rat anterior pituitary cells described by Vale et al. (Endocrinol. 1972, 91,562). After three days of incubation the cells were stimulated for 24 hours with IL1β alone or in association with dexamethasone or indomethacin. At the end of the stimulation the culture media were collected and frozen at -20°C until radioimmunoassay was performed for ACTH, prostaglandin E (PGE_2) and cAMP.

Between 0.5 and 50 ng/ml IL1β stimulated in a dose dependant-manner the release of ACTH and PGE_2 with a maximum secretion of respectively 1.5 and 3 times the control value. This secretion was not accompanied by any changes in cAMP concentration. The association of IL1β with dexamethasone (50 nM) inhibited both the PGE_2 and the ACTH secretion induced by IL1β whereas the association of IL1β with indomethacin (10 μM) inhibited only the PGE_2 production without affecting significantly the ACTH release.

In conclusion, IL1β stimulates ACTH release from normal rat anterior pituitary cell in culture. The stimulation is inhibited by dexamethasone and the cellular transduction mechanism involved in this ACTH release, requires neither cAMP nor PGE_2.

NEUROPEPTIDE Y (NPY)-INDUCED SUPPRESSION OF MALE SEXUAL BEHAVIOR: NEURAL LOCI 328

J.T. Clark, S.P. Kalra, P.S. Kalra
Dpt. OB-Gyn, Univ. Fla. Col. Med., Gainesville, FL 32610

NPY stimulates feeding and suppresses sexual behavior following intraventricular administration. We have now attempted to identify neural sites mediating the suppression of male sexual behavior by intracerebral injection at various diencephalic sites. Sexually vigorous males were implanted with unilateral cannulae under pentobarbital anesthesia. Each male was tested for sexual behavior in the dark phase of the light cycle as follows: 3 and 7 days post-surgery after no experimental treatment; 10 days post-surgery following intracerebral injection of 120pmol NPY or the saline vehicle (0.5 μl); and 14 days post-implantation following injection of NPY or vehicle. The two experimental tests were conducted using a counterbalanced design. When injection sites were located within the medial preoptic area (mPOA, n=14), NPY induced a suppression of sexual behavior as evidenced by increased latencies to intromission (saline: 1.6±0.9 vs NPY: 4.6±1.2 min), to ejaculation (4.8±0.7 vs 6.2±0.9 min) and to the post-ejaculatory intromission (5.2±0.2 vs 5.7±0.2 min). Also observed was an increased number of mounts preceding the ejaculation (6.3±1.4 vs 12.5±3.0) and 2/14 males failed to display any copulatory behavior after NPY, but all behaved normally after saline injection. Injection of NPY into sites other than the mPOA were not as effective in altering behavior. Injection into the lateral POA was without any discernible effect (n=7). Injection into sites anterior and lateral to the mPOA decreased intromission frequency (n=4) whereas injection into sites dorsal to the mPOA decreased ejaculation latency as well as intromission frequency (n=5). Paraventricular nucleus - anterior hypothalamic area injections increased intromission latencies (n=7). These studies demonstrate that unilateral injection of NPY into the mPOA causes major decrements in male sexual behavior. Thus, we suggest that the mPOA may be one of the central sites mediating NPY-induced suppression of male sexual behavior in the rat. (Supported by NIH grant HD 11362 and a postdoctoral fellowship HD 06660).

DIET-INDUCED THERMOGENESIS (DIT) IN DEPRESSION: EFFECT OF IMIPRAMINE TREATMENT. 329

M.H. Fernstrom, M. Massoudi, and D.J. Kupfer. Department of Psychiatry and Center for Neuroscience, University of Pittsburgh School of Medicine, Pittsburgh, PA USA.

Reductions in appetite and weight are common symptoms of major depression. During antidepressant (AD) treatment, such symptoms disappear, and weight is restored to normal. However, AD treatment can be associated with unwanted, excessive weight gain in 10-30% of patients. Weight gain can reflect an increase in caloric intake, a reduction in caloric expenditure, or both. The present studies focus on changes in resting metabolic rate (RMR) [the best index of caloric expenditure] in depressed patients, before and during antidepressant treatment. We have previously observed a reduction in RMR of patients treated with tricyclic ADs (Biol. Psychiat. 20:688, 1985). Our present study examines DIT (the naturally-occurring increase in RMR after food consumption) in normal and depressed subjects. We also compared the DIT response of a depressed patient (#4) before and during imipramine (a tricyclic AD) treatment for 2 weeks. In these preliminary findings, we found no differences in DIT between normal and depressed subjects. A large decrease in DIT (32% reduction) was observed in Patient #4 during AD treatment.

Normal	DIT (%)	Depressed	DIT (%)
#1	16%	#3 - Drug-free	19%
#2	19%	#4 - Drug-free	22%
		- + Imipramine	15%

DIT is caused at least partly via sympathetic nervous system (SNS) activation, mediated predominantly by beta receptors: an increase in DIT reflects increased metabolic activity and decreased caloric storage. Because chronic imipramine treatment reduces overall SNS activity, such a decrease might explain the reduced DIT (ie, a reduced metabolic activity and increased caloric storage). If so, such changes in caloric expenditure, related to SNS activity, may be important in understanding the cause(s) of weight gain during chronic AD treatment.

(Supported by MH30915, and the John D. and Catherine T. MacArthur Research Foundation on the Psychobiology of Depression.)

ROLL OF SEPTUM AND PREOPTIC AREA IN MASCULINE AND FEMININE SEXUAL BEHAVIORS IN MALE RATS. 330

Y. Kondo, A. Shinoda, *K. Yamanouchi, *Y. Arai
Department of Psychology, Faculty of Letters, Gakushuin University, Tokyo, and *Department of Anatomy, Juntendo University School of Medicine, Tokyo, Japan.

It has been suggested that septum plays a strong inhibitory role in regulating feminine sexual behaviors in female and androgenized female rats, because of lordosis facilitation by surgically disfunctioning the septum. In this report, effects of septal or preoptic lesions on both masculine and feminine sexual behaviors were examined in male rats.

The medial, lateral septum (MS or LS) or the medial preoptic area (POA) were lesioned in orchidectomized rats. A number of rats without brain surgery received orchidectomy and served as controls. Three weeks later, animals received subcutaneous implantation of Silastic tubings containing testosterone. Masculine behavioral observations were carried out 5, 10, 15, and 20 days after the implantation. After the end of masculine behavioral tests, Silastic tubings of T were removed. Two weeks later, all males were implanted with Silastic tubings containing estradiol-17β(E_2) in order to observe feminine sexual behavior. Tests were carried out 5, 10, and 15 days after the implantation of E_2. Progesterone were given 3 - 5 hrs prior to each feminine sexual behavioral test.

Male animals with bilateral medial POA lesions or with bilateral LS lesions showed low masculine sexual activity, whereas MS-lesioned males showed normal levels of the activity when compared with that of controls. On the other hand, only LS-lesioned males displayed lordosis in feminine sexual behavioral tests. The males of the MS-lesioned, POA-lesioned and control groups showed low lordotic activity. These results suggest that the lateral septal area plays the role to facilitate masculine sexual behaviors and to inhibit feminine sexual behaviors. The medial preoptic area may exert only a facilitatory influence on masculine sexual behaviors in the male rats.

VASOACTIVE INTESTINAL POLYPEPTIDE (VIP) IN HUMAN CEREBROSPINAL FLUID OF DEMENTIA WITH CEREBRAL ATROPHY IN JAPAN. 331

K. Nakamura,[1)] H. Kaneko,[1)] M. Hayashi,[1)] T. Shimizu,[1)] T. Ihara,[1)] S. Kanto,[1)] M. Kusakabe,[1)] J. Itoh,[1)] C. Yanaihara,[2)] N. Yanaihara,[2)] and M. Irie.[1)]
[1)]Toho University School of Medicine, Tokyo 143,
[2)]Shizuoka College of Pharmacy, Shizuoka 422, Japan

Fahrenberg et al have documented that VIP in cerebral fluid (CSF) tended to be decreased in brain atrophy, suggesting that VIP has, as one of neuropeptides in brain, connection with emotion. The aim of the present study was to investigate human CSF for the presence of VIP with special reference to its association with dementia. The subjects were categorized as follows: (Group A) 12 controls without brain atrophy nor dementia: mean age 32.2 years for 6 as a young age group(A-1) and 67.9 years for 6 as an old-age group(A-2); (Group B) 14 patients with brain atrophy and without dementia: mean age 79.2 years; and (Group C) 14 patients with both brain atrophy and dementia: mean age 79.8 years. The degree of intellectual impairment was assessed by Hasegawa's method. CSF was obtained by lumbar puncture. VIP concentration in CSF was determined by a radioimmunoassay using antiserum R504, synthetic VIP as standard and (125)I-synthetic VIP as labelled antigen. The dilution curve of human CSF in the radioimmunoassay was paralled to the standard curve of VIP. In gelfiltration analysis on Sephadex G50, immunoreactive VIP (IR-VIP) in CSF was found to coelute as a single component with synthetic VIP. IR-VIP in CSF from Group A-2 (286.8 ± 22.6pg/ml, mean ± S.D.) was lower ($p < 0.05$) than that from Group A-1 (334.3 ± 16.8). Group B showed a lower ($p < 0.05$) level of IR-VIP in CSF (241.0 ± 18.0) than Group A-2, but IR-VIP in CSF from Group C (123.6 ± 20.0) was most significantly ($p < 0.01$) lower than those from any other groups. VIP also differed among the classifications of dementia. It is suggested that VIP concentration in CSF is associated with the level of intelligence; these data also suggest a possible function of VIP in the regulation of the behavior of those suffering dementia.

NOREPINEPHRINE STIMULATES AND DOPAMINE INHIBITS PULSATILE LHRH RELEASE IN VIVO IN OVARIECTOMIZED RHESUS MONKEYS 332

E. Terasawa, C. Krook, G.A. Davis, G. Watanabe
Wis. Reg. Primate Research Ctr., Univ. of Wisconsin, Madison, WI 53715-1299

Although numerous studies in rodents indicate that catecholamines play a role in controlling LHRH release, the information available in primates is extremely limited and evidence is indirect. In the present experiment we obtained direct evidence for this topic by monitoring simultaneous changes in pulsatile LHRH release and the release of catecholamines and their metabolites from the stalk median eminence of unanesthetized female rhesus monkeys. A push-pull cannula was inserted into the stalk-median eminence in ovariectomized female monkeys, a modified Krebs-Ringer solution was perfused through the cannula and a 200 µl fraction of perfusates was collected every 10 min. After 2 h of baseline sample collection, norepinephrine (10^{-6} to 10^{-5}M) or dopamine (10^{-5}M) or amphetamine (10^{-6} to 10^{-4}M) was applied for 10 min through the cannula, and sample collection was continued. LHRH in perfusates was measured by RIA and catecholamines and their metabolites were measured by HPLC. Before catecholamine or drug application LHRH release was pulsatile with interpeak intervals of 50-60 min, peak amplitudes of 3-6 pg/ml and nadirs of 1-2 pg/ml. Application of norepinephrine induced a LHRH release of 2.5-4 fold peak amplitude, while dopamine and amphetamine resulted in clear suppression of LHRH release. HPLC analysis indicated that amphetamine application induced an increase in dopamine and its metabolites in the stalk median eminence. Therefore, these results suggest that an increase in norepinephrine concentration in the median eminence stimulates and an increase in dopamine in the median eminence inhibits pulsatile LHRH release from LHRH neuroterminals of ovariectomized rhesus monkeys. (Supported by NIH grants HD15433 and RR00167).

EPINEPHRINE & ESTRADIOL PRETREATMENT ENHANCE NOREPINEPHRINE-MEDIATED SECRETION OF GnRH BY RAT HYPOTHALAMIC CELL CULTURES. 333

A.T.W. Lim, F. Petraglia and W. Vale.
The Clayton Foundation Laboratories for Peptide Biology, The Salk Institute, La Jolla, CA.

Increasing evidence suggests that in vivo epinephrine (Epi), norepinephrine (Norepi) and gonadal steroids work in concert to modulate hypothalamic GnRH release. Employing long term monolayer cell cultures, we have examined the effects of the catecholamines and gonadal steroids on the immunohistochemical staining and the secretion of GnRH-like immunoreactivity (LI) from cultured rat hypothalamic cells. Hypothalamic tissues removed from 2-3 d old Sprague-Dawley rats were enzymatically dissociated, counted and resuspended in culture media. Following 10d plating at 5x10 6 cells/well in 10% fetal calf serum enriched B-PJ media, culture media were replenished and supplemented with vehicle, Epi (10-9 to 10-5M) or 10-9M E2 alone or in combination and incubated for further 24h. Employing rabbit antiserum raised against synthetic [Lys8]-GnRH, indirect immunofluorescence staining of GnRH-LI was found predominantly in cell bodies and proximal processes of untreated or E2 only treated cultures. 10-5M Epi pretreatment markedly enhanced GnRH-LI staining in distal neuronal processes and the effect was intensified by concommitant E2 but not Prog administration. The secretory responses to various agents over a 1h period were determined by using a double antibody GnRH RIA with routine sensitivity of 0.5pg/sample. Norepi (10-7M and 10-5M) consistently stimulated significant GnRH-LI release (1.6+0.3 and 2.4+0.4 respectively; control <0.5, GnRH-LI pg/well, n=4, mean+s.e.m.) from cultures primed 24h with both Epi (10-5M) and E2 (10-9) together but not with either of them alone. Replacement of Epi with forskolin (10-4M) or dibutyryl cyclic AMP (10-4M) produced parallel results but substitution of Prog (10-9 to 10-7M) for E2 promptly abolished subsequent Norepi stimulated GnRH-LI release. We conclude that in hypothalamic cell cultures (i) Epi, Norepi and E2 interact in a specific and concerted manner to induce GnRH-LI release and (ii) the priming effect of Epi, may in part, involve adenylate cyclase-cAMP system.

CRF INHIBITION OF LH IS MEDIATED BY OPIOIDS: ROLE OF TESTOSTERONE. 334

K.E. Nikolarakis, O.F.X. Almeida & A. Herz, Department of Neuropharmacology, Max-Planck-Institut für Psychiatrie, D-8033 Martinsried, West Germany.

CRF (0.2nmol, icv) given to male rats castrated for 5d caused a 70% inhibition of LH levels within 30 min. This effect was partially reversed (30% inhibition) when the opiate antagonist naloxone was infused (9.6mg/kg/d) starting 2d prior to CRF testing, implicating that the action of CRF was mediated via endogenous opioids. This was confirmed in superfusions of hypothalamic slices with CRF in vitro: within 20 min. of presentation, CRF doses between 10^{-12} and 10^{-8}M caused significant increases in ß-endorphin from the slices.

From our own work and that of others, we know that the LH-suppressive effects of opiates are diminished in long-term (>2 weeks) male castrates, and we exploited this model to obtain further evidence that opioids may be involved in the CRF inhibition of LH secretion. CRF (0.2 nmol, icv) resulted in a reduced inhibition of serum LH levels in rats castrated for 8 weeks compared with those castrated for 5d (30% vs. 80%).

To investigate the possibility that castration might influence the magnitude of the CRF inhibition of LH by altering ß-endorphin synthesis and/or release, we measured the in vitro basal release rate of ß-endorphin from hypothalamic slices obtained from castrated rats that were substituted with varying amounts of testosterone in Silastic capsules at the time of gonadectomy (castrations were performed 5d prior to killing). We observed that the amount of ß-endorphin release increased with increasing doses of testosterone replacement.

We conclude from the above experiments that testosterone modulates the CRF inhibition of LH through effects upon hypothalamic ß-endorphin synthesis and release.

Supported by SFB 220 of the Deutsche Forschungsgemeinschaft, Bonn.

ESTROGEN-DEPENDENT EFFECTS OF NOREPINEPHRINE ON HYPOTHALAMIC GnRH RELEASE IN THE RABBIT 335

K.-Y.F. Pau and H.G. Spies, Oregon Regional Primate Research Center, Beaverton, Oregon 97006

In the rabbit, either coitus or intraventricular administration of norepinephrine (NE) induces luteinizing hormone (LH) release and ovulation. These stimuli activate the hypophysial-gonadal axis by initiation of a neuronal process that may involve both catecholaminergic and peptidergic neurons. This study compared the simultaneous release of gonadotropin-releasing hormone (GnRH) from the mediobasal hypothalamus (MBH) and gonadotropins from the pituitary in ovariectomized (OVX) and estradiol-treated OVX does (OVX/E_2) during intrahypothalamic perfusion of NE. All does were fitted with push-pull (PP) cannulae directed into the MBH and subsequently subjected to PP perfusion at a flow rate of 20 µl/min for 6 h to measure hypothalamic GnRH release. Five OVX/E_2 and seven OVX does received NE that was added directly to the PP medium at the rate of 2.5 µg/min for 2 h during the 6 h of MBH-PP perfusion. In addition, six OVX/E_2 does were given intrahypothalamic perfusion of homovanillic acid (HVA), a metabolite of the adrenergic system, to serve as controls. All PP samples were collected at 10-min intervals, and blood samples were obtained at 20-min intervals. The GnRH, LH, and follicle-stimulating hormone (FSH) were measured by radioimmunoassays. In OVX/E_2 does, intrahypothalamic perfusion of NE, but not HVA, stimulated a tenfold increase in peak values of hypothalamic GnRH within 30 min, and a threefold increase in peak values of plasma LH within 40 min. Thereafter, both GnRH and LH levels returned to basal values by the end of the NE perfusion. In contrast, the same NE treatment failed to stimulate GnRH and LH release in OVX does. Changes in plasma FSH after NE treatment were not observed in any of the 3 groups of rabbits. These results indicate that the NE-stimulated neuronal discharge of GnRH that is accompanied by an increase in plasma LH is estrogen dependent. The results further support the hypothesis that GnRH is the neuropeptide that mediates the NE-stimulated LH release and ovulation. Supported by NIH grants RR-00163, HD-16631, and HD-18185.

CENTRAL EFFECTS OF LHRH ANALOGS INDICATE AN INHIBITORY ROLE OF LHRH TO MODULATE ITS OWN SECRETION. 336

M. Valenca, M. Ching, and A. Negro-Vilar, Reprod. Neuroendo. Sec., Lab. Reprod. Dev. Tox., NIEHS-NIH , Res. Tri. Pk., NC 27709.

Previous work from our laboratory [J. Androl. (Supp.) 6:41, 1985] indicates that LHRH agonists can negatively affect endogenous LHRH secretion when given in a regimen that induces testicular regression. Administration of a highly potent LHRH agonist ([D-Ala^6, Des-Gly^{10}] LHRH ethylamide) immediately after orchidectomy (ORDX) significantly attenuates the rise of LH from days 2 through day 10 after ORDX. Measurement of LHRH levels in hypophyseal portal blood 10 days after ORDX combined with daily agonist treatment (100 ng/day/animal) revealed a significant decrease in LHRH values in portal plasma when compared with ORDX controls. Arcuate-median eminence (ARC-ME) fragments obtained from ORDX rats that had received in vivo the LHRH agonist daily for 5 days showed a decreased basal secretion of LHRH and also a diminished response to K^+ stimulation when compared with similar fragments obtained from ORDX, saline-treated controls. These two sets of experiments, therefore, provide direct in vivo and in vitro evidences suggesting that part of the antigonadal activity of LHRH agonists is exerted by central inhibition of endogenous LHRH release. In order to evaluate whether a tonic LHRH inhibitory activity is operative within the median eminence, additional experiments were performed in which median eminence fragments from adult male rats were incubated in vitro in the presence of two different and potent LHRH antagonists ([D-pGlu^1,D-Phe^2,D-Trp^{3,6}]LHRH and [D-Phe^2, Pro^3, D-Phe^6] LHRH). Both antagonists significantly enhanced the basal secretion of LHRH over two consecutive 30 min periods. The latter results suggest that LHRH antagonists may enhance LHRH release perhaps by interacting with LHRH receptors playing an inhibitory role on the endogenous secretion of the decapeptide. These observations coupled with the anatomical evidence showing LHRH fibers making contact with LHRH neurons strongly suggest a tonic inhibitory or modulatory role of LHRH neurons to regulate their own function.

PREOVULATORY LH SURGE IN THE RAT: PULSE ANALYSIS AND ADVANCEMENT BY OPIOID RECEPTOR BLOCKADE. 337

L.G. Allen, D. Caton, S.P. Kalra
Depts. of OB-Gyn and Anesthesiology, Univ. of Fla. Col. of Med., Gainesville, FL 32610

The LH secretory profile was characterized by PULSAR in blood samples (50 µl) collected at 3 min intervals between 1430-1730 h of proestrus starting from low undetectable levels (< 1 ng/ml), LH hypersecretion occurred in 3 distinct phases, each displaying episodic LH release: basal phase (1.32 ± 0.46 pulses/h), ascending phase (1.23 ± 0.75 pulses/h) and plateau phase (1.5 ± 0.73 pulses/h). The ability to detect LH episodes during the ascending phase depended on the slope of LH rise, distinct pulses were seen in cases of less steep ascension. The LH secretory pattern was analyzed in proestrous rats infused intravenously with naloxone hydrochloride (2 mg/h) between 1100-1400 h. LH levels rose in a similar three-step fashion (basal phase: 1.32 ± 0.56 pulses/h, ascending phase; 1.10 ± 0.46 pulses/h, and plateau phase: 3.0 pulses/h). There were 4.33 ± 1.14 pulses/3 h in naloxone-treated rats (N = 6). Finally, LH secretion was analyzed in response to unvarying LHRH pulses (10 ng/ pulse) delivered between 1200-1700 h at 20 or 30 min intervals in pentobarbital-blocked rats. The LH rise was minimal after 2 pulses (basal phase), followed by a steep ascending phase and a plateau phase. Although the time course of the LH rise was similar, higher plateau LH levels were attained by 20 min (14.62 ± 3.83 ng/ml) than by 30 min LHRH pulse frequency (9.82 ± 2.53 ng/ml); LH levels of spontaneous or naloxone-induced LH surges also were within this range. These studies show that the spontaneous and naloxone-induced LH surge on proestrus is pulsatile in nature and that it can be reproduced by exogenous LHRH delivered at a frequency of 20 or 30 min as seen in ovariectomized rats. Therefore, LH hypersecretion on the afternoon of proestrus may be a consequence of a decrease in opioid tone resulting in acceleration of pulsatile LHRH output. (Supported by NIH HD 08634).

EVIDENCE AGAINST A COMMON RELEASE SIGNAL FOR PROLACTIN AND LH IN WOMEN. 338

L.A. Marshall , M.C. Martin , R.B. Jaffe
U of Calif, San Francisco, San Francisco, CA.

It has been suggested that a common mechanism may control both LH and prolactin (PRL) daytime pulsatile discharge. Little is known about nocturnal LH and PRL secretion and regulation. This study was undertaken to examine the relationship between LH and PRL pulses, during the day and night. We previously showed that estradiol (E_2) administration increases daytime PRL pulse frequency; therefore, studies were performed in the early follicular phase (EFP), and after chronic E_2 administration. Six cycling women were studied for 24 h, on d 2-4 of the cycle, and again 1 wk later, after daily injections of 1 mg E_2 benzoate achieving E_2 levels of 390 ± 80 pg/ml. Serum LH and PRL were measured every 15 min. Pulses were defined as increments greater than 3 coefficients of variation (c.v.) above previous nadirs, with c.v. determined using pooled samples. LH and PRL pulses were considered concordant if initiated within the same 15 min interval. In the EFP, a total of 62 LH and 17 PRL daytime pulses were detected for all 6 subjects; 11 of these were concordant. At night, out of 15 LH and 23 PRL pulses, only 3 were concordant. After E_2, 42 LH and 36 PRL daytime pulses occurred; 14 were concordant. At night, out of 7 LH and 22 PRL pulses, only 2 were concordant. Diurnal variation of both PRL and LH secretion was observed. In 5 of 6 EFP studies, there was a significant increase in nocturnal LH interpulse interval over daytime patterns. E_2 administration was associated with marked nocturnal PRL surges (to 86 ± 25 ng/ml) and coincident suppression of LH pulsatile secretion at the onset of sleep. After a long LH pulse-free interval (305 ± 50 min), LH pulses, often high amplitude, were restored in early morning hours. Thus, our data do not support a common release signal for LH and PRL under these conditions. Concordance of pulses occurred occasionally in daytime studies and only rarely at night, both in the EFP and after E_2. The consistent suppression of LH pulses coincident with nocturnal pulsatile PRL release following E_2 provides further evidence against a common release signal for the 2 hormones.

OVARIAN FACTORS ANTAGONIZE THE SELF PRIMING ACTION OF LUTEINIZING HORMONE RELEASING HORMONE (LH-RH) 339

J. de Koning, A.M.I. Tijssen, G.W. Hilberath, H. Kamsteeg, G.P. van Rees
Dept. of Pharmacology, Univ. of Leiden, The Netherlands

During continuous exposure of pituitary glands of dioestrous rats to LH-RH a clear biphasic luteinizing hormone (LH) response is displayed: a first phase of low LH release is followed by a second phase of dramatically increased LH release. During two intermittent exposures to LH-RH, 1 h apart, this phenomenon expresses itself in the so-called self-priming effect of LH-RH. In intact animals the self-priming effect wears off when the interval between LH-RH stimulations exceed 1 h. The latter process is prevented when the ovaries have been removed prior to the first injection of LH-RH, or when priming is generated in vitro (a functional ovariectomy). However, when during the interval between the two LH-RH exposures in vitro a steroid-free ovarian extract is added to the media, the primed state wears off again.

Following withdrawal of ovarian influences in vivo or in vitro, the initial pituitary LH response to LH-RH increases spontaneously with time: priming in the absence of LH-RH. Moreover, after long-term ovariectomy LH-RH-induced LH release during the two phases have become equally high. These processes are reversed in vivo when ovaries are implanted under the kidney capsule, or in vitro by the addition of ovarian extracts.

Manipulation with ovarian influences (in vivo: ovaries auto-implanted into the spleen; in vitro: use of extracts of ovaries selected during the oestrous cycle or of ammonium sulphate-precipitated ovarian extracts) enabled us to demonstrate that the ovarian activity described above is not inhibin, although it might be present in bovine follicular fluid. Like inhibin, these factors are inactivated during heat or methanol treatment and are not extracted with charcoal or chloroform/ether.

Summarizing the results, it can be concluded that ovarian factors antagonize or neutralize the priming action of LH-RH. These factors may play a role in processes which keep the pituitary gland in a phase of low LH responsiveness to LH-RH during the oestrous cycle.

MODULATION OF ß-ADRENERGIC STIMULATION OF GROWTH HORMONE RELEASE BY STIMULATORY AND INHIBITORY INTERCELLULAR COMMUNICATIONS 340

M. Baes and C. Denef
Laboratory of Cell Pharmacology, School of Medicine, University of Leuven, Belgium

Adrenergic catecholamines have been shown to exert a direct stimulatory effect on GH release at the pituitary level. This was first described by Cronin et al. using superfused dispersed pituitary cells and confirmed by us using superfused pituitary cells cultured as reaggregates. In the present study we provide evidence that this ß-adrenergic stimulation is modulated by intercellular communications of somatotrophs with other pituitary cell types.

Pituitary cell aggregates composed of a somatotroph-enriched population (65% somatotrophs), obtained by separating pituitary cells of adult male rats on a velocity sedimentation gradient, displayed a very low responsiveness to epinephrine (E) (10 nM) even when these aggregates were cultured in the presence of 80 nM dexamethasone. In these culture conditions secretory responses of aggregates composed of the total pituitary population were at least 10 times higher. When the cells of the somatotroph-enriched population were mixed and co-aggregated with a population of small-sized cells obtained from the sedimentation gradient of adult male or adult female rats (all with very low GH secretory potential) ß-adrenergic responsiveness of the somatotrophs significantly increased. Coaggregating a gonadotroph-thyrotroph enriched population with the somatotrophs did not affect the responsiveness of the latter to E. In contrast, addition of a folliculo-stellate (FS) cell enriched population (66% FS cells) to the total population of adult males significantly reduced the stimulatory effect of E in the latter population.

We conclude that stimulatory intercellular signals originating in a small-sized cell type as well as inhibitory signals originating in FS cells modulate the responsiveness of somatotrophs to ß-agonists. Preliminary results indicate that secretory responses to the well established growth hormone releasing factor peptide (GRF) are similarly inhibited by FS cells. Stimulatory interactions also occur but are less dramatic compared to those involved in E-stimulated GH release.

EVIDENCE THAT GH DEPLETION AND N_s UNCOUPLING BOTH CONTRIBUTE TO THE DESENSITISATION OF GH RESPONSES TO GRF 341

C. Dieguez, C.A.E. Edwards, J.R. Peters, R. Hall, M.F. Scanlon
Neuroendocrine Unit,
University of Wales College of Medicine, Cardiff.

Recent data suggest that the GH response to GRF is reduced following prior exposure to high concentrations of GRF. However, it is unknown whether this is due to alterations in GRF receptors, adenylate cyclase activity or the size of a GRF-releaseable storage pool of GH. In order to clarify these questions we have compared the effects of GRF pretreatment (10^{-8} M every 2 hrs for 12 hours) with those of SS (10^{-6} M), Forskolin (10^{-5} M) and GRF + SS (10^{-8} M and 10^{-6} M added together) pretreatment on the subsequent GH responses to GRF (10^{-12} M to 10^{-8} M), cholera toxin (CT, 10^{-8} M), IBMX (10^{-4} M) and Forskolin (10^{-5} M). Experiments were performed on 4 day monolayer cultures of rat anterior pituitary cells. The cells were pretreated with test substances every 2 hrs for 12 hours and incubated with GRF on Forskolin for 3 hrs. GH was measured in the medium by RIA.

Bmax GH responses to GRF (10^{-8} M) were reduced after both GRF pretreatment (control, 173% of basal vs GRF 25% of basal, $p < 0.001$) and Forskolin pretreatment (control 173% of basal vs GRF 89% of basal, $p < 0.005$) but were increased after SS pretreatment (control 173% of basal vs GRF 246% of basal, $p < 0.02$). However GH responses after pretreatment with GRF + SS were not significantly different to control. The ED_{50} for GRF action was unaltered by SS pretreatment (control $4.85 \times 10^{-11} \pm 0.92$ vs 1.4×10^{-10} M ± 0.38, $p > 0.05$) or by Forskolin pretreatment (1.4×10^{-10} M + 0.7, $p < 0.05$) but was increased by GRF (9×10^{-10} M ± 4.4, $p < 0.05$) and GRF + SS pretreatment ($1.01 \times 10^{-9} \pm 7.3$, $p < 0.01$). GH responses to Forskolin (32% of basal vs 121% of basal, $p < 0.01$), CT (40% of basal vs 106% of basal, $p < 0.025$) and IBMX (95% of basal vs 133% of basal, $p < 0.025$) were also decreased after GRF pretreatment in comparison to controls.

Reduction of Bmax GH responses to GRF, CT, IBMX and Forskolin by GRF pretreatment and the reversal of this action by combined SS + GRF pretreatment suggests that depletion of the GRF-sensitive releaseable pool of GH may contribute to the desensitisation phenomenon. In addition however, the increase in ED_{50} of GRF following GRF or GRF + SS pretreatment as compared to control or SS pretreatment alone, supports the view that uncoupling of the N_s protein also plays a role in this phenomenon.

RELEASE OF IMMUNOREACTIVE GROWTH HORMONE-RELEASING FACTOR (GRF) AND SOMATOSTATIN FROM INCUBATED HYPOTHALAMUS IN YOUNG AND OLD MALE RATS 342

M. Ono, N. Miki, K. Shizume. Department of Medicine, Institute of Clinical Endocrinology, Tokyo Women's Medical College, Shinjuku-ku, Tokyo 162, Japan.

In order to study the neuroendocrine mechanism(s) involved in age-related decline in growth hoemone (GH) secretion, we compared content and in vitro release of hypothalamic GRF and somatostatin between young (3 months old) and aged (20-24 months old) male Wistar rats. Hypothalamic tissues were obtained by decapitation, homogenized in 1 N AcOH and lyophilized. In vitro studies were carried out by incubating 3 hypothalami per vial in Krebs-Ringer bicarbonate buffer containing 0.5 mg/ml bacitracin, 0.1 % BSA and 11 mM glucose (KRBG), pH 7.4, under 95 % O_2-5 % CO_2. After 30 min-preincubation, tissues were incubated in fresh KRBG for 30 min (basal release) followed by an another 30 min-period of incubation in high K^+ (50 mM) KRBG (K^+-stimulated release). Serial dilutions of hypothalamic extract and incubated media were parallel to the standard curve of rat GRF and somatostatin RIAs and their immunoreactivities coeluted with synthetic peptides on Sephadex G-50 superfine column. GRF level in whole hypothalamus was significantly less in old (N=6) than in young rats (N=6) (455.5±36.8 vs 657.5±28.5 pg, p<0.001), whereas somatostatin content was significantly greater in old as compared to that in young animals (31.0±2.0 vs 24.4±1.4 ng, p<0.025). In vitro, old rat hypothalami exhibited 55 % reduction of basal GRF release (N=6) as compared to that (N=6) in young rats (15.7±0.9 vs 34.8±6.4 pg/30 min, p<0.01), and moreover K^+-evoked increase in GRF release was only 27 % of that observed in young rats (38.1±2.5 vs 138.5±13.4 pg, p < 0.0001). Basal release of somatostatin was also significantly less in old than in young rats (54±18 vs 143±45 pg, p< 0.05), but there was no difference in K^+-stimulated release of somatostatin between old and young rats (479±45 vs 551±33 pg). These results indicate that aging is associated with attenuated secretion of hypothalamic GRF, which may contribute to the diminished pulsatile GH release in old male rats. Physiological significance of decreased somatostatin secretion in old rats remains unknown.

MECHANISMS UNDERLYING THE EFFECTS ON GROWTH HORMONE SECRETION OF PHARMACOLOGIC MANIPULATION OF α-ADRENOCEPTOR OR CHOLINERGIC RECEPTOR AGONISTS AND ANTAGONISTS IN THE NEONATAL RAT. 343

V. Locatelli, S.G. Cella, V. De Gennaro, W. Wehrenberg, E.E. Müller
Department of Pharmacology, University of Milan, Italy, and Department of Health Sciences, University of Wisconsin, Milwaukee U.S.A.

Growth hormone (GH) secretion is under a dual regulatory control exerted by somatostatin (SS) and GH-releasing hormone (GHRH). SS and GHRH are in turn under control exerted by a family of neurotransmitters, among which catecholamines and acetylcholine play a major role. Our aim was that of evaluating whether in neonatal rats, as in adult animals, adrenergic and cholinergic systems are fully operative to stimulate or inhibit GH secretion and, possibly, of singling out the respective contribution of GHRH and SS.

α_2-Adrenergic receptors - In 10-day-old rats of either sex, activation of α_2-adrenoceptors by clonidine (CLON, 150 µg/kg BW, i.p.) stimulated GH release, while, conversely, α_2-adrenoceptor blockade by yohimbine (YOH, 10 mg/kg BW, i.p.) decreased baseline GH levels. Administration of a GHRH antiserum (100 µl/rat, i.p.), completely abolished the stimulatory effect of CLON, while a SS antiserum (200 µl/rat, i.p.) potentiated the GH-releasing effect of CLON. The inhibitory effect of YOH on GH levels was abolished by pretreatment with SS-antiserum. These data indicate that while α_2-adrenoceptor stimulation releases GH via endogenous GHRH, blockade of α_2-adrenoceptors lowers GH levels via SS.

α_1-Adrenergic receptors - Methoxamine (METHOX, 10 µg/rat, i.p.), a α_1-adrenoceptor agonist, significantly reduced plasma GH concentrations, an effect which was abolished by pretreatment with SS antiserum. These data indicate that stimulation of α_1-adrenoceptors reduces GH secretion via SS.

Cholinergic muscarinic receptors - Pilocarpine (4 mg/kg BW, i.p.), a cholinergic muscarinic agonist, did not modify basal GH levels, while atropine (0.5 mg/kg BW, i.p.),a muscarinic antagonist, significantly decreased plasma GH. Pretreatment with SS antiserum prevented the inhibitory effect of atropine. These data demonstrate that the cholinergic system regulates GH secretion via SS.

Supported by Special C.N.R. project "Oncology" grant N. 85. 02266.44

EXOGENOUS GROWTH HORMONE (GH) INHIBITS BOVINE BUT NOT MURINE PITUITARY GH SECRETION 344

S.M. Rosenthal, B.L. Silverman, W.B. Wehrenberg*, A. Baird+, S.L. Kaplan, M.M. Grumbach
Dept. of Pediatrics, Univ. of California-San Francisco, San Francisco, CA; *Dept. of Health Sciences, University of Wisconsin-Milwaukee, Milwaukee, WI; +Laboratories for Neuroendocrinology, The Salk Institute for Biological Studies, La Jolla, CA.

Research has demonstrated that the administration of GH leads to diminished pituitary GH content, blunting of the GH response to provocative stimuli, and decreased pulsatile GH secretion. These results have led to the hypothesis that GH may regulate its own secretion by a short-loop negative feedback mechanism. To test this hypothesis, we evaluated the effects of biosynthetic methionyl human GH (hGH, provided by Genentech, Inc.) on basal and growth hormone-releasing factor (GRF) stimulated GH secretion. Dissociated cell cultures of rat and bovine pituitaries were prepared by standard procedures and incubated for 3 days in DMEM supplemented with 10% FCS. On the third day cells were washed with serum free medium and 20 µg/ml hGH was added to some wells (chronic GH exposure). Cells, 24h later, were washed and treated with GH (acute exposure) or GRF (10^{-9} M) applied in a 2^3 factorial design. Medium was collected 4h later and GH was measured by species specific RIAs. Both acute and chronic exposure of bovine pituitary cells to exogenous hGH significantly (p<0.01) reduced GH secretion. Acute treatment resulted in GH secretion declining from 579±24 to 500±17 ng/ml/4h (X±SEM, n=24), while chronic treatment resulted in GH declining from 595±21 to 483±17. In contrast, exogneous hGH had no effect on rat pituitary GH secretion; concentrations varied between 340±30 and 380±30. As expected, GRF treatment caused a significant increase (p<0.01) in GH secretion in both the bovine (489±18 to 590±21) and rat (250±30 to 470±30) systems. The presence of acute GH, chronic GH or both had no effect on GRF stimulated GH secretion. These results demonstrate that there are species specific differences in the ability of GH to have a direct effect on its own secretion at the level of the somatotrope.

ARE HYPOTHALAMIC GRF AND SRIF INVOLVED IN HYPOTHYROIDISM-INDUCED GROWTH FAILURE ? 345

N.Miki, M.Ono, T.Tsushima, K.Shizume, Dept. of Medicine, Tokyo Women's Medical College, Tokyo 162, Japan

To study whether thyroid hormone deficiency impaires growth hormone (GH) secretion via the hypothalamus, we studied in rats sequential changes after thyroidectomy in content and release of hypothalamic GRF and SRIF, pituitary GH content and responsiveness to GRF and serum IGF-I level as an index of integrated GH secretion. Release of immunoreactive GRF and SRIF was observed in vitro 2, 4 and 8 weeks after thyroidectomy (Tx): three hypothalami were incubated in Krebs-Ringer bicarbonate solution (KRB) containing 0.5mg/ml bacitracin and 0.1 % BSA for 30 min (basal release) followed by an another 30 min-period of incubation in 50 mM K^+-KRB (K^+-stimulated release). Pituitary GH content and in vivo response to rat GRF (1 µg/kg BW) under nembutal anesthesia and serum IGF-I level in Tx rats measured 1, 2, 4, 6 and 8 weeks after operation all started to decrease significantly at 1 week and then progressively to less than 1, 2.3 and 8.4 % of sham-operated (SO) rats, respectively, at 8 week post-operation. Hypothalamic content of GRF and SRIF was similarly reduced but later than these parameters: GRF began to decline at 4 week (-22 %, P<0.05) and SRIF at 6 week (-31 %, P<0.01). Treatment of Tx rats with T_4 (2 µg/ 100 g BW) for 7 days partially but significantly restored all the above parameters at 8 week except hypothalamic GRF and SRIF contents. In vitro, alteration in GRF and SRIF release was observed prior to the change in their hypothalamic contents: K^+-stimulated GRF release was more than 1.5 fold greater in Tx than in SO rats at 2, 4 and 8 weeks, while K^+-evoked SRIF release was increased in Tx rats at 2 (+33 %,P<0.01) and 4 (+20 %, P<0.01) but not at 8 weeks post-operation. Basal GRF, but not SRIF, release was also enhanced at all the stages tested (P<0.05-0.01). Thus, the synthesis and release of pituitary GH were decreased in spite of an increased GRF secretion in Tx rats. These results indicate that thyroid hormone deprivation acts primarily to depress the function of somatotrophs and change in GRF secretion may be secondary to pituitary GH deficiency. Increased secretion of SRIF may also contribute to the decreased GH release observed at an early stage of hypothyroidism.

COMPARISON OF THE EFFECTS OF ACUTE GROWTH HORMONE (GH) AND CLONIDINE (CLON) ADMINISTRATION ON THE GH RHYTHM. 346

M. Zorza and L.C. Terry, Univ. of Mich. and VA Medical Centers, Ann Arbor, MI.

Clon apparently provokes release of growth hormone-releasing factor (GRF) (Endocrinol. 114:1950, 1984). However, a delay of the first spontaneous GH pulse following the clon-induced GH burst in rats has also been reported (Neuroendocrinol. 38:1, 1984). This study was undertaken to determine if GH suppression following initial clon stimulation of GH release is due to GH autofeedback regulation.

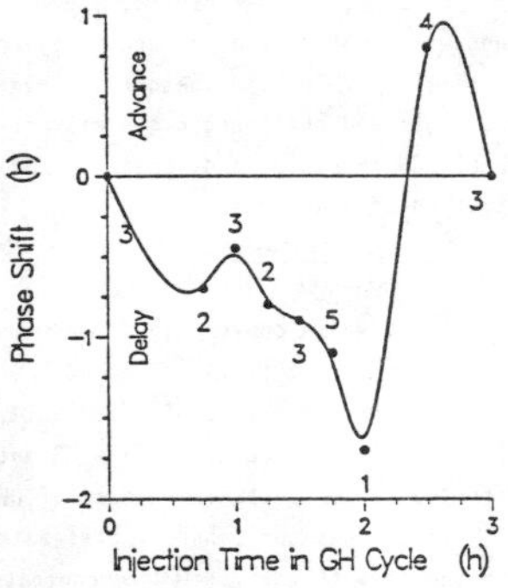

Chronically cannulated, adult, male rats were sampled from 800 to 2000 h. Either saline, 35ug human (h) GH, or clon (5-40 ug) was injected iv at 1200 h. hGH, depending upon the phase of the GH cycle in which it was delivered, either phase advanced or delayed the GH rhythm compared to saline controls (Right). The normal period of GH release was resumed after the delay or advance indicating that a true phase shift of the underlying GRF oscillator had been effected. Injection of clon dose dependently suppressed GH release for up to 6 h following the initial stimulated GH surge. This effect cannot be due to GH autofeedback regulation alone because (a) phase delays were induced independently of the phase of clon injection, (b) no phase advances were observed, and (c) although the clon-stimulated GH surge was smaller than that following hGH injection, the duration of the phase delay was markedly extended. In a second experiment, rats were pretreated with rGRF antiserum, which does not crossreact with hGRF, to suppress endogenous GH pulsatile release. Injection of clon, compared to saline, significantly reduced the GH response to a 1 ug hGRF injection 2 h later. These results suggest that (a) GH exerts phase control over the GRF oscillator and (b) clon stimulates release of GRF and somatostatin.

EFFECT OF TESTOSTERONE ON GROWTH HORMONE (GH) SECRETION IN FEMALE RATS DURING A CONTINUOUS INFUSION OF GH-RELEASING FACTOR (GRF) 347

H. SUGIHARA, I. WAKABAYASHI, S. AKIRA, S. MINAMI, F. TAKAHASHI, A. MOTOYAMA, N. LING*
Nippon Medical School, Tokyo, Japan and *The Salk Institute, San Diego, U.S.A.

We have observed the effect of testosterone on GH secretion in unrestrained female rats given continuous infusion of human GRF [1-44] NH_2 after they had received ovariectomy.

Adult female Wistar rats were used throughout the study. Some rats were ovariectomized 6 weeks previously. Two mg testosterone propionate was injected sc daily for 21 days starting 3 weeks after the ovariectomy. Four to 5 days prior to use, all rats were provided with two indwelling cannulae; one in the right atrium for undisturbed blood collection and the other in the inferior vena cava for vehicle or GRF infusion. Vehicle or GRF was administered by infusion pump (0.6 ml/h) at a dose of 50 ng/kg BW/min for 6 h. Serial blood specimens were obtained every 20 min.

During 6-h vehicle infusion, pulsatile GH secretion was observed at 1-2 h intervals in intact female rats. When they received 6-h GRF infusion, pulsatile GH secretion occurring at 1-2 h intervals was evident and striking elevations of trough GH values were observed. GH secretory profiles during vehicle and GRF infusion among ovariectomized rats were similar to those observed in intact female rats. Dramatic changes in pulsatile GH secretion was observed among ovariectomized rats that had received testosterone. In these rats, pulsatile GH secretion occurred regularly every 3.2 h during vehicle infusion and trough GH values were less than 10 ng/ml. Continuous GRF infusion to the rats that had received ovariectomy + testosterone augmented significantly the amplitude of pulsatile GH secretion occurring every 3.2 h without altering trough GH values.

Results suggest that testosterone modulates the release of somatostatin that mediates intermittent tonic inhibition of GH secretion during GRF infusion in female rats.

REGULATION OF TH GENE TRANSCRIPTION IN THE FEMALE RAT HYPOTHALAMUS 348

M. Blum[+o], B.S. McEwen[o], J.L. Roberts[+]
[+]Columbia University, College of Physicians & Surgeons, and [o]Rockefeller University, New York, NY

The tuberoinfundibular dopaminergic (TIDA) neurons of the hypothalamus release dopamine into the portal vasculature after which it is carried to the anterior pituitary where they inhibit the release of prolactin (PRL) from the lactotrophs. About 50% of the TIDA neurons have been shown to concentrate radioactive estrogen (E) and indeed several research groups have shown that E treatment effects dopamine turnover. Our interest is to determine whether E modulates the expression of the gene encoding for the rate limiting enzyme for catecholamine biosynthesis, tyrosine hydroxylase, in a parallel manner to DA turnover. E treatment in a 3wk ovx rat for 20' or 60' elicits a dramatic decrease in TH gene transcription which gradually returns to 70% of control values within 4d. In order to test the hypothesis that the return towards control levels after E treatment was due to a positive feedback of PRL on the TIDA neurons, we analyzed the effects of E in a HYPOXed animal. E elicited an immediate rise in TH transcription in the HYPOXed rat which was maintained throughout the 4d paradigm. This rise in the absence of the pituitary was unexpected. Since removal of the pituitary also inhibits adrenal steroid secretions, the results may have been due to altered adrenal function. Thus, we followed up these studies by analyzing animals which had been OVX and ADX prior to the E injection paradigm. In these studies E had the same effect that it had in the HYPOXed animals. However, to our suprise, in the OVX/ADX animal, E caused a decrease in the rate of PRL gene transcription in the anterior pituitary. Serum levels of PRL were measured by RIA from the OVX/ADX animals. Basal levels of PRL were found to be high. Acutely E did elicit a decrease in circulating levels of serum PRL, in agreement with the observed transcriptional effects of E in this system. Thus, it appears that the response of the TH gene in the TIDA neurons and the PRL gene in the anterior pituitary lactotrophs to E is influenced by adrenal function. Whether or not the effects of the adrenal secretions are directly on the TIDA or indirectly through other neuronal systems is not clear.

POST-TRANSLATIONAL PROCESSING OF CRF IN THE OVINE MEDIAN EMINENCE 349

J.W. Funder, A.I. Smith, F.J. Morgan, M. Fullerton, I.J. Clarke, D. Engler.
Medical Research Centre, Prince Henry's Hospital and St. Vincent's Institute of Medical Research, Melbourne, Australia 3004.

Corticotropin-releasing factor (CRF1-41) is synthesized in the hypothalamic paraventricular nucleus (PVN), transported to the external zone of the median eminence (ME), and released into hypophysial portal blood. With an antiserum against synthetic oCRF1-41 and ^{125}I-Tyr^{o}-oCRF1-41 as tracer, concentrations of ir-CRF (pg/mg wet weight, mean ± SE, n=5) were: PVN, 11.7±2.5; ME, 2276±296; anterior pituitary (AP), <0.5; neurointermediate lobe, 10±2.2. Analysis of the ir-CRF in these areas by Sephadex G-75 chromatography showed two peaks - a 'major' peak coeluting with CRF1-41 and a 'minor' peak eluting eight fractions later; on HPLC, the 'minor' peak eluted before CRF1-41.

Since CRF contains Arg35-Lys36, we tested the hypothesis that the 'minor' peak represented product(s) of proteolytic cleavage at this site. CRF36-41 and 37-41 were prepared from Tyr^{o}-oCRF34-41 and identified by amino acid analysis. In the CRF1-41 RIA, both fragments gave non-parallel displacement curves; parallelism was obtained with ^{125}I-Tyr^{o}-oCRF34-41 as tracer and Tyr^{o}-oCRF34-41 as standard. Both fragments migrated in the 'minor' peak area in acetonitrile/TFA, but when heptafluorobutyric acid was substituted for TFA, 5 ir-species were seen in the ME, 4 corresponding with CRF16-41, 36-41, 37-41 and 1-41, and one presently uncharacterized. The combined molar concentration of CRF36-41 and CRF37-41 in ME was 1.5 times greater than CRF1-41 in normal sheep, and 10 times greater in sheep given dexamethasone (1 mg, bd IM, 10 d), which markedly reduced CRF1-41 and increased CRF16-41 and CRF37-41.

We conclude that 1) ir-CRF in ovine ME consists of 5 species of which CRF1-41 is a minor component; 2) glucocorticoids exert a negative feedback at the hypothalamic level to increase the conversion of CRF1-41 to CRF16-41 and CRF37-41; 3) this conversion may represent a physiological control of levels of bioactive CRF; 4) the presence of these fragments in ME suggests the possibility of additional physiological role(s).

CHARACTERISATION OF CALCITONIN GENE-RELATED PEPTIDE RECEPTORS IN RAT NERVOUS SYSTEM 350

S.J. Wimalawansa, H.R. Morris* and I. MacIntyre
Royal Postgraduate Medical School, London; * Imperial College, London.

Calcitonin gene-related peptide (CGRP) is a 37 amino acid product of the calcitonin (CT) gene which has been shown to have a potent effect on the cardio-vascular system and smooth muscle. CGRP has been shown to co-localize with substance P and with acetylcholine in certain situations. The present study was undertaken to demonstrate the presence of CGRP-specific binding sites in the rat nervous system, using a specific and sensitive radioreceptor assay.

Binding studies were performed on rat cerebellar membrane preparations (2 mg/ml protein) at pH 7.5 in 50 mM Tris buffer containing 1% BSA, using 125-I-(His)CGRP (human α-CGRP) as the label (specific activity of 1900 Ci/mmol). The binding of 125-I-CGRP was rapid, reversible, temperature dependent and linearly related to membrane protein concentration up to 4 mg/ml.

High concentrations of 17 different peptides and peptide hormones (1 nmol/tube) were unable to displace receptor bound CGRP. Furthermore, 7 different fragments of human α-CGRP similarly had no effect. Salmon CT (30% homology to CGRP) and human CT (19% homology) were able to displace receptor bound CGRP, but only at 10^4 and 10^5 molar excess, respectively. Rat CGRP, human α-CGRP and human β-CGRP were equipotent.

Scatchard analysis showed two distinct binding sites, one with high affinity, low capacity (Kd 2.5 x 10^9 M^{-1}, Bmax = 10.2 fmol/mg protein) and the other with low affinity, high capacity (Kd = 8.0 x 10^8 M^{-1} and Bmax = 150 fmol/mg protein). High concentrations of specific binding sites were demonstrated in hypothalamus, pituitary, medulla and adrenal gland. CGRP binding was found to be highest (2.366 fmol/mg protein) in cerebellum where the immunoreactive CGRP content was minimal (1 pmol/g), whereas the dorsal half of the spinal cord had high concentration of CGRP (370 pmol/g) and its receptor binding sites (1.631 fmol/mg protein). These findings are consistent with a role for CGRP in sensory neurotransmission and in cerebellar function.

PROOPIOMELANOCORTIN (POMC) GENE EXPRESSION AND PEPTIDE PROCESSING DURING EARLY STAGES OF RAT PITUITARY DEVELOPMENT 351

J.E. Pintar, A.S.Liotta, and D.I.Lugo.
Columbia P&S and Mt. Sinai Medical School,NYC,10032.

The extent of POMC processing and the location of cells containing POMC mRNA in the fetal rat pituitary from embryonic ages e13 to e17 were studied. Following peptide extraction of isolated fetal pituitaries from these ages, POMC-derived peptides were identified by RIA following gel chromatography and HPLC separations. Equimolar amounts of B-endorphin (1-31) and desacetyl-a-MSH, but little B-LPH, were detected and indicate that extensive cleavage of the ACTH and B-LPH POMC domains occur at these ages.

Although immunostaining with B-endorphin antisera confirmed previous observations that cells in the ventral portion of the anterior lobe are the first to become immunoreactive during development, it was necessary to determine whether other cells could be synthesizing POMC peptides that might be lost during preparation of sections for ICC. Thus pituitary cells containing POMC mRNA during early development were identified by *in situ* hybridization. Rat fetuses were fixed with 4% formaldehyde containing DEP, cryostat sectioned, hybridized with 3H-POMC cRNA (synthesized from probes provided by Drs. James Roberts and Beth Schachter), and exposed for 1-3 weeks. Radiolabelled cells were found only in the ventral portion of the anterior lobe at the earliest stages examined thus far (e13.5).

Taken together, these observations demonstrate that POMC gene expression during early rat pituitary development occurs only in a subpopulation of cells in the anterior lobe, and thus that proteolytic cleavages of the ACTH and B-LPH domains, which is complete in the adult intermediate lobe but occurs to only a limited extent in the adult anterior lobe, predominate in the anterior lobe at early stages of pituitary development. This suggests a possible transient activation of an adult intermediate lobe specific processing enzyme durng early stages of anterior lobe differentiation.

DOUBLE IMMUNOFLUORESCENCE REVEALS PARTIAL COLOCALIZATION OF UROTENSINS I AND II IN A TELEOST CAUDAL NEUROSECRETORY SYSTEM 352

B.A. Larson, H.A. Bern, R.J. Lin, R.S. Nishioka
Wichita State University, Wichita, KS 67208 and University of California, Berkeley, CA 94720

A double immunofluorescence technique was devised to investigate the distribution of urotensins I (UI) and II (UII) in the caudal neurosecretory system of *Gillichthys mirabilis*. Individual caudal spinal cord cryostat sections were incubated sequentially with anti-CRF serum (which cross-reacts with UI), anti-IgG-fluorescein, biotin-conjugated anti-UII, and avidin-rhodamine conjugate. Two patterns of immunoreactivity were found. UI and UII appeared to coexist in some perikarya, but most appeared immunoreactive only for UI. However, the vast majority of fibers and terminal endings in the urophysis displayed immunoreactivity for both peptides. No convincing evidence of immunoreactivity only for UII and rare examples of non-immunoreactive cells whose neurosecretory status is doubtful were found.

The numerical discrepancy between perikaryal and fiber staining types, combined with a lack of topographical segregation of the two immunoreactive cell types, variability in immunofluorescence intensity for CRF/UI, and apparent differences between species found by others lead us to speculate that all caudal neurosecretory cells may synthesize both peptides. Immunoreactive differences may reflect different states of cellular activity. However, the presence of a small minority of fibers and perivascular axonal endings in the urophysis apparently immunoreactive only for CRF/UI does not support this hypothesis.

The sequential double immunofluorescence method offers several advantages over other techniques and is especially useful for colocalization studies when primary antisera from different species are not available.

(Supported by NSF grant PCM 84-05249 and NIH NRSA 5 F32 NS07260-02 BNS-1 to B. A. L.)

FURTHER EVIDENCE THAT SOMATOSTATIN-14 IS A GROWTH HORMONE RELEASE-INHIBITING FACTOR IN THE GOLDFISH 353

T.A. Marchant, J.G. Dulka, R. Fraser, and R.E. Peter
Department of Zoology, University of Alberta, Edmonton, Alberta, Canada T6G 2E9

The relationship between somatostatin-14 (SRIF-14) and growth hormone (GH) release in the goldfish was studied using several experimental approaches. First, it was found that SRIF-14 caused a rapid and dose-dependent decrease in GH secretion from goldfish pituitary fragments *in vitro*; the half-maximal effective dose of SRIF-14 was approximately 5.0 nM. This demonstrates that SRIF-14 inhibits GH release by acting directly on goldfish somatotrophs. In a second experiment, lesioning the preoptic region of the goldfish forebrain resulted in a decrease in immunoreactive SRIF-14 present in the pituitary, with a concomitant increase in blood levels of GH. This suggests that the preoptic region regulates GH secretion through a SRIF-14 projection to the pituitary. Finally, seasonal changes in pituitary content of SRIF-14 were examined in the goldfish. An inverse relationship between pituitary SRIF-14 content and seasonal changes in blood levels of GH was evident. These results provide further support for the hypothesis that SRIF-14 is a GH release-inhibiting factor in teleosts, and indicates that this action of SRIF-14 has been highly conserved during vertebrate evolution. Supported by Alberta Heritage Foundation for Medical Research and Natural Sciences and Engineering Research Council of Canada.

STEREOSPECIFICITY OF DOPAMINE INHIBITION OF GONADOTROPIC HORMONE GtH SECRETION IN GOLDFISH (*Carassius auratus*) IN VIVO. 354

R.J. Omeljaniuk, S.H. Shih, R.E. Peter
Dept. Zoology, Univ. Alberta, Edmonton, Alberta, CANADA.

In goldfish, pituitary gonadotropes are innervated by dopaminergic neurons and several lines of evidence indic ate that dopamine (DA) acts as a GtH-release inhibitory factor to modulate spontaneous release and GtH-releasing hormone (GnRH)-stimulated release of GtH. This study examined the DA-receptor specificity of inhibition of GtH secretion in goldfish by testing the effects of various DA-receptor antagonists on GtH secretion *in vivo*.

Goldfish, of mixed sex acclimated for 1 week at 12° C and 16 h photoperiod, were injected intraperitoneally with DA-antagonists with or without GnRH, then serum samples were taken at various intervals and evaluated for GtH by RIA. Domperidone, pimozide, fluphenazine, and metoclopramide all potentiated the action of a super-active analogue of teleost GnRH (tGnRH-A) but only domperidone and pimozide significantly increased serum GtH levels. In time-course studies, maximal serum GtH levels occurred at 24 h post-injection of pimozide plus a superactive mammalian GnRH (LHRH-A), or domperidone plus LHRH-A. Furthermore, domperidone significantly increased serum GtH and potentiated the action of tGnRH-A in a dose-related fashion; domperidone significantly reduced the ED_{50} for tGnRH-A. Domperidone is a specific DA:D2 receptor antagonist which does not cross the mammalian blood:brain barrier. It is likekly that in the goldfish domperidone blocks pituitary DA:D2 receptors to mediate increased spontaneous GtH-release and pontentiates GnRH action. This hypothesis is supported by the stereospecificity of DA-antagonist mediated elevation of serum GtH levels in the goldfish. Intraperitoneal injection of (-)-sulpiride, a specific DA:D2 receptor antagonist, increased serum GtH levels in a does-related fashion whereas (+)-sulpiride, the inactive stereoisomer, was without effect.

These data indicate that in goldfish the inhibition of GtH secretion is mediated by a pituitary DA:D2 receptor. Supported by NSERC and AHFMR.

PROLACTIN SECRETION IN RAINBOW TROUT : EFFECT OF OSMOTIC PRESSURE AND CHARACTERIZATION OF A HYPOTHALAMIC PRL RELEASING ACTIVITY. 355

P. PRUNET, F. GONNET, INRA, Laboratoire de Physiologie des Poissons - Campus de Beaulieu 35042 RENNES FRANCE.

The development of an *in vitro* superfused technique of anterior pituitary fragments associated with a homologous RIA for salmon prolactin (PRL) allow us to study factors which control PRL release in rainbow trout *Salmo gairdneri* : both osmotic pressure (known to be important in others fish species) and hypothalamic factors were investigated. Hyperosmotic medium (400 mOsm/l) induced 30 % decrease of PRL secretion by trout perfused pituitaries whereas hypoosmotic environment (220 mOsm/l) resulted in an increase of PRL secretion. However similar results were obtained with gonadotrophin and lower variations of osmotic pressure (closer to natural variation of fish plasma osmotic pressure) does not induce modification of PRL release. Moreover hypoosmolarity only induce a short term burst of PRL secretion which is also obtained when isotonicity follows hyperosmolarity or hypoosmolarity. Theses results indicate that OP is not a major factor controlling directly pituitary PRL secretion in rainbow trout and that changes in hormone secretions initially observed may result of physical modification of the outer cell membrane.

Using this superfusion method with an isoosmotic medium it was possible to test crude hypothalamic extracts : a dose-dependent stimulation of PRL release was obtained, the equivalent of one hypothalamus inducing a 150 % stimulation. When hypothalami spent media was tested similar results were observed. In attempt to identify the releasing principle (s) we further tested a possible direct action of serotonin on PRL cells. A dose related (10^{-9} to 10^{-5}M) increase in PRL release was observed when serotonin was used and the addition of a serotonin antagonist (pizotifen 10^{-5}M)prevented the stimulatory effect. Moreover addition of pizotifen (10^{-5}M) to hypothalamic extracts induced a 60 % reduction of the hypothalamic stimulation. TRH was also shown to stimulate PRL release in a dose dependent manner. Theses results indicate that rainbow trout PRL cells can be directly stimulated by serotonin and that PRL releasing activity of trout hypothalamus involves serotonin and possibly TRH effects.

EFFECTS OF ADRENERGIC RECEPTOR AGONISTS AND ANTAGONISTS ON THE SECRETION OF PROLACTIN (PRL) IN RATS. 356

J. Jurcovicova, T. Le, E. Vijayan, L. Krulich
Southwestern Medical School, Dallas, Texas 75235

The influence of the central NE system on the secretion of PRL remains controversial because NE receptor agonists as well as antagonists have been shown to stimulate PRL release. In an attempt to resolve this dilemma we first tested the effects of graded doses of a series of NE receptor agonists and antagonists with differential affinities for the multiple NE receptors on basal PRL secretion in conscious male rats bearing right atrial cannulae. Neither activation (IVT isoproterenol, 4 or 40 µg) nor blockade (i.v. propranolol, 1 to 10 mg/kg) of the β receptors had any influence on basal PRL levels. The preferential α_2 receptor agonists clonidine or UK 14304 stimulated PRL release with an identical potency (0.125 to 0.5 µM/kg), but the preferential α_2 antagonists yohimbine or rauwolscine also had a stimulating effect, whereas the more selective antagonist idazoxan was ineffective. The α_1 agonist ST587, claimed to penetrate into the CNS, slightly evevated PRL levels however, the α_1 antagonists corynanthine, WB4101, and to a lesser extent prazosin, also elevated PRL levels. Subsequent experiments showed that the PRL-releasing effect of UK14304 was inhibited by idazoxan but only weakly by prazosin. In contrast, UK14304 did not consistently counteract the PRL-stimulating action of rauwolscine nor did ST587 counteract the effect of corynanthine. The PRL-releasing effects of all α antagonists persisted despite a large depletion of hypothalamic NE following blockade of NE synthesis with FLA63.

Conclusions: 1) No evidence was obtained for an influence of the β receptors on PRL release. 2) The role of the α_1 receptors is uncertain but activation of the α_2 receptors seems to have a stimulating effect. 3) The PRL-releasing effects of the α-receptor antagonists cannot be correlated with their respective affinities for the α receptor subtypes and are probably not derived from their blockade. This may explain the seeming paradox we set out to study.

Index

Z